Having Twins

A Parent's Guide to Pregnancy, Birth, and Early Childhood

Elizabeth Noble

Second Edition

with Leo Sorger, M.D., F.A.C.O.G., Medical Consultant

Foreword by Louis Keith, M.D., F.A.C.O.G.

Illustrated with line drawings by Maya M. Jacob

Houghton Mifflin Company   Boston

To
Julia
and
Carsten

Library of Congress Cataloging-in-Publication Data

Noble, Elizabeth, date.
    Having twins : a parent's guide to pregnancy, birth, and early childhood / Elizabeth Noble with Leo Sorger ; foreword by Louis Keith ; illustrated with line drawings by Maya M. Jacob. — 2nd ed.
        p.   cm.
    Includes bibliographical references and index.
    ISBN 0-395-51088-0
    1. Twins.   2. Pregnancy, Multiple.   3. Prenatal care.   4. Birth, Multiple.   5. Infants (Newborn) — care.   I. Sorger, Leo.   II. Title.
RG567.N62   1990
618.2'5 — dc20   90-38969
                                  CIP

Printed in the United States of America

CRW 10 9 8 7 6 5 4 3 2

This publication is meant to serve as a guide for achieving the maximum comfort and health for women having multiples — from conception through early childhood. Because each individual has her own particular medical history, the reader should consult her physician before beginning any regimen described in this book.

Having
Twins

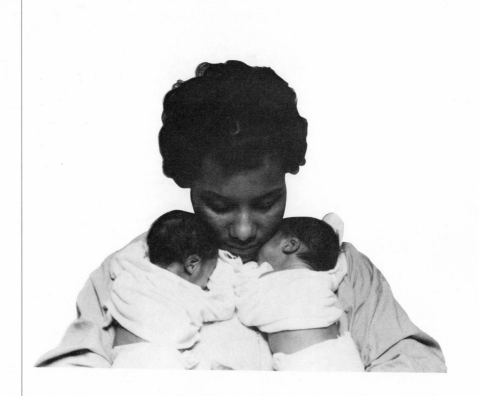

Books by Elizabeth Noble

Having Twins
Essential Exercises for the Childbearing Year
Childbirth with Insight
Marie Osmond's Exercises for Mothers-to-Be
Marie Osmond's Exercises for Mothers and Babies
Having Your Baby by Donor Insemination

Acknowledgments

THE FIRST EDITION of *Having Twins* owed its creation primarily to the requests and contributions of parents of twins and other multiples, because at that time there was no guide for the prenatal and birth experience of twins. Countless parents, twins, triplets, physicians, psychologists, psychiatrists, teachers, nurses, and researchers shared their insights, experiences, and photographs. Contributors to that edition included Suzanne Arms, Jerry Armstrong, Rudolph Ballentine, Gail Sforza Brewer, Tom Brewer, Jason Birnholz, Oliver Cope, Don Creevy, Labib Habashy, Judy Hagedorn, Agnes Higgins, Daniel Hubbard, Donald Keith, Louis Keith, Helen Kirk, Janet Kizziar, Charles Mahan, Paulo Parisi, Jean Roma, Rosemary Theroux, Josephine Tingley, Fran Ventre, Gregory White, and Grace Wyshak.

I am grateful to the following people who kindly made contributions or improved one or more chapters of the revised edition: Jeannine Parvati Baker, Ron Benzie, Janet Bleyl, Charles Boklage, Elizabeth Bryan, Vito Cardone, David Cheek, Linda Cooper, Linda and Chris Degnan, Robert Derom, Karen Dietz, the staff of DoubleTalk, Denise Duncan, Roger Evenson, Graham Farrant, Beth Fine, Lisa Fleischer, Helga Grützner, Helen Harrison, David Hay and the LaTrobe Twin Study, Rhia Hughes, Sherokee Ilse, Yoko Imaizumi, Janet Kalhally, Helen Kirk, Shirley Maag and the National Organization of Mothers of Twins Clubs, Pat Malmstrom and the staff of Twin Services, Marion Meyer, Christopher Millar, Kim Millar-Jones, Lynn Moen, Christiane Northrup, Michel Odent, MaryEllen O'Hara, Bob Orenstein, Marilyn Riese and the Louisville Twin Study, Hanspeter Ruch, Nancy Segal and the Minnesota Center for Twin and Adoption Research, Selma Taffel, Tufts New England N.I.C.U., Cape Cod M.O.T.C., Barbara Unell, Carlo Versi, Elizabeth von der Ahe, Andrew Wilkinson, Teresa Wolding, Diony Young, and *Twins* magazine.

I wish to express my deep appreciation to Louis Keith, who not only wrote the foreword but skillfully edited the material in style and content twice; first as it was written chapter by chapter, and then as a complete manuscript.

My family has been truly long-suffering during these two years of lengthy revisions. Thank you, Julia, for being so patient and understanding, and Carsten, for nursing to the click-click of the computer. Special thanks to Leo, who shared his broad clinical experience on all the medical issues in the book and put up with my very late nights.

Contents

Foreword

I WAS PLEASED and honored to be asked to write the Foreword to this, Elizabeth Noble's revised and expanded version of her early book. In the years that followed the publication of the first edition, much has changed about our perceptions of twins and supertwins. Not only has public interest in multiple births increased enormously, but that interest has been matched by additional concern on the part of physicians. Indeed, some people have also suggested, with good reason, that we are in the midst of an epidemic of multiple births. The exact causes of this epidemic are not totally clear but many include the increased use of assisted reproductive technologies or fertility-enhancing agents and the delaying of childbirth into the third and fourth decade by women in at least some developed countries.

Although some of my prior observations no longer are germane, specific principles regarding the care of twin (and higher-order) pregnancies remain exactly where they were almost a decade ago. The most important of these is the fact that all multiple gestations represent potentially high-risk pregnancies and that the survival rate of multiples is less than that of singletons. Having said this, I continue in my admiration and respect for Elizabeth's point of view, that is, to provide the mother with the necessary information to have an informed and enlightened pregnancy that hopefully will have an excellent outcome. It is unfortunate but true that even the best prenatal care and strict adherence to the principles of obtaining appropriate nutrition and adequate rest and gaining what many physicians would call "excessive weight" cannot forestall all of the complications of multiple gestation. However, as Elizabeth so aptly points out, they can forestall many of the "morbid events" and make for an easier pregnancy that may go closer to term.

As the readers of this book soon will come to know, preterm delivery remains the single most vexing problem to parents of multiples and physicians who take care of them. Thus, the clinical challenges for physicians, patients, and health educators remain exactly as they were years ago: (1) early diagnosis; (2) institution of intensive prenatal, intrapartum, and postpartum care to improve survival for the newborns and lessen the potential for complications; and (3) reduction of the likelihood of serious illness or death in the first month of life for the newborns.

Reading this book as an obstetrician/gynecologist, I soon came to recognize that it provided a body of information that generally is not available in traditional medical textbooks. The author and the publishers kindly acceded to my request to provide me with the manuscript in sufficient time to read every word of it. Prior to this, Elizabeth had sent me numerous chapters, which I commented on, often in great detail. Her point of view is always pro-patient and generally proactive. However, for Elizabeth Noble, "proactive" does not mean only avoiding unnecessary intervention on the part of the physician but also assisting the mother and her partner to develop an attitude that allows them to properly prepare for the pregnancy.

One of the major features of this book is Elizabeth's ability to educate and inform the reader from the point of view of parents-to-be. Her research for this volume has been extensive. She has read many of the articles and textbooks that are on my desk and that I would normally provide my patients and students. In addition, she is familiar with a wealth of supporting literature in a variety of fields. Clearly, her quotations give the reader the benefit of many diverse opinions. Perhaps even more important, she has provided a reading list, a resource section, and references that make this volume even more valuable.

Some chapters — such as the discussions of sharing space and bonding — are unique. Others, such as "Emotional Consequences of Twin Loss," are extraordinarily insightful. The entire book provides a wealth of information for first-time mothers as well as for parents who already have children. The chapter on nutrition is particularly important as the American medical establishment slowly comes to the opinion that it has neglected this important aspect of prenatal care and that there may be serious deficits in the types of information that we routinely provide to our patients.

As Elizabeth was preparing for this volume, I was busy reading for my own research projects and to further my activities as president of the Center for the Study of Multiple Birth. Conversations with Professor Emile Papiernik of the University of Paris convinced me of the importance of rest. At the same time, discussions with Barbara Luke of the Section of Maternal and Fetal Medicine of the Department of Obstetrics and Gynecology at the Johns Hopkins Medical School in Baltimore made me acutely aware of the importance of maternal nutrition as it relates to the so-called optimal weight gain of pregnancy. The sum of my impressions and my reading allows me to endorse Elizabeth's position on these three subjects even more wholeheartedly.

It is unfortunate that the United States has yet to provide the means for working mothers and new mothers to obtain rest during and after their birth. The very morning that I am writing this (March 15, 1990), a lengthy article in the *Chicago Tribune* describes a bill before Congress that would give a one-year maternity leave to all women.

The American public must face the fact that adequate prenatal care (including nutrition and rest) is not available to all women. The reasons are variable and include poverty, ignorance, and a host of other social ills that prevent all women, regardless of social class, from obtaining medical care. In the coming decade, our country must address this issue with vigor if it hopes to improve the lot of our newborn children and their mothers.

When my brother and I founded the Center for the Study of Multiple Birth some fifteen years ago, we hoped to raise the consciousness level of the general public and the medical profession about the risks of multiple pregnancy as we saw them at that time. Happily, the general level of awareness has increased. In addition to our efforts, many other research and support organizations have emerged, both in the United States and abroad, as can be seen from the resources listed in this book. Nonetheless, it is worth reflecting on comments made directly to me by Professor Papiernik several years ago. He said, "The care given to the mothers of multiples is a mirror of the interest that society takes in women and children." How true this statement was and still remains.

Elizabeth Noble's book *Having Twins* will help all members of society give the parents of multiples the care and support they need. By reading the book and adhering to its concepts, mothers of singleton pregnancies will also benefit. I am sure that this was Professor Papiernik's wish and one that is shared by Elizabeth, her medical consultant, Dr. Leo Sorger, my identical twin brother, Donald M. Keith, and me.

Louis G. Keith, M.D., F.A.C.O.G.
Professor, Obstetrics and Gynecology, Northwestern
University Medical School and Prentice
Women's Hospital & Maternity Center
President, the Center for the Study of Multiple
Birth, Chicago, Illinois
Former Co-Vice-President, International Twin
Association

Introduction

UNTIL RECENTLY, the books and pamphlets designed for general reading about twins have concentrated on their care, psychology, and development — once they have arrived. Little has been available to inform and guide the couple who learn in pregnancy that they are to become parents of twins.

Statistically, one in every forty-five people is a twin — hardly the "obstetric abnormality" that twinning is termed in some medical texts. In fact, plural birth rates have been rising steadily since 1980, when *Having Twins* was first published; in 1985, 13 percent more multiple births occurred in the United States than in 1980.

Because of advances in obstetrics, more twins are being diagnosed prior to birth. Also, the diagnosis is being made earlier in the pregnancy and the health and survival of multiple infants is continuing to improve. Hormone treatment for infertility and the new reproductive technologies are associated with increased occurrence of twins. Many studies have shown that older women conceive more twins, and today the trend is for women to postpone childbearing. Caesarean birth is on the rise for women over thirty and for presentations other than headfirst; such presentations occur frequently with twins. The average childbirth educator or maternity care provider has little information that is relevant and helpful to the multiple birth experience. For all these reasons, a comprehensive resource for those giving and receiving prenatal care and preparation for twinbearing is essential.

The thrill of carrying twins is often outweighed by concern for the potential hazards. Expectant parents are soon warned, by strangers as well as friends, family, and physician, that multiple births involve high risk. The risks include premature delivery, smaller babies, and a higher chance of disability or death occurring from birth through the first year of life. The research I undertook in the 1970s for the first edition of this book convinced me that many of these problems can be prevented or alleviated by *really good* prenatal care, that is, by the mother's commitment to a vigilant program of nutrition, exercise, rest, and preparation in addition to regular checks at the doctor's office or clinic. In the decade since the first edition, evidence has mounted to support this view. The focus of *Having Twins*, then and now, is the physiological and psychological dimensions of twinning. Learning from mothers who successfully carry normal-birth-weight babies to term empowers other women to do the same. While I acknowledge and discuss hazards and their management, I also stress strategies for prevention so that complications and interventions will be less likely to occur among readers of this book.

This edition deals, much more than the first, with complications and medical interventions that result from all the new prenatal tests and obstetric procedures. By attempting an adequate description for the parents who will confront them, I do not wish to imply my endorsement. I have played devil's advocate wherever I believe there is questionable safety and efficacy, but often the long-term effects of a test or procedure are still unknown. I have read hundreds of studies for this book and I quote from many of them, but I know that in a few years any or all of them could be contradicted by other studies. (Such was the case, for instance, with the association between oral contraceptives and twinning.)

Walking the tightrope between providing comprehensive information and at the same time making commonsense recommendations has not been easy. Mothers who have lost a multiple tend to advocate total surveillance, even routine Caesarean (with which many of their physicians would be in happy agreement). In contrast, those who enjoyed healthy pregnancies and birthed their babies naturally feel that describing complications, disability, or loss only makes parents fearful and sets them up to anticipate problems.

My position has been to inform parents of all possibilities and at the same time encourage them to keep their trust in nature. After all, we all hear about and see car accidents, but most of us still feel confident to drive on the roads. My personal bias is always toward natural birth and against intervention unless medically necessary — which even then may lead to an ethical dilemma, such as when parents' wishes for their babies' well-being conflict with the recommendations of the staff.

Having worked with childbearing couples for more than twenty years, I can no longer sit on the fence about issues that I believe are important. In this book I tackle controversies rather than avoiding them by suggesting that readers consult their doctors (who may have little experience with multiples). At the expense of so-called objectivity, I am sharing with readers my best opinions — the truth as I see it. I am also very much an advocate for the unborn and newborn babies.

Being pregnant today, especially if the pregnancy is "high risk," is full of challenges of which our grandmothers never dreamed. More than ever before, parents need to be *thoroughly* informed and empowered to make choices and take responsibility for their decisions. They need guidance and support to confidently face the months and years ahead.

One of the drawbacks of gaining knowledge and insight is that feelings of guilt can emerge over actions taken prior to acquiring that knowledge. "If only . . . " is a natural reaction, although not a constructive one. Sometimes premature labor, for example, is caused by an undetected infection, or it can result from deep ambivalence about the pregnancy. It never hurts — I venture to say it always helps — to explore all the dimensions of dysfunction and disease. This is not to suggest that problems are "all in the mind," because, in fact, the evidence is clearly in the body! I feel that meditation, visualization, hypnosis, and counseling are as valid as drugs in many cases and are certainly without the side effects of drugs (an additional important consideration when tiny babies are involved). Often individuals can recognize and resolve their attitudes on a conscious self-help level, such as by consulting Louise Hay's book *Heal Your Body: The Mental Causes for Physical Illness and the Metaphysical Ways to Overcome Them.* Evidence has convinced me also of the value of natural remedies such as homeopathy and Bach flower essences for treating both the emotional and physical aspects of medical problems.

People usually remain stuck in guilt feelings until they genuinely (not rhetorically) ask, "Why me?" At some point the need develops to take personal responsibility for an experience or alternatively to rationalize it as a random event within a person's concept of the universe. Self-exploration is still a path toward the second conclusion.

Issues of guilt inevitably arise when mothers hear recommendations for natural childbirth, breast-feeding, and avoidance of circumcision, for example, especially for those who did otherwise and now regret their decisions. Always, some women won't care and some women will feel remorse. But in the attempt to spare women guilt feelings, many health care professionals give inadequate support for practices that are clearly best for mother and babies. I call this the "white bread" philosophy. This is, whole grain bread is much better for us than white bread, but it is not widely available. Therefore, the philosophy goes, let us reassure the people who get the inevitable white bread in the store, restaurant, hospital, and so on, that it is just as good. By analogy, the "white bread" philosophy underlies the reassurance that bottle-feeding is the equivalent of breast-feeding, that the "abdominal birth canal" (Caesarean section) is just another way to give birth, and so on. Unfortunately, such well-intentioned attempts at equalization have backfired; more women than ever are having intervention, and breast-feeding has not been increasing with any significance. And women feel guiltier than ever!

I, like everyone else, have had to learn from mistakes, mishaps, and losses. The best way I can support others in similar situations is to acknowledge that I, too, made the same mistake — not that it wasn't a mistake in the first place. What women feel in their hearts cannot be denied, and facilitating the acknowledgment of those feelings is the first step to healing. I fully appreciate the statement by parents that they would rather be less wise and compassionate and have a living baby. But it is my personal belief that destiny, karma, or whatever name you give to it does play a role in our lives. Such lessons are agonizing but nevertheless are necessary in some cosmic plan yet to be comprehended.

People outside families of multiples often misunderstand the facts about twinning. It is up to parents, teachers, and others who live and work with multiples to provide education and help reduce twinism. Society needs to support a sense of self-worth for each individual independent of the twinship. Pregnancy, if not before, is the best time to begin learning and sharing information. Certainly expectant mothers of multiples cannot remain aloof from the myriad questions and comments they will hear.

I wrote the first edition of *Having Twins* in response to all those parents whose questions clearly showed the need for information and guidance about the experience of pregnancy and the birth of multiples. The book owes its creation to the suggestions, hints, and anecdotes provided by such parents as well as to an extensive review of the twin literature and medical research. To write this guide for parents, I also interviewed multiples and their families, attended twin births, twin conventions, twin club meetings, and conferences on twin studies, and I visited schools with twin students.

This second edition is greatly revised and expanded. I have added seven chapters and up-to-date statistics and new information on prenatal communication, bonding, the experience of twinship in utero, prenatal screening, nutrition, the experience of loss, and guidelines in the event of loss.

Whether the conception of twins is felt by parents to be a miracle or an accident, education for the prenatal and perinatal period helps allay anxiety and assists in preparation for a healthy pregnancy, satisfying birth experience, and a happy family.

Having
Twins

1 The Fascination of Multiple Births

SINCE HUMANKIND'S earliest days, explanations have been sought for the phenomenon of twins. Religious beliefs, cults, rituals, and superstitions have developed around these "instant siblings" in almost every culture. Myths and legends about twins emphasize aspects, often bizarre and mystical, that set them apart from the general population. Amazing coincidences, chance meetings of twins separated at birth, and other newsworthy events satisfy today's demand for fascinating stories about twins. Whether the occurrence of twins is considered inspiring or threatening, twins and other multiple births always arouse curiosity.

While history records births of multiples other than twins, sets of more than three had little chance of survival until this century. More than three hundred complete sets of quadruplets are living in the United States. The oldest living set is the Perricone males from Texas. Anthony, Bernard, Carl, and Donald, born in 1929, are quadrazygotic (arising from four eggs). The first known quadruplets to survive were reported in France in 1915. The St. Neot quadruplets were born in Britain in 1934, the same year that the Dionne quintuplets made headlines in Canada. All five Dionne babies were delivered at home and survived, although their total combined weight was just over 11 pounds (three were still alive in 1990). Their later life, however, was less than happy, as fame led to exploitation. Between 1980 and 1990 three sets of quintuplets were born in Canada, the first there since the Dionnes. In the United States there are at least twenty-six sets of quintuplets with all five living. The oldest living female triplets in the United States are Faith, Hope, and Charity Cardwell in Texas, age ninety-one, and the oldest male triplets are eighty-nine-year-old Clarence, Claude, and Clyde Rees in Minnesota. There are at least nine sets of sextuplets worldwide with all six living and an additional nine sets that have five survivors. The largest naturally occurring multiple pregnancy was nonuplets.

A few remarkable American women have truly experienced the

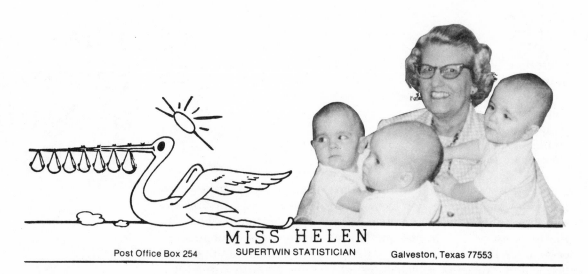

MISS HELEN
SUPERTWIN STATISTICIAN

Post Office Box 254   Galveston, Texas 77553

COLLECTOR OF

BITS 'BOUT

MULTIPLES

Helen Kirk, "supertwinologist," has made a lifetime hobby collecting "bits 'bout multiples."

singular phenomenon of multiplicity. A Texas mother bore quintuplets, quadruplets, three sets of triplets, and nine singletons. In North Carolina a woman, by the age of thirty-one, had delivered twenty children. Only one was a singleton; the rest were quintuplets, quadruplets, two sets of triplets, and two sets of twins! Eight of these children were alive in 1960 when the last triplets were born. Nebis Ramos, in Chicago, gave birth to four consecutive sets of twins, although she never took fertility drugs. A woman in South Africa bore two sets of triplets within ten months in 1960. A Chilean woman who in 1981 produced her fifty-fifth child had five sets of triplets (all boys!). Another woman conceived and lost a set of triplets but within two years had birthed another set.

Such memorabilia are collected by a "supertwinologist," Helen Kirk of Galveston, Texas. She has been gathering "bits 'bout multiples" for more than forty years, ever since the birth of the Badgett quadruplets started her on this hobby. A national resource, Kirk shares her knowledge and statistics with experts throughout the United States and the world. Kirk has corresponded with thousands of multiples and has a regular "birthday file." She hopes that one day her amazing collection will be displayed in a museum.

Horatio H. Newman, an early twinologist, wrote that "everyone is interested in twins, or they should be." Twins always arouse public interest, and some gain widespread fame. Probably the best known in history were Chang and Eng, the conjoined twins from Thailand who were the origin of the term *Siamese twins*. Although these twins were joined at the chest, their union did not prevent them from marrying and fathering a total of twenty-two children. As entertainers and curiosities, they traveled all over with Barnum's circus until their almost simultaneous deaths.

Shakespeare was the father of fraternal* twins; he used twins as a dramatic device in many of his plays, particularly in *A Comedy of Errors* and *Twelfth Night*. Playwright Peter Shaffer scored a Broadway hit with *Equus*, as did his identical twin, Anthony, with *Sleuth*. Elvis Presley was a twin, but his brother died at birth. Other famous twins include Maurice and Robin Gibb of the Bee Gees rock group, Ann Davis of "The Brady Bunch," Anita Bryant, Heloise, Muhammad Ali, and the late Shah of Iran. Ann Landers and Dear Abby are twins who chose the same career of consoling lonely hearts. Famous parents of twins include Cybill Shepherd, Debby Boone, former "Today" show host Jane Pauley and her husband, Gary Trudeau, Congressman Joe Kennedy of Massachusetts, and the late Ingrid Bergman. British Prime Minister Margaret Thatcher delivered her twins between the two parts of her bar examination. *Big Business*, a 1988 comedy film starring Bette Midler, deals with mistaken identities of two sets of twins mixed at birth. *The Man in the Iron Mask*, a film based on the novel by Dumas, describes the banishment of the twin brother of Louis XIV. Ross and Norris McWhirter were twin founders and compilers of *The Guinness Book of World Records*, which, of course, has many amazing entries on the subject of multiple births. Scholastic and sporting achievements of twins, particularly in the United States, may be found in Amram Scheinfeld's book *Twins and Supertwins*.† *Twins: Nature's Amazing Mystery* by Kay Cassill is also a wonderful source of twin lore.

Twins are conceived more commonly than other multiples and suffer less from the hazards of sharing one uterus than do larger multiples. There are more than 125 million twins in the world. In the United States during 1987, almost 82,000 twins and other multiples were born, nearly 12,000 in California alone. They often arouse am-

---

* See the Glossary for definitions of types of twinning and Chapter 2 for a complete discussion.
† The term *supertwins* refers to triplets, quadruplets, and other higher-order multiples.

Two nations are in thy womb, And two manner of people shall be separated from thy bowels; and the one people shall be stronger than the other people; and the elder shall serve the younger.
GENESIS 25:23

And the first came out red all over like an hairy garment; and they called his name Esau.

And after that came his brother out, and his hand took hold on Esau's heel and his name was called Jacob.
GENESIS 25:25–26

And Isaac loved Esau, because he did eat of his venison, but Rebekah loved Jacob.
GENESIS 25:28

And it came to pass, when she travailed, that the one put out his hand; and the midwife took and bound upon his hand a scarlet thread, saying, This came out first. And it came to pass, as he drew back his hand, that, behold, his brother came out: and she said, How hast thou broken forth? this breach be upon thee: therefore his name was called Pharez.
GENESIS 38:28–29

bivalent feelings of fascination and fear. The pastor in the town where the Dionne quintuplets were born announced that they were God's answer to those who advocated birth control. For couples undergoing infertility treatment with hormones, the conception of higher-order multiples may be a mixed blessing.

Multiple birth has always evoked surprise and curiosity about the laws of nature. Primitive societies that were unaware of the biological facts of multiple conception considered twins the work of God, the devil, or both. The birth of twins has been afforded special significance in myths, legends, cultural taboos, sanctions, and rituals throughout the world. Our heritage of twin folklore continues to exert some influence today, affecting even modern scientific research. Experts are concerned with the differences between twins, their negative and positive characteristics, and their problems of dependency and attachment — the stereotypes of the love-hate relationship. Some writers have observed that the Old Testament emphasizes the differentiation and competition between twins, whereas harmonious bonds are stressed in Greek mythology. Current views of twinship fluctuate between these two traditions.

Biblical Twins

Jacob and Esau are probably the best-known twins in the Bible, and their story reveals hostility and division within the family. The dispute over who would be first-born began in the uterus. Esau was actually born first, but Jacob sought his revenge at the deathbed of their blind father. Dressed as Esau, Jacob received his father's blessing on the first-born. He was helped in this deception by his mother, as he was her favorite twin. Identifying the first-born is still an item of interest, if not an issue of primogeniture, as any twin today can testify. Recent studies have shown that mothers tend to favor and protect the weaker twin or the second-born — whoever is the underdog. The priority of birth, of course, depends not on superiority of strength but on convenience of position, and this is reversed in Caesarean birth.

Pharez and Zarah are another pair of biblical twins whose struggle began in the uterus. Pharez was born first, although the midwife had already seen and identified the hand of Zarah. Considered the second-born, Pharez became the father of King David, while his twin brother did not distinguish himself. Thus, it is not always the first-born in literature who rises to fame, but often the second twin achieves his destiny after heroically surmounting obstacles.

Interestingly, a French survey found that half the parents of twins considered the first-born the elder, while the other half regarded the first-born as younger. In Japan the second-born is considered the elder, as he or she was mature enough to let the other twin be born first.

Greek and Roman Mythology

Castor and Pollux were the most famous twins in Greek myths, which also included Apollo the sun god and his sister Artemis the moon goddess and Hercules and his twin brother Iphicles. Castor and Pollux are the two main stars in the constellation Gemini (which means "twins") and the third sign of the zodiac. Their myth caught the imagination of Leonardo da Vinci, whose painting *Leda and the Swan* hangs in the Louvre in Paris. Actually, Castor and Pollux were members of two different sets of twins conceived and carried within one pregnancy. Pollux and Helen were fathered by the god Zeus, who disguised himself as a swan to seduce the virtuous Leda. However, the same night another pair of twins, Castor and Clytemnestra, were also begotten by a mortal father, Leda's husband. Four children resulted from these two separate matings and were hatched from two

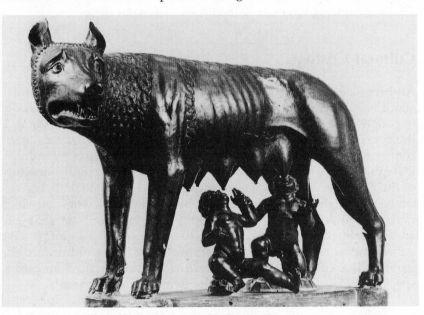

Romulus and Remus, twin founders of Rome.
Courtesy of Carlo Verdesi, Rome.

eggs. This myth plays down the human levels of twinning as it explores the fantasies of divine paternity and dual conception.

Another Greek twin myth concerns Narcissus, from whom the term *narcissistic,* meaning self-love and self-absorption, derives. The most common account of the legend is that Narcissus was so vain that he fell in love with his own reflection in a pool. However, another interpretation explains that Narcissus had an identical twin who died, and thus it was his brother's image that he constantly sought. Twin likeness and intimacy lend themselves to exaggeration in modern fiction. Recent novels have explored the themes of narcissism, homosexuality, and even murder between identical twins.

The Greek myth of Amphion and Zethus is similar to the better-known Roman legend of Romulus and Remus, twins who were abandoned at birth and raised by a female wolf. Zeus was the father of the twins Amphion and Zethus, but this time he took the form of a satyr in impregnating their mother, Antiope. Romulus and Remus owed their divine heritage to their father, the god Mars. In both tales the twins survived a hazardous beginning, abandoned in the countryside until rescued by a shepherd. In later life both sets of twins founded a famous city, Thebes in the Greek version and Rome in the Roman one. The Forum in Rome contains a temple built in honor of Romulus and Remus, and the standards of weights and balances — symbolizing the balancing forces of twinship — were kept there.

Cultural Customs

Anthropologists have documented many attitudes and customs about twin births that have arisen in various cultures and times out of people's need to explain phenomena that they can't understand. If the conception and paternity of a single child are beyond a culture's comprehension, then all the more so is the arrival of two individuals. Different peoples' interpretation of twin birth relates to the structure of their society, into which such births must be assimilated. The relevance and rights of birth order may be shaken in societies for which rank is significant. Two persons who may look and act alike can arouse feelings of suspicion or even dread. Some social groups have viewed twins as punishment; others welcome twins and reward the parents. If a culture believes that twins are reincarnated ancestors, special privileges are extended to the twins and their parents.

In many primitive societies the birth of two infants suggested two fathers, and the tradition of the particular group established whether the extra father was evil or divine. Archaic customs pertaining to twin sacrifice have been recorded in literature. If twins were considered to have violated the incest taboo, both were sacrificed. In other cases, one twin was selected and sacrificed. Sometimes one or both twins were sacrificed, either because the father was considered an evil sorcerer or because, as offspring of divine paternity, they were considered beyond the claim of earthly parents. In some cultures the first-born was chosen, in others the second-born. The sex of the twins may also determine their fate. In the Pacific island of New Britain, both twins were permitted to live if they were the same sex — if they were not, the girl was killed. In New Guinea, however, it was the boy who was unacceptable. In parts of Africa, less drastic measures were taken to diminish the twinship. One of the twins was sent away to live with relatives, or sometimes both were confined together and excluded from certain tribal activities.

Twins may be viewed with disapproval from a social as well as a religious point of view. Double paternity in some societies was evidence of adultery and of intercourse during pregnancy. In societies that held a taboo against intercourse during pregnancy, twins were sacrificed. Because animals generally give birth to litters (more than one offspring in one birth), a mother with twins may be held in very low esteem in some cultures. Sanctions may operate against the parents, the twins, or the whole family. The Australian tribal aborigines live within a complex structure of myths, known as "dreamtime," that regulate every aspect of their daily living. Twins pose a threat to their secret and sacred traditions and invoke great fear of the supernatural.

The economic conditions of social groups also influence the customs that define twinning. Among the Australian aborigines, where resources are scarce, one twin is frequently killed. For similar reasons, the Eskimos formerly killed one twin of a pair as well as members of the older generation who became a burden. Sometimes one of the twins was given away, but childbearing and childrearing necessarily had to be kept to the bare minimum.

The incidence of twinning in an ethnic group appears to have little significance in influencing social attitudes. In Asia, where the fewest number of twins are born, they have not always been welcomed. The Tunguses of Manchuria apparently held twins in such distaste that they felt that ill luck would result if anything were bought or borrowed from the mother. Even in modern Japan the birth of twins can bring shame on a family, as in former times when the paternity was not understood and the arrival of twins was viewed

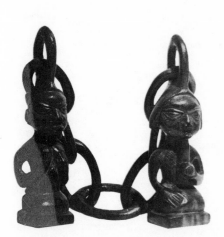

Twin images are used in West African rituals to ensure the health of twins. They are placed at the door of a house, and gifts of oil and beans are put in a small dish in front of them. In the event of a death, the mother will carry the images in her skirt band. These wooden images from Dahomey (Benin) are carved from one piece of mahogany without joints. The male twin smokes a pipe.
Courtesy of Professor E. G. Parrinder, London.

with both fear and awe. In Indonesia the father of twins may request an amulet from the priest to guard against the subsequent birth of twins.

In Africa, where twinning rates are the highest in the world, especially among the Yoruba in Nigeria, elaborate customs prevail to deal with the high number of twin births and, in the past, deaths. Apprehension and dread of twins is expressed in some areas by the ominous curse "May you be the mother of twins," also signified by two outstretched fingers. In other parts of Nigeria twins are esteemed; outside Lagos a temple is dedicated to the twin deity for twin pilgrims and their parents.

The most fascinating customs surrounding twins are found in the Ibeji cult in Africa. *Ibeji* means "to beget two" and is also the linguistic term for twins. If one or more Ibeji twins should die, carved effigies are created. The wooden statues are fashioned in the likeness of the dead twin or twins and are suitably clothed. They are cared for, offered food, and adorned during certain rituals. The images serve as companionship for the surviving twin or the family, provide a refuge for the dead spirit, and protect the living against torment. The mother cares for the statues as if they were a real child until the surviving twin is able to take over their care.

The placenta is accorded special significance in some primitive societies. It may be viewed as a lost twin and buried with appropriate ceremony. The custom of fixed names was found in at least seventy-five African tribes by one researcher. The first- and second-born twins and the elder and younger siblings each have a name that describes their family position. These names are the same in every family with twins. Among the Yoruba, the first-born is considered the younger — sent ahead by the elder twin to check out the world. Pediatrician Elizabeth Bryan describes in her book *Twins in the Family* a Nigerian mother who brought her twin daughters to a clinic. They were called Taiwo ("The One Who Has First Taste of the World") and Kainde ("Who Lags Behind"). They had several pairs of twin cousins also called Taiwo and Kainde. Idi Amin, the former dictator of Uganda, included in his lengthy self-chosen list of titles "Father of All Twins."

In Africa and India and among the Indian tribes of the West Coast of North America, twins were believed to have power over the elements. In cultures where such power was considered threatening, twins were killed to prevent natural disasters, or elaborate purification rituals were required, as in Bali, to restore the balance of natural forces. Where their power over nature was considered beneficial, twins were highly regarded. The Mohave Indians believed that twins were the incarnation of immortals or an older person returned to earth in a double form. They held that twins could cause thunder, lightning, and rain; in a drought, they would pour water over the graves of twins. In this society twins were treated with deference and respect. The Kwakiutl Indians in British Columbia regarded twins as a sign of plenty, and their birth heralded a good year of hunting and fishing. These tribes believed that the wind is the ''breath of twins'' and that disease could be cured by twins, who used the wooden rattles from their birth ceremonies. Some Hindus in India believed that crops could be saved from hail and rain if the buttocks of a twin were painted black and white and then faced toward the elements. Parents of twins in Africa were called upon to perform rites to stimulate reproduction in livestock and agriculture.

Sometimes women enjoy emancipation as a result of bearing twins. In one African tribe the mother of twins is identified by having half her face and legs painted red and white and half her hair shaved. Held to be the incarnation of clan fertility, she is obeyed by all and allowed the privilege of joining in men's conversations and making jokes.

Superstitions around twins exist in Western European tradition. Warnings about eating a double grain of rice or double nuts and fruits are described in the French literature. A well in Scotland was endowed with the power to cause the conception of twins if a woman drank more than half a cupful of its water. Today twins provide interesting anecdotes of parallel clairvoyance, when they feel each other's illnesses, accidents, and traumas.

An indication of a positive attitude toward twins in Western society is the number of social and research organizations (discussed later) and periodicals that promote the welfare of multiples. In 1875, Sir Francis Galton, writing in the anthropological literature, first proposed the use of twin studies to examine the still controversial questions of heredity and environment, or ''nature versus nurture.'' Much of the current medical and genetic research is complex and seeks to improve the outcome for the babies as well as the mothers; half a century ago the mothers were considered at greater risk than the babies. Emphasis is also shifting from postpartum events to the importance of the prenatal environment, and investigators are becoming aware of factors operating even before conception, such as the mother's health and nutrition.

Astrology is one mechanism for explaining the coincidences of life and death. The horoscopes of individuals born close together are of interest to astrologers, who claim to explain the differences and the similarities between such individuals through interpretation of the stars and planets. Twins, therefore, can be different even though identical. Astrologers explain that the ascendant star influences the individual characteristics, and the star changes frequently.

It is not uncommon for birthdays to repeat themselves in one family. (See "Family Time" in Chapter 6.) Brothers or sisters born years apart often share the same month of birth and occasionally the exact birthday. Sets of twins may also have common birthdays. Nancy Sutherland, one of the founders of the New Zealand Federation of Parents Centres, conceived three sets of twins in the month of May. While the appropriate sign of the zodiac (Gemini) operates from May 21 to June 21, twins are not born in greater numbers at this time.

Accounts of amazing coincidence between total strangers born at the same hour and latitude may be found in the astrological as well as the twin literature. Such people are considered twins by fate, if not by genetics. Similarly, there are stories of twins separated at birth by adoption into different families whose lives nevertheless run on an almost parallel track. When these individuals find they have a twin, they may confess to having experienced feelings of incompleteness. Sometimes such twins die of the same cause at the same time, thousands of miles apart.

For years I had the same dream, about playing as a child in a silver pond. The dream always ended with a man in a black cloak who stole my companion. When I traced my natural mother I learned that she had miscarried a twin when she was pregnant with me.

Twin Studies and Organizations*

In March 1979 a pair of identical male twins was brought together for study by Professor Thomas Bouchard of the University of Minnesota Department of Psychology. The men had been separated at three weeks of age and met again for the first time thirty-nine years later. The similarities in their separate existences were remarkable. Each man had been named James by his foster parents, each worked in law enforcement, and each married a woman named Linda for his first marriage and a woman named Betty for his second. Each twin had a son named James Alan, and the twins drove the same make of car. After they met, they were able to switch roles and speak to the other's wife on the telephone without arousing suspicion about their identity. In the decade since this unique study began, the Minnesota Center for Twin and Adoption Research has interviewed more than one hundred twin pairs reared apart.

* See the two Resource chapters at the back of the book for further information about the organizations mentioned in this section.

Such studies shed light on the influence of heredity and environment. The genetic factors appear more significant when the twins have been separated; and one expert, René Zazzo of Paris, France, considers that genetic effects, especially the twin bond, tend to be erased by the influence of the environment when twins live together. For certain traits of personality, identical twins reared together were actually less similar than identical twins reared apart. The nongenetic factor is inherent in twins raised together, and Zazzo criticizes twin studies that focus on twin pairs without taking into account that they are a couple. Almost all twin research is limited to the view that twins are an identical pair — duplicates of each other. The environmental situation, however, is more complex. The twins interact with each other and with society as part of a unique bond, but not as perfect replicas. The relationship is more like that of a married couple than a simplistic model of duplicate organisms performing in the same way. Even if twins are physically identical, they are not psychologically identical, and they experience different emotional effects from their duality.

Twin studies make a valuable contribution to research on health, disease, and social and psychological development, especially anatomical, environmental, and genetic questions. Ongoing research involving diabetes in identical twins, begun by Dr. J. Stuart Soldner in 1966 at the Joslin Diabetes Center in Boston, has enabled researchers

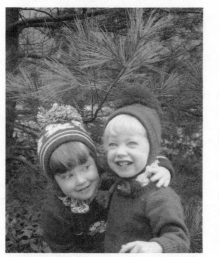
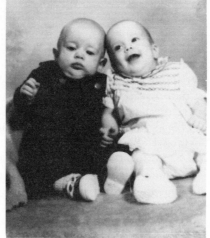
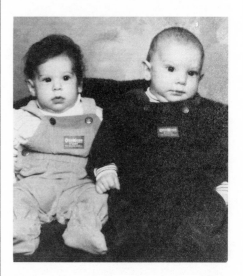

"Invisible twins": most twins look dissimilar.

to better understand the types of diabetes, to predict onset, and to explore preventive measures. The methodology in studying twins is as important as the content of the research. Some of the research on mental and psychological ability, for example, is biased with built-in comparisons. Many researchers seem to set out with a negative orientation. They focus on behavior problems, delayed development, stuttering, left-handedness, and so on.

Proper scientific investigation is important not just to society but for twins themselves, as they suffer from stereotyping that an occasional sensational report can facilitate. Several organizations have been set up to conduct studies scientifically and to provide support for twins and their families. Some groups focus on gemellology (the study of twins), other groups are formed for twins themselves, and yet others for relatives of twins.

The Gregor Mendel Institute of Medical Genetics and Twin Studies in Rome was named after the founder of genetics, who made his early discoveries with botanical twin pairs of sweet peas. This institute provides free medical and dental care for more than fifteen thousand twin pairs and produces a journal (*Acta Geneticae Medicae et Gemellologiae*). The International Society for Twin Studies (ISTS), an international, nonpolitical, nonprofit, multidisciplinary scientific organization, fosters scientific research and encourages social action in all fields related to twins and twins studies. Members include twin researchers, twins, parents of twins, and others. Collective membership is granted to official groups such as Twins Clubs and Mothers of Twins Clubs. In addition to sponsoring an international congress every three years, the ISTS conducts special working groups on obstetrics, standardization of twin data collection and analysis, and behavioral research. The Working Party of Obstetrics of the ISTS, which meets every three years when the parent body is not in session, held its first U.S. meeting in Chicago in 1988. Periodic newsletters and announcements are offered as well as a journal. The founder and president of the ISTS, Luigi Gedda, is the author of *Twins in History and Science* (1961). A twin foundation, the Luigi Gedda Institute, was established in Jerusalem in 1980.

The International Twins Association (ITA) was founded in 1934 by Reverend Edward Link of Silber Lake, Indiana. It is a nonprofit, family-oriented organization that promotes the spiritual, intellectual, and social welfare of twins. The club grew rapidly since its first reunion for twins and was renamed the International Twins Association in 1937. Current membership totals more than a thousand sets of twins, and an annual convention is held every summer.

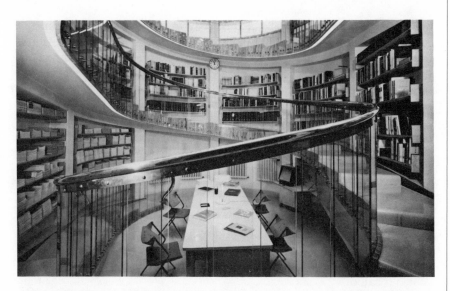

The Gregor Mendel Institute in Rome is devoted to the study and care of twins. Pictured here is the library on medical, genetic, and twin studies. *Courtesy of the Gregor Mendel Institute.*

The annual Twins Day Festival is held in Twinsburg, Ohio, which is situated between Cleveland and Akron and was named in honor of a pair of twins, Moses and Ariel Wilcox, who donated land and funds toward the town's first school. More than two thousand twins and supertwins attend the yearly festival, which includes a parade, games, contests, exhibitions, entertainment, and fireworks.

The Twins Foundation in Providence, Rhode Island, is building the country's first comprehensive twin registry and has almost ten thousand names, including a Twins Hall of Fame for celebrities. The founder and president is Kay Cassill, author of *Twins: Nature's Amazing Mystery*.

Twin registries are very important for collecting data not just about multiples but on heredity, environmental influences, family diseases, and so on. The Vietnam Era Twin Registry was established by the Veterans Administration to study various health-related issues as part of the Vietnam Experience Twin Study (VETS). These issues include correlations between exposure to agent orange and incidence of infertility, spontaneous abortion, and birth defects in veterans' offspring.

The National Academy of Sciences, Kaiser Permanente, a health maintenance organization in northern California, and the University of Minnesota in Minneapolis also have twin registries. The Minnesota Twin Family Registry is one of five major projects associated with the Minnesota Center for Twin and Adoption Research. The Minnesota Twin Family Registry hopes to identify a minimum of five hundred families composed of the twin pair, both spouses, and at least one adult child of each. The registry will look at the influences of genetic and environmental factors on such features as physical appearance, personality traits, interests, occupations, and attitudes. The researchers are particularly interested in emergenesis, or how genes may influence a physical or behavioral feature in one generation that has not been previously observed.

In 1988, two million dollars were donated by Carl Kroch to establish, in the memory of his wife, the Jeanette Kennelly Kroch Center for Twin Studies. Studies will be conducted within the Prentice Women's Hospital and Maternity Center of the Northwestern Memorial Hospital of Chicago, where the Center for the Study of Multiple Birth is also located.

The Center for the Study of Multiple Birth in Chicago was organized in 1977 by twin brothers Donald and Louis Keith. One twin is an obstetrician-gynecologist and the other works in private industry. The purpose of the center is to stimulate and foster medical and social research into multiple birth and to help mothers with the special problems they and their offspring will encounter. The center also sponsors scientific conferences on the care of twins and other multiples and encourages funding for the support of medical and social research. An additional resource for the public is the twin bookstore, which specializes in books for parents of multiples, such as the center's own publication *The Care of Twin Children: A Common Sense Guide for Parents*. Major concerns of the center include improvement of clinical standards, early diagnosis of multiple pregnancy, better care through the childbearing year, and a reduction of maternal and fetal complications. The first institution of its kind in the United States, the center has become a leader in the field of multiples. Social and psychological issues, such as the rights of minority groups, are also a concern.

The Louisville Twin Study at the Child Development Unit, University of Louisville School of Medicine, Kentucky, was organized in 1957 by Frank Falkner, M.D., a pediatrician interested in twins. The current director (and president of ISTS) is Adam P. Matheny, Jr., Ph.D. Topics of research include psychological development of personality, temperament, intelligence, language and reading ability, and physical growth. The study draws from all segments of society to ensure a sample that is representative of the general population.

About six hundred pairs of twins have participated in the study, with recent subjects followed since infancy. The twins are tested in the laboratory several times a year for the first few years of life and yearly thereafter. Because researchers think that the progressive development of intelligence and personality may be intimately related to the structure and lifestyle of each family, parents are interviewed about typical behavior patterns of the twins at home and a social worker observes the twins at home. Information is also obtained from teachers about the twins' behavior in school. Both identical and fraternal twin pairs and siblings are studied to identify the features of personality and mental development most sensitive to genetic control. In recent years, follow-up studies have been made of the twins as young adults, and second-generation twins are being recruited as the original participants have twins of their own.

Other Louisville studies concentrate on prenatal influences, including the effects of prematurity on subsequent development, while evaluations in the newborn period have looked at constitutional and genetic influences on newborn behavior and the relation of newborn behavior to later development.

The European Multiple Birth Study (EMBS), with headquarters at the Catholic University of Leuven, Belgium, studies the management of pregnancy and labor with emphasis on the prevention of preterm delivery. The EMBS encourages accurate determination of type of twinning (discussed in detail in Chapter 2) so that twin studies can be used by researchers in related fields such as genetics. The EMBS also maintains a databank with detailed information about several thousand twin pairs. Placental tissue can be sent for genotyping, a process discussed in Chapter 2.

The LaTrobe Twin Study of Behavioral and Biological Development began in Melbourne, Australia, in 1978 and studies twins and their siblings and cousins. This long-term research with more than eight hundred families involves detailed questionnaires and a wide range of behavioral and language tests to shed light on cognitive and social development. A chief concern is the early identification and remediation of language and reading problems. David Hay and colleagues at LaTrobe are also researching the effect of twins on siblings and on postpartum depression in mothers.

The National Organization of Mothers of Twins Clubs (NOMOTC), formed in 1960, is a resource for mothers, grandmothers, godmothers, and legal guardians of multiples. Its official motto is "Where God Chooses the Members." Membership now numbers in the thousands with hundreds of Mothers of Twins Clubs spread through every state.

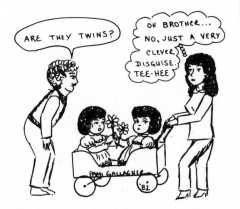

Reproduced with permission from DoubleTalk.

I have been to the last ten national conventions and I just love it. My husband is really happy for me to get away, and I have seen more of this country through the Mothers of Twins Club than I ever would have otherwise.

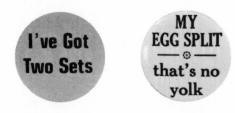

Buttons and bumper stickers display the pride of parents.

The NOMOTC distributes a quarterly newspaper, *MOTC's Notebook*, a publication called *Your Twins and You*, and bibliographies of literature on twins, child care, and current research projects involving multiples. As part of its aim to further education and communication about all aspects of twin life, the NOMOTC hopes to unite all its clubs into one network to allow all to be active participants in national medical and educational research and to facilitate a broader interchange of information. A cope/outreach department serves members in isolated areas without easy access to a MOTC group and provides support to those with emotional and medical difficulties. Bereavement support is offered, and a pen pal program provides communication with those in similar circumstances. The research department actively screens and supports all legitimate research proposals to be sent to members. The screening and development of a contract is quite important because not all research is bona fide.

The NOMOTC annual convention is held in July and has crisscrossed the nation from Orlando to Anaheim. Numerous workshops cover twin research, childrearing, and women's issues. One of the lighthearted activities of the convention is the "Show, Tell, and Sell" night, when each member club displays its T-shirts, buttons, bumper stickers, booklets, and other creations.

Philanthropic endeavors of Mothers of Twins Clubs are also impressive. Many state organizations actively raise money for college scholarships, since college expenses are often a burden for families with multiples. Club members frequently donate blood for use during multiple births. They generously volunteer their time to complete questionnaires for hospitals, graduate students, government agencies, and twin researchers. Some of the studies benefit the rest of society. For example, research with voice printing of twins has helped the FBI draw up guidelines for lie detection tests. Medication studies with twins have helped reveal the side effects of drugs. Some states offer training for workshops, conventions, and other phases of club work.

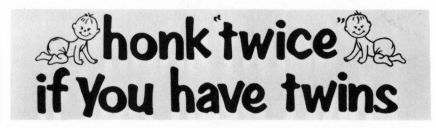

Readers who are mothers of twins are requested to contact the national executive office of the NOMOTC for the multiple birth data form. The information you supply will be fed into the Multiple Birth Data Bank at the national headquarters, which stores information from thousands of mothers of twins and supertwins.

Guidelines are available for starting a local Mothers of Twins Club chapter if one is not available in your area. Local groups consist of a dozen or more members who provide moral support, parenting hints, and recycling of clothes and equipment. The emphasis of the meetings varies with the clubs. Many groups are primarily social and provide outings for the mothers in the form of committees, fundraising projects, raffles, bazaars, and banquets. Others are more oriented to education and invite guest speakers such as geneticists, pediatricians, and psychologists. Frequently the members are asked to complete research questionnaires for various studies on a wide range of issues, including diabetes, congenital defects, speech development, sibling relationships, school policies, and allergies.

Member clubs have their own newsletters, with such titles as *Reflections, Twinette Gazette, Twinsville, Double Dilemma, Double Delight, Twincerely Yours, Doubly Blessed, Double Exposure, News of Twos,* and *Twofolders,* which offer child care tips, recipes, and birth announcements for mothers and their "twinfants."

Twin Services is a nonprofit health education and social service agency dedicated to improving the health and family functioning of parents and expectant parents of multiples. To make sure that families have the information and timely support they need to cope with the stresses of birthing and rearing twins and triplets, trained counselors answer questions on a free telephone counseling service, the Twinline, every weekday from 10:00 A.M. to 4:00 P.M. California time. Topics raised by callers range from the symptoms of preterm labor, breast-feeding, and teaching twins to sleep through the night to why toddlers bite, how to place twins in school, and how to deal with competition in the teen years. A quarterly newsletter and a series of more than thirty-five handouts give parents current information about twin development and care. Training and technical assistance are offered for health and family service providers. For parents in the San Francisco Bay area, the group sponsors classes, a clothing and equipment exchange, and a respite care program for low-income families in crisis.

British author and pediatrician Elizabeth Bryan, with the Twins and Multiple Births Association (TAMBA), established several twin clinics in London at Queen Charlotte's and Chelsea Hospital. Parents

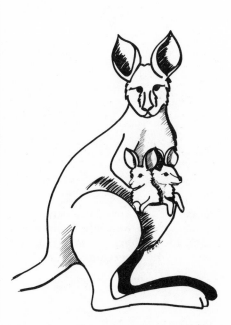

Logo of the Cape Cod (Massachusetts) Mothers of Twins Clubs, designed by Trish Hastings.

The club was a real lifesaver for me. We had just moved and I knew no one. With triplets you are so tied down anyway.

It is so reassuring to meet others in the same situation. You think you are the only one who feels that you can never give your twins as much love as one child. But then you realize others have those same feelings of guilt.

Unless you have had twins you just can't really know what it is like. My local club has helped me keep my sanity.

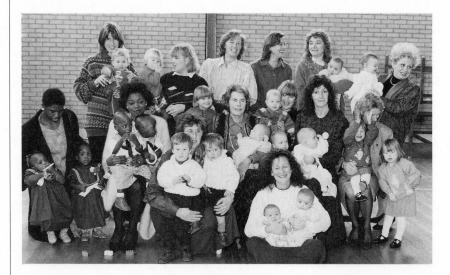

London pediatrician Elizabeth Bryan, founder of the Multiple Births Foundation in London, enjoys a gathering of twins with Lady Mountbatten.

come with their twins to a children's clinic for routine assessments of language, behavior, growth, disabilities, and testing for type of twinning. Monthly prenatal talks are given to expectant parents. The clinics also serve as a teaching forum for professionals, and volunteer research opportunities are available. In the TAMBA support room volunteers provide practical help, information, advice, and refreshments and can look after other children so parents can talk with a pediatrician. Special clinics are held every three months for supertwins, twins with special needs, and families suffering the loss of a twin. Bryan also established the Multiple Births Foundation for professionals.

In other countries, similar organizations concerned with "twindom" include the Australian Multiple Birth Association (AMBA), Parents of Multiple Births Association (POMBA) in Canada, and South African Multiple Birth Association (SAMBA) and TAMBA in Great Britain. An umbrella organization, Combined Multiple Birth Association (COMBA), is headquartered in London. In Australia the mothers of multiples obtained a grant from the country's Department of Maternal and Child Welfare to provide a postpartum domestic service. Free household help is available from women who are themselves mothers of twins or triplets and have completed a training course in hygiene management and baby care. These helpers share their experience and give advice as well as help with housework and feeding sessions. Twin and triplet buggies are lent free to members of the association and sale or rental of other equipment is also offered.

$\mathcal{2}$ How Are Twins Formed?

IN THE ANIMAL KINGDOM, multiple births are rare in large, long-lived animals whose pregnancy lasts more than 150 days, and mammals with two breasts characteristically give birth to singletons. The human being, the horse, and the elephant are mammals that typically produce only one offspring. The Texas armadillo consistently bears four identical quadruplets, all arising from one egg. Fraternal twins are the usual offspring for the marmoset and are not uncommon in sheep.

There are two types of multiples: those with identical genes and those with different genes. Twins may be either of these types, and triplets and higher-order multiples are more commonly a combination of types. The incidence of *identical* twins, who have identical genes and always look alike, is fairly uniform throughout the world. The biology of this type of twinning is not well understood. Twins whose genes are not identical and who look no more alike than brothers and sisters are called *fraternal*.* This more usual type results from double ovulation, the causes of which are partly understood, and its incidence varies with race, geography, and maternal age.

Clearly, if twins are of opposite sex, they cannot be identical, although many people don't understand this fact (how often mothers of twins are asked whether Linda and Dustin, say, are identical!). In the case of twins of the same sex, the type of twinning may be obvious at birth, but sometimes microscopic examination of the placenta, blood groups, or even DNA may be necessary.

---

* The terms *identical* and *fraternal* are familiar labels, but they describe only the external appearance of twins and not their anatomical origin, or *zygosity*. Furthermore, the labels encourage stereotyping of the individuals. *Identical* favors the prejudice of duplication — that twinship is a bond of two equal halves. *Fraternal*, meaning ''brotherly,'' is equally imprecise; it would make more sense to describe unlike twin sisters as ''sororal.'' In this book I will use the more precise labels of zygosity (*monozygotic* and *dizygotic*), which is discussed in detail a little later in this chapter.

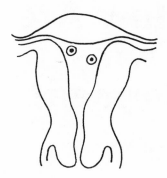

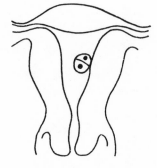

One or more eggs may be fertilized to produce a multiple pregnancy.

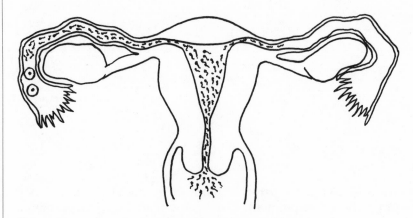

Fertilization occurs in the outer third of the Fallopian tube.

Fertilization

In a normal menstrual cycle the female ovary releases an egg (a phenomenon called *ovulation*), which travels through the Fallopian tube to the uterus. If unprotected intercourse takes place around the time of ovulation, millions of microscopic sperm make their way through the female reproductive tract. When one sperm successfully penetrates the egg, fertilization — the union of male and female cells — is achieved. Timing is important, as fertilization must occur when the egg is viable — when it is in the outer third of the tube and within about 24 hours of ovulation. The fertilized egg becomes a union of cells that divides and grows as it travels down the tube to seek a spot in which to implant in the wall of the uterus. If the egg is not fertilized, it travels into the uterus and is shed with the preparatory lining of the uterus during menstruation, and the cycle is repeated.

Geneticist Charles Boklage of the East Carolina University School of Medicine estimates that twinning occurs in one-eighth of all natural conceptions (not all the twin pairs survive to term, however; see the vanishing twin syndrome in Chapter 4) and 8 percent of all births. (Natural conceptions are those that occur without hormonal stimulation of ovulation.) The twinning rate is more than 1 in 30 miscarriages, according to Uchida and his colleagues in a 1983 study. Identical twins are thought to arise from a delay in the cell division process. As this is a deviation from the normal sequence of events, identical twin pregnancies are more frequently miscarried than fraternal twin pregnancies.

Identical Twins (Monozygotic)

The events of fertilization determine the type of twins that develop. Monozygotic (identical) twins result from the union of one egg and one sperm. The cause of monozygotic twinning remains a mystery — some chance factor favors a delay in the division process of the fertilized single egg or favors a delay in implantation. As a result the chromosomes, which carry the genes and are fixed in quantity (46), double in number and the egg splits into equal halves. Each twin develops from an identical half of the original fertilized egg. The term *monozygotic* means "one-cell union" (the term *monovular*, "arising from one egg," is also sometimes used).

Monozygotic twins are always the same sex and have identical features — hair and eye color, blood groups, body scent, dental impressions, and so on. They also have very similar electroencephalograms and cardiovascular measurements.

About one-third of all twins are monozygotic, with an equal distribution of male-male and female-female pairs, although recent Dutch and Swedish figures indicate a relative increase of monozygotic over dizygotic. About one-quarter of monozygotic twins are "mirror twins" because certain features are related as in a mirror image — on the opposite side: a whorl or cowlick, a birthmark, or even internal organs such as the appendix may be on reverse sides of the twins. In addition, one mirror twin is left-handed and the other right-handed, and they tend to cross their thumbs, arms, and legs in opposite ways.

Genetic endowments are laid down at the moment of conception, but prenatal and postpartum influences may lead to differences in size, appearance, and psychological development. Sometimes one twin develops at the expense of the other within the uterus (a phenomenon called twin transfusion syndrome, explained fully in Chapter 7), resulting in an imbalance of birth weights. Birth trauma may involve only one twin. In childhood and later life, environmental factors can modify weight, height, the development of certain skills, and emotional characteristics.

Modern science tends to think of twins as a dichotomy. Physicians and psychologists classify, compare, and contrast the larger and the smaller, the first-born and the second-born, the extrovert and the introvert. These common considerations, unfortunately, affect parents and their perceptions of their twins. This in turn alters parental interaction with the children, even when the twins may have been diagnosed as monozygotic. In fact, monozygotic twins may differ considerably in size at birth and may look even less alike in the beginning than dizygotic twins. Whatever the type of twinning, the notion of a pair is a narrow definition of the twin experience. Rather, it is more like the experience of a married couple, who are individuals even as they see themselves as one entity and interact with their community largely as a couple.

Fraternal Twins (Dizygotic)

The more common type of twinning is dizygotic (fraternal). Two eggs, which may be from one or both ovaries, are fertilized by two different sperm, just as one egg is joined by one sperm in a singleton pregnancy. Two separate unions, or zygotes, are formed; hence the term *dizygotic* (also called *binovular*, "arising from two eggs").

Dizygotic twins may or may not look alike, as with any brothers or sisters. This type of twinning is simply a double birth, as commonly happens in other species. Dizygotic twins are siblings with the same birth date who shared the same uterine environment. It is possible for their conception date to differ, although this is unusual.

Approximately half of dizygotic twins are same-sex pairs and half are male-female (although in Holland and Sweden same-sex dizygotic twins occur 10 to 15 percent more often than male-female pairs). The percentage of females increases with the number of multiples. For example, females are 48.4 percent of singleton births, 49.2 percent of twins, and 50.5 percent of triplets. The incidence of mixed-sex twins, which are clearly identified as dizygotic, solves the problem of definition of zygosity in about one-third of twin births.

Twin types break down as follows:

Male-Male		Male-Female	Female-Female	
Monozygotic	Dizygotic	Dizygotic	Monozygotic	Dizygotic
$\frac{1}{6}$	$\frac{1}{6}$	$\frac{1}{3}$	$\frac{1}{6}$	$\frac{1}{6}$

Although age is one key factor shared by dizygotic twins, it is nevertheless possible for slight differences in age to occur. As long ago as the second Talmud, the phenomenon of *superfecundation* was acknowledged. During one reproductive cycle, two eggs may be released that can be fertilized on two different occasions. As the conceptions will be only a week or so apart, such a slight difference in age and growth may well pass unobserved at birth. It is also possible for each twin to have a different father, as in the myth of Leda and the swan (described in Chapter 1). A case of double ovulation and superfecundation was reported in Germany in 1978, where the subsequent twins were clearly of different parentage — one was black and one white. The mother had sexual intercourse with two different men a short time apart but within one menstrual cycle. Another report concerned a mother who claimed that her twins were fathered by two different men, which blood typing indeed confirmed. *Parade* magazine reported a case in 1983 of a Nigerian mother and a Caucasian father who had dizygotic boys, one black and one white; however, this was not a case of superfecundation but simply genetic potluck.

Superfetation occurs when a second egg is fertilized in a following reproductive cycle. Marked difference in the weight of the twins at birth may indicate such an occurrence. Superfetation is theoretically possible anytime in the first three months of an established pregnancy, but it is rare because the hormones produced once a pregnancy becomes established usually prevent ovulation. Therefore, it is thought that low hormone levels at the beginning of such a pregnancy do not adequately suppress ovulation. Genetic research has indicated possible involvement of a gene that acts to reverse the normal suppression of ovulation.

Although most twin births today occur in hospitals where the second twin is delivered within minutes of the first, there are exceptions. Some cases have been reported in which days, even months, elapsed between the two births. In Texas a mother actually gave birth to her twins in different years, as one was delivered in December 1966 and the other in January 1967. These are not necessarily instances of superfetation, however, as one twin is sometimes born prematurely, or is even miscarried, while the other is carried to term uneventfully.

Geneticist Charles Boklage believes that both monozygotic and dizygotic twinning are variations of the cellular events that occur when a single embryo develops. Some factors that may be involved are abnormal timing of conception rhythms (such as conception after a period of abstinence) or the relative timing of ovulation and intercourse. Boklage further claims that there is "no sound evidence of a two-egg origin for natural dizygotic twins." He suggests that the cellular events of monozygotic and dizygotic twinning are part of the same process and postulates that dizygotic twins occur before fertilization and monozygotic after and that both types may occur in daughter cells of the same egg.

My dates were vague and even after the pregnancy test I had a sort of period. All through the pregnancy I just felt that one twin was very different. I know the second one wasn't ready to be born — he squirmed like a squirrel and didn't want to come out.

Third Type of Twin: Third Phase of Egg/"Polar Body Twinning"

A third type of twinning has been mentioned from time to time. Elizabeth Bryan writes that it is "likely to happen that occasionally a single ovum would divide and each half would be fertilized by different sperm." Charles Boklage is studying this type of twinning, which he calls a tertiary oocyte — an egg in its third phase of division.

It is possible for two sperm to fertilize two egg cells derived from a single secondary oocyte (the cell that is usually fertilized). The secondary oocyte has two half-sets of chromosomes, one more than is necessary to go with the sperm's half-set to form a functional zygote. The extra set usually goes into a small accessory cell called the second polar body immediately after fertilization. For several reasons, including delay of fertilization, the secondary oocyte may divide without fertilization. In that case, a roughly equal division occurs instead of the very asymmetric division that usually produces the zygote and the much smaller second polar body, yielding two cells that may now be fertilized by different sperm.

This twinning process has been seen to occur in the rat and the mouse, and natural human situations analogous to those experiments do raise twinning rates. According to Boklage, the half dozen or so studies seeking this kind of twinning in humans have been limited by one of two factors: (1) In several studies, the researchers were looking for twins identical for all maternal genes, which is impossible after the mixing of genes produced by recombination during the egg cell's development. (2) Some researchers knew that much but still lacked the technology to ask the question properly. With the specific exception of DNA sequences in or very near each chromosome's centromere (the part of the chromosome involved in chromosome sorting during cell division), there is no expectation that such twins would differ in their resemblance patterns from any pair of nonidentical siblings. Only within the past few years has it become possible to study centromeric sequences directly.

To research this type of twinning, Boklage is seeking dizygotic twins or triplets who are "a pair and a spare" (monozygotic twins plus a single), which is the most usual type of triplet combination. He requires blood samples from them and their parents and pays the costs incurred. (His address can be found in Resources.)

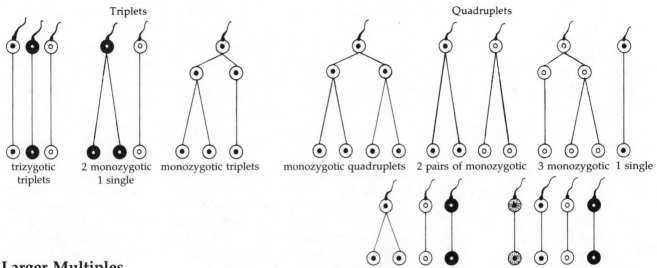

Triplets

trizygotic triplets   2 monozygotic 1 single   monozygotic triplets

Quadruplets

monozygotic quadruplets   2 pairs of monozygotic   3 monozygotic   1 single

2 monozygotic   2 dizygotic   quadrazygotic quadruplets

Larger Multiples

Triplets, quadruplets, and other multiple births may occur as a combination of monozygotic and dizygotic twinning or as just one of these types. The Dionne quintuplets were monozygotic, the result of one egg splitting into five divisions after fertilization. Monozygotic triplets may also occur, although it is the least frequent type. More commonly, triplets arise from three separate eggs or a combination of monozygotic twins and one singleton. (It is also possible that the pregnancy began as two pairs and that one embryo of one of the pairs "vanished." See Chapter 4.)

The use of hormones to stimulate ovulation as a treatment for infertility inflates the number of births of twins and larger multiples beyond the normal incidence. Multiple births that result from hormone therapy for infertility are commonly dizygotic, but with two particular types of therapy (in vitro fertilization and GIFT, discussed under "Reproductive Technology" in Chapter 3) there is an unexplained increase in monozygotic twins. (While the armadillo always has monozygotic quadruplets, the phenomenon is rare in humans.)

Twin deliveries average 1 in 90 of all live births (about 2 percent of all live babies) and 97 to 98 percent of all plural deliveries.* Prior to the use of fertility drugs, triplets occurred once in 90 × 90, or 8,100, pregnancies, according to Hellin's rule,† and quadruplets once in 90

"Supertwins" can develop in a multitude of ways.

---

* In 1987 in the United States, twins occurred at a rate of 1 in 83, if fetal deaths were included, and 1 in 92 of all live births.
† If the number of twins in a population is known, then the approximate number of triplets will be n^2 and of quadruplets n^3, where n is the number of twins.

× 90 × 90, or 729,000, pregnancies. The ratio of these multiple births per 1,000 total live births reached a thirty-year high in 1985: 21.0 for all U.S. women of childbearing age. In 1987, almost 3 percent of plural births were triplets or higher-order multiples.

Pregnancy Anomalies

It is possible, but extremely rare, for an *ectopic* twin pregnancy to occur. In such cases the egg does not reach the uterus but grows, for only a short while, outside the uterus, usually in the Fallopian tube. Combinations of one ectopic and one uterine pregnancy have happened. Women have also miscarried a twin, sometimes without realizing it, but delivered the other baby at term. Once in a while evidence of an undeveloped twin compressed into the placenta is observed at birth or can be found later in a tumor.*

Placenta and Membranes

During the first week after fertilization, the fertilized egg reaches the uterus and the *placenta* begins to develop in the wall of the uterus. The placenta, composed mostly of maternal and some fetal tissue, grows to be at least six inches across and a couple of inches thick. The function of this important organ is to transfer nutrients and waste products between the fetal and maternal circulations. The transfer is achieved by tiny fingerlike projections called villi, which are bathed by the mother's blood and together form a surface area of more than 150 square feet. The fetal blood vessels within the villi, if linked together, would be about thirty miles long. The fetus is attached to the placenta and thereby to the mother's circulation by the umbilical cord. Adequate development and function of each placenta are essential to fetal growth and well-being.

The developing fetus is contained within a membranous sac filled with fluid that provides freedom for growth and movement, acts as a shock absorber, and maintains an even temperature. The sac consists of two *membranes* that arise from the edge of the placenta. The outer membrane is the *chorion* and the inner layer is the *amnion*. The cell division that results in monozygotic twins usually occurs within the first week following fertilization, before the amnion devel-

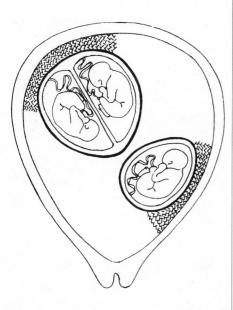

Triplets may be a combination of monozygotic twins and one single.

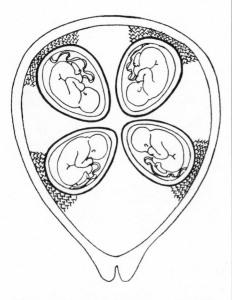

Quadruplets are commonly formed from four separate eggs (quadrazygotic).

* *Fetus papyraceus*, or *compressus*, is the medical term. Occasionally incomplete development appears as a hydatidiform mole.

ops (about day 9); therefore, each monozygotic twin almost always grows in his or her own separate inner sac. The chorion (outer sac) is formed around day 4; monozygotic twins developed before that time will also be enclosed in separate chorions.

Attention to the type of placenta and to the combination of placentas and membranes can reveal much about zygosity, or type of twinning, although not all obstetricians or pathologists are skilled in evaluating placentas. But the placenta should always be carefully examined at birth and samples sent for zygosity testing if the evidence is not clear.

The chorion or outer membrane is more opaque than the amnion, it contains blood vessels, and it is fused to the underneath surface of the placenta. A ridge felt on that surface of the placenta indicates the attachment of the chorion. When two chorions attach to the placenta, there is an obvious line where they join. The amnion is a clear shiny membrane with no blood vessels. It can be easily pulled away from the placental surface of adjacent membranes.

Placentas are described in amniotic and chorionic terms (*di-* for more than one placenta, *mono-* for a single placenta). A monochorionic placenta proves monozygotic twins. Two separate placentas occur rarely in monozygotic twins if the twinning process begins on the fourth day after fertilization. Dizygotic twins usually have two entirely separate placentas, but the placentas are sometimes fused. (This is a racially determined characteristic and is most common in African blacks.) Careful attention in such cases reveals that there are two amnions and two chorions without any connecting blood vessels. The dividing septum on the fetal surface of fused placentas has to be carefully examined for two or four layers.

It is thus not reliable to assume that twins of the same sex with what appears to be a single placenta are monozygotic, any more than to assume that separate placentas indicate dizygotic twins. If, on closer examination, the inner layers can be eased apart with no evidence of the outer chorionic tissue between them, one outer sac and one original egg — monozygotic twins — are suggested. However, sometimes microscopic analysis reveals chorionic tissue sandwiched between two amnionic layers.

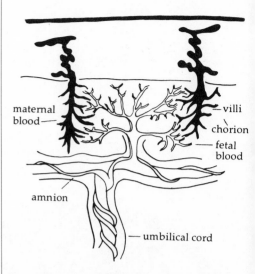

The babies' development depends on the growth and development of the placenta. Although the maternal and fetal circulations never mix, nutrients and waste products are exchanged through the villi.

Monoamnionic Twins

Twins formed after the first week of fertilization will be contained within one common inner sac and one outer sac. Only 1–2 percent of

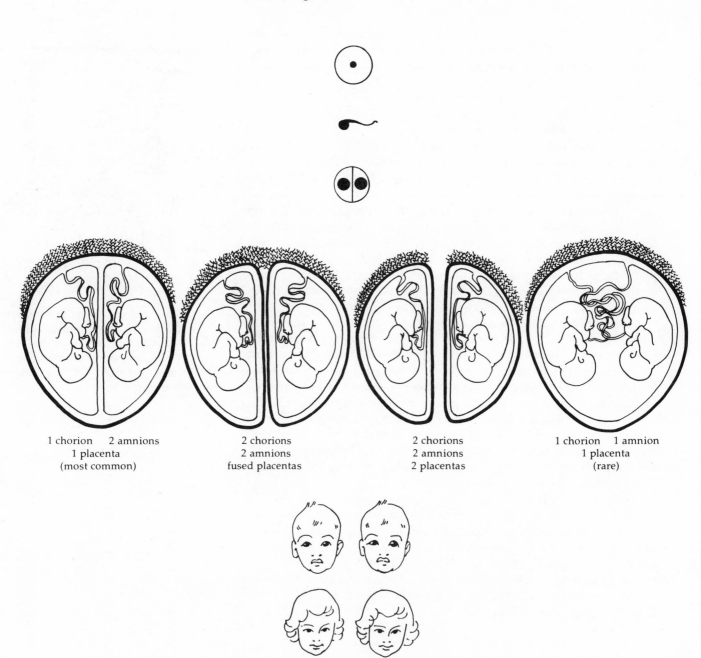

1 chorion   2 amnions
1 placenta
(most common)

2 chorions
2 amnions
fused placentas

2 chorions
2 amnions
2 placentas

1 chorion   1 amnion
1 placenta
(rare)

Monozygotic twins
are always the same sex.

Monozygotic twins result from the union of one egg and one sperm.

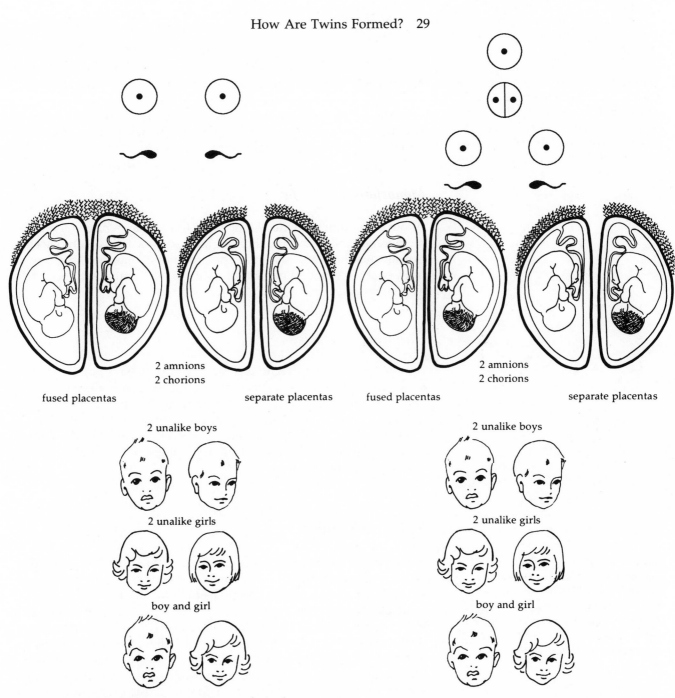

2 amnions
2 chorions

fused placentas

separate placentas

2 amnions
2 chorions

fused placentas

separate placentas

2 unalike boys

2 unalike girls

boy and girl

2 unalike boys

2 unalike girls

boy and girl

About 50% of dizygotic twin pairs are of mixed sex.

Dizygotic twins result from the fertilization of two eggs by two sperm.

"Polar body twinning": twins result from one egg and two sperm.

As triplets, we always thought we were one fraternal and two identical twins. Only when we were in our forties and all had blood tests because of a special illness that one of us developed did we find out that we were three fraternals.

monozygotic twins are monoamnionic. They can be diagnosed prenatally by ultrasound and amniocentesis (see Chapter 8).

Anomalies such as a single artery in the umbilical cord instead of two and insertion of the cord into the membranes instead of directly into the placenta are associated with monoamnionic twins.

Monochorionic Twins

About 60 percent of monozygotic twins have their own separate inner membranes and share one chorion. Monozygotic twins with one chorion always share one placenta. The presence of one chorion at a twin birth enables about 20 percent of twins to be identified immediately as monozygotic.

Dichorionic Twins

Another possible combination is for each twin to have both his or her own inner and outer sac. This is always the case with dizygotic twins and occurs in about 25 percent of monozygotic twins. Twins with separate chorions and amnions always have separate placentas, although in some cases the placentas can become fused. See the figures on pages 28 and 29 for a description of all possible combinations of placentas and membranes.

Zygosity Testing

Everyone had always thought we were fraternal twins. After four pregnancies I developed severe kidney disease and my sister and I underwent tests to see about a transplant. After three decades we learned that we were identical after all. Now I have one of my twin's kidneys.

Some people regard zygosity as unimportant unless there is going to be an organ transplant, but twins and their parents do not always know when the information might be helpful, and then it may not be available. For the twins' and their family's interest, as well as for medical research, it would be helpful if zygosity were established routinely and paid for by health insurance. Mothers who have lost twins often say they didn't "bother" to find out what type their twins were, but if they conceived multiples again they usually wished they had a way of knowing the zygosity of the first pair. Testing is necessary in only 25 percent of twin deliveries as different sex of the twins and type of placenta can usually determine the twin type.

Another method for determining zygosity is to test the blood from the umbilical cords. If the blood groups are different, then the twins are clearly not monozygotic. Blood testing beyond routine determination of blood type and Rh factor costs about $200 and examines other factors in the blood. These tests are about 85 percent accurate for white Americans, according to Boklage. HLA typing, which is done for paternity tests, is not useful in the case of twins because any siblings match in 25 percent of cases.

Physical appearance and skin color provide important evidence of zygosity as the twins grow older. (At birth, even monozygotic twins may look very different if they have been subject to the twin transfusion syndrome, discussed in Chapter 7.) Dental characteristics are also identical for monozygotic twins.

The handprints and footprints of monozygotic twins are similar, but the fingerprints are always unique. One study found errors in almost a quarter of the cases where twin typing was determined on the basis of fingerprints, but when information about hair and eye color was given, the error was reduced to 13 percent. The late Dr. H. W. Kloepfer, a geneticist at Tulane University in New Orleans, did extensive evaluations of handprints and footprints from hundreds of twin pairs to provide 95 percent accuracy in the determination of twin types.

The ultimate zygosity test is DNA "fingerprinting," which has nothing to do with hands. Any sample of human tissue may be sent to a genetics lab for analysis — blood is the most common sample, but this typing has been done even on a few hair roots. There is only one chance in 16,000 that all the markers in a set of chromosomes will match another person's DNA. This test costs about $600 and is required only for same-sex dichorionic twins whose zygosity cannot be established by other methods.

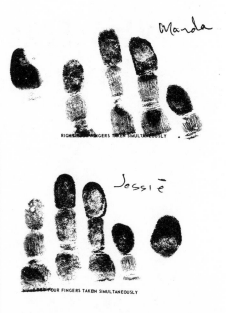

Not even monozygotic twins have the same fingerprints.

Who Has Twins?

3

BIRTHS OF TWINS and other multiples are recorded by statisticians and analyzed in population studies. Many of the statistics are difficult to decipher and compare, however, partly because of differences in the populations catalogued, discrepancies or uncertainties in collecting and reporting the data, and variances in the way data are classified and analyzed. The picture is further confused by undetermined zygosity (type of twinning) in many cases and lack of information about artificial versus spontaneous conceptions. With the use of fertility drugs and reproductive technology today, it is no longer possible to discern true characteristics of the twinbearing population. In addition, many studies rely on volunteers and self-administered questionnaires, so standardizing and comparing twin data are difficult.

Twinning peaks vary at different times in the same population and in different populations. They may depend on the mother's age of menarche (onset of menstruation) or the age at which the mother had her first child or even sociolegal circumstances such as the availability of abortion. The content of the diet as well as adequacy of nutrition may play a role in predisposition to twinning and may explain geographical and ethnic differences in the incidence of twins.

In discussing the incidence of twinning, statistics deal only with the birth of twins, but we now realize that many more twins are lost than we ever knew before — from induced abortions, miscarriage, and the vanishing twin syndrome (discussed in Chapter 4). Likewise, stillbirths are often excluded from the twin tally, and it is not always clear that twins are counted if there is only one survivor (discussed in Chapter 6).

Some statistics, however, can give us an insight into the types of people who are more likely than others to have multiple pregnancies. The factors causing monozygotic twins are not understood, but the incidence of this type of twinning is almost the same among different races and cultures. Trends have been observed with dizygotic twins that depend on race, age, family size, seasons, geography, hormones, and heredity. Some of these factors may coexist. For example, if an increase in twin births is related to both maternal age and the use of oral contraceptives, societies in which women postpone child-bearing by taking the pill may show a higher number of twins in the older age group. It is not uncommon for women to ovulate twice a month, as can be learned from basal temperature charts, and geneti-cally more women inherit the likelihood of bearing twins than ac-tually do.

Race

Twinning rates, zygosity, and types of placenta vary considerably with race. The greatest number of twin births occur among the Nige-rians, particularly the Yoruba — about 45 per 1,000 births. The fewest numbers of twins are born to Asians. Twins occur among Japanese and Chinese at the rate of about 4 per 1,000 births. However, while dizygotic twins are more common than monozygotic twins in gen-eral, among the Japanese there are two sets of monozygotic twins for

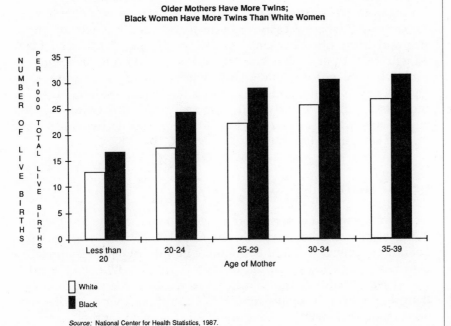

**Older Mothers Have More Twins;
Black Women Have More Twins Than White Women**

NUMBER OF LIVE BIRTHS — PER 1000 TOTAL LIVE BIRTHS

Age of Mother: Less than 20, 20-24, 25-29, 30-34, 35-39

☐ White
■ Black

Source: National Center for Health Statistics, 1987.

Twinning is more common in blacks than in whites.

every set of dizygotic. For a mixed group of Asians, such as Chinese, Malays, and Indians, the rate is 8 per 1,000 births. The incidence in Europeans and white Americans falls between these two extremes: 25.3 per 1,000 for black Americans and 20.4 per 1,000 for whites. This racial factor is thought to have a hormonal basis, as higher levels of circulating hormones that stimulate egg production in the ovary are found in blacks and mothers of twins generally. The rate for multiple nonwhite births in 1960 was 36 percent higher than that for white multiple births, but in 1985 the difference between the races decreased to 24 percent. In contrast, monozygotic twins occur with almost uniform frequency in all racial groups — between 4 and 5 per 1,000 births. The rate is always less than that of dizygotic twins except in Asia, where they are about the same. The chance of a triplet pregnancy for white Americans has been calculated at 1 in 8,400 and for black Americans 1 in 9,800.

Age

It has long been understood that the older the mother, the more likely she is to have twins. This theory is based on the indication that with increasing age the female body produces higher levels of gonadotropin hormones, which predispose more eggs to mature and be released from the ovaries (see "Hormones" later in this chapter). In 1987, the incidence of twinning peaked between the ages of thirty-five and thirty-nine for white Americans (27 per 1,000), and black Americans (31 per 1,000). The rate after age forty diminishes except for black women, for whom the incidence of twins increases through age forty-nine. Although there is a general decrease in twin births for mothers age forty to forty-four, this age group had twice as many supertwins in 1987 as in 1980. In 1971 there were 18 twins per 1,000 births; the figures rose to nearly 22 per 1,000 by 1987.

Sexual Activity

Despite the common correlation between maternal age and the incidence of twins, other research has found that twins are most frequently conceived within the first three months of marriage, presumably because of higher levels of sexual activity. Likewise, a post-World War II study found that twins were conceived more promptly than singletons as veterans returned home. The observation has also been made that twins occur more often in unwed mothers, and the

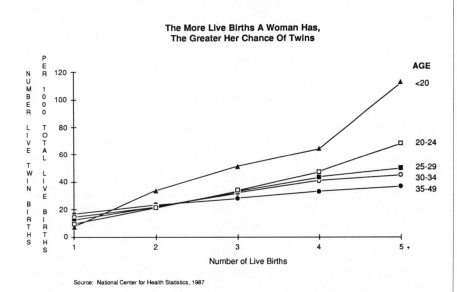

The More Live Births A Woman Has,
The Greater Her Chance Of Twins

Source: National Center for Health Statistics, 1987

Older mothers have more twins.

explanation may involve the irregularity of sexual intercourse. (I know of several cases in which a single woman conceived twins with one sexual encounter.) The twinning rate in one Swedish study was 40 percent higher for unwed than for married mothers.

Another Swedish study reported that mixed-sex dizygotic twins were more common in younger mothers, who engaged in intercourse more frequently than older women. The investigation assumed that the sex of the offspring is related to the phase of the menstrual cycle when fertilization occurs. This idea has been publicized by Dr. Landrum Shettles in his guide to timing intercourse to favor the conception of the preferred sex (*Your Baby's Sex: Now You Can Choose*). Human ovulation, as in the rabbit, can be triggered by sexual activity, particularly by female orgasm, as well as influenced by higher centers in the brain; indeed, some women have willed their egg to split or consciously desired to release two eggs, according to Australian psychiatrist Graham Farrant.

Family Size

Twinbearing families are more fertile, and statistics show that the more children a woman has, the greater her chance of conceiving twins. However, because an increase in family size also parallels an increase in maternal age, the two factors are associated. The number of prior live births, however, is the more significant influence, according to unpublished 1988 data from the National Center for Health Statistics.

Seasons

Twin births do not usually occur under the sign of Gemini. Actually, the reverse was found in a 1976 survey in England: the probability of a twin birth was lowest in May and highest in November. Many researchers found no significant seasonality, while others have found peaks in different months. Twins conceptions in the Northern Hemisphere are generally highest in February and March, as the days become longer and lighter. Some interesting random facts emerge out of a considerable body of research. For example, in Italy increased twinning has been observed when the mother was born between January and May and when the grandmother was born in winter; also, mothers born in the summer produce fewer mixed-sex twins.

Geography

Although Scandinavians record twinning rates similar to those of Europeans and Caucasian Americans, some Finnish island communities have had a very high incidence. The rate was 15–20 per 1,000 until the 1960s, when it began to decline, compared with 7–11 per 1,000 for Europe in general. A possible explanation is that the exposure to light of certain glands, such as the pineal and pituitary, following the long northern winters stimulates double ovulation. The decline in multiple births in these formerly isolated communities over the past thirty years is attributed to population increase, urbanization, and changes in marriage and migration patterns.

Like seasonality, the literature on twinning and geography reveals a mixed bag of conclusions. In Rumania, high twinning rates similar to those of blacks in the United States have been observed. One study in California found that the frequency of twinning was higher there than in the rest of the country, but a more recent study noted an increased rate among whites in the northeastern states.

Twinning has always been more common in rural than in urban areas. Explanations include the larger stature and superior physical fitness of rural women as well as better diet and less environmental pollution. Population characteristics and social customs of marriage and childbearing are also associated with geographical differences.

Hormones

Mothers of dizygotic twins, especially Nigerians, who have the highest rate of twinning in the world, show high levels of gonadotropin hormones, which stimulate the ovaries. The normal ovary has about half a million eggs, but only about four hundred actually mature in the thirty-to-forty-year span of a woman's reproductive life. Gonadotropins such as follicle-stimulating hormone (FSH), human chorionic gonadotropin (HCG), and the drug Pergonal stimulate ovulation, as does clomiphene citrate (Clomid, Serophene), a synthetic agent that affects hormone function. All have been used successfully to treat human female infertility and in animal husbandry to increase litter size.

Sometimes hormone therapy can produce very-high-order multiples. Nonuplets (nine babies) were conceived by women in Sydney, Australia, in 1971, in Birmingham, England, in 1976, and in Naples, Italy, in 1979, as a result of hormone therapy. In 1988, twelve fetuses were miscarried by a woman in Switzerland. These large multiples caused considerable distress for the parents. As higher doses and frequent administration of hormones are more likely to result in a multiple birth, hormone therapy is now carefully monitored and such mishaps are less common.

Clomiphene citrate is the most widely used fertility drug, and it leads to the conception of twins in about 7 to 10 percent of the women who take it. Pergonal, a more powerful drug prepared from the natural hormones in the urine of postmenopausal women, encourages the egg to mature, but ovulation itself requires an injection of another hormone, HCG (human chorionic gonadotropin). (A test for this same hormone in pregnant women aids in the diagnosis of twins, discussed in Chapter 4.) Approximately 20 percent of the pregnancies achieved with Pergonal turn out to be multiples, most of them twins.

These kinds of infertility therapy have caused a greater number of multiples to be born than would occur naturally within a given population.

Studies attempting to link oral contraceptives and twinning have been largely inconclusive: they have shown that the use of oral contraceptives increases the chance of a twin pregnancy, makes no difference, or even causes a decline in twinning rates!

Grace Wyshak, a biostatistician at Harvard Medical School, has shown that mothers of multiples have an earlier onset of menstruation, shorter menstrual cycles, and earlier menopause than mothers of singletons. Research by others on Orthodox Jewish women indi-

I took Clomid for my first pregnancy and we had only one baby. I thought the same thing would happen again, but I had quads.

I had tried to get pregnant for fifteen years. Clomid did nothing for me, so the doctor resorted to Pergonal. Conceiving triplets means we will have quite a large family after a long wait.

cates that women who conceive late in their ovulatory cycle have a threefold chance of bearing twins.

Reproductive Technology

In addition to hormonal stimulation of the ovaries, new surgical techniques have increased the number of multiple births. In vitro fertilization (IVF), gametes intra-Fallopian transfer (GIFT), and embryo transfer (ET) are invasive and expensive undertakings, and to increase the likelihood of a successful pregnancy two or more embryos may be transplanted.

The process of IVF involves removing one or more eggs from the stimulated ovary and mixing them with sperm in a glass dish (not a test tube). After fertilization, the resulting embryos are placed in the uterus. In GIFT, the eggs and sperm are mixed together and then placed in the Fallopian tube, where conception would have occurred naturally. Embryo transfer involves IVF with a donor egg in cases where a woman has diseased or absent ovaries.

Heredity

If a mother has already borne dizygotic twins, her chances of conceiving another set are quadrupled. Mothers of dizygotic twins often show more than one egg ripening in a reproductive cycle. Wyshak has done extensive research on the inheritance of genetic factors in twinning, using the excellent records kept by the Mormon Church in Salt Lake City, Utah. She found that the gene favoring dizygotic twins passes along the female line. If a woman has a history of dizygotic twins in her family on her mother's side or if she is a twin herself, her chances of conceiving twins are increased. However, not all the women who are genetically capable of bearing twins actually do so, for some of the reasons discussed in this chapter.

The influence of heredity through the paternal line, or with monozygotic twinning, is unclear. While it is generally acknowledged that the incidence of monozygotic twins is uniform for all groups, since the 1970s the monozygotic rate has increased by more than 50 percent in Sweden and northwestern Europe. Some intriguing cases of monozygotic twinning have been reported. Four sets of monozygotic twins were discovered in one extended family, and there are cases in which a mother had monozygotic twins by two different husbands. Similarly, a man had monozygotic twins with two different wives. There are also cases in which monozygotic twins have had monozygotic twins.

The genetic component in twinning is modified by environmental factors. These factors include psychological stress, nutrition, climate, and intercourse after sexual abstinence, which may stimulate hormone production. Environmental influences may affect the egg, the uterine environment, or both.

Nutrition and Physical Characteristics

Older, heavier, and taller women with several children have the greatest tendency to bear twins. Denmark, Norway, and the Netherlands have the most twins among whites — 20.48 per 1,000 births. Africans have more twins than Asians, who are smaller. Women who conceive twins weigh more for their height prior to pregnancy than women who bear singletons.

Since twinning rates fall during wartime, the influence of nutrition is considered significant. Evidence of this fact has been shown in animal husbandry: if sheep are fed a better diet, more twins are born. With the use of fertility drugs, small-framed women often conceive twins or higher-order multiples and have difficulty gaining and comfortably carrying adequate weight.

African women who were themselves twins or children of twins were not found to be more likely to bear twins than women with no family history of twinning. As this is contrary to statistics in white populations, environmental causes were sought. Diet, particularly yams (sweet potatoes),* has been suggested as an explanation. The incidence of twinning is higher — 62 per 1,000 — in the classes of African society where a native diet is consumed and lower — 15 per 1,000 — in the upper strata, whose members eat a more Western diet.

It is clear that the causes of twinning are many and complex. The chances of having twins are not increased just because twins "run in the family." A woman's age, hormone levels, nutrition, emotional state, sexual activity, and environmental conditions (including season and latitude) all play a role along with inheritance. Even if dizygotic twins have occurred in the mother's family, she may never conceive dizygotic twins or, by a stroke of fate, may actually have monozygotic twins.

* Apparently yams contain a hormone-like substance that plays a role in twinning.

How to Tell if There Are More than One

4

THE DETECTION of multiple pregnancy is not difficult, and medical technology continues to develop resources for diagnosis. A common problem in twin pregnancies is that twins are simply not suspected. Even if the mother herself queries her doctor or midwife, the idea is often dismissed with the remark "Oh, it's just a big baby." Although ultrasound is used more often now in routine prenatal care, twins still go undetected, especially in rural areas. However, the situation has greatly improved since 1962, when the Mothers of Twins Clubs in Illinois surveyed its 2,631 members and found that only 510 knew of their twins in advance. A Twin Services study in the San Francisco Bay area in 1981 found a 75 percent diagnosis rate of twins prior to birth. A 1984 POMBA survey in Canada found that 82 percent were diagnosed before birth. In a 1986 study with 80 Massachusetts volunteers, the figure was 89 percent. In all cases the diagnosis was made by ultrasound.

Every pregnant woman, at some time during her nine-month pregnancy, wonders if she is carrying twins as she contemplates her astonishing abdomen. If there is a history of twins in the family, relatives are usually the first to suggest this possibility to an expectant couple.

Some couples just have an uncanny feeling and are often proved right. One woman, only in her third month and not obviously pregnant, was amazed when a complete stranger approached her in a nightclub and declared that she was carrying twins. She laughed off the comment at the time, but a few weeks later her doctor confirmed the psychic's intuition.

Confirming a multiple pregnancy is important for medical reasons as well as for allowing the couple time to get over the surprise and make adequate physical and psychological preparations.

Twin pregnancy is frequently associated with exaggeration and earlier onset of the customary signs and normal discomfort of the pregnant state — what medical texts call a "high suspicion index." The uterus may be very large for the stage of pregnancy, assuming

I became suspicious when I needed to be in maternity clothes at three months.

I had gained 70 pounds by the time I was seven months pregnant. I couldn't find maternity clothes to fit. If I tried on a size 13 or 14 it would fit my legs and bottom, but forget my belly. I couldn't pull the pants anywhere near it. Then if I found anything to go over my waist, my legs would be swimming in it.

an accurate menstrual history. Marked weight gain is another indicator, particularly at the beginning of pregnancy. In a 1987 survey by *Twins* magazine, 37 percent of respondents who suspected they were carrying multiples thought so because of weight and abdominal size. Physical changes are more apparent in subsequent pregnancies than during the first, but growth with twins is much faster in the early weeks than with a singleton.

Weight Gain

The pregnant woman's weight gain relates to the baby's weight gain, so a woman carrying twins may gain about twice what she would carrying one baby. This is a necessary, positive, and healthy sign. The *Twins* survey found that weight gains ranged from less than 30 pounds to more than 80 pounds. Most mothers, especially those who breast-fed, quickly lost the extra weight after birth. Adequate nutrition and its associated weight gain are of vital importance for the future mental and physical development of the babies, for the mother's own physical requirements, and for the successful outcome of the pregnancy.

Body size is not always an indication of twins, however, as some mothers gain less with twins than others do with singletons. If they eat an excellent diet with adequate protein, the needs of their unborn babies may be met, but an expectant mother who is poorly nourished and does not gain enough weight risks having her multiple pregnancy escape detection, leading to serious consequences for the survival and health of her babies. It has been found that twins diagnosed during pregnancy were heavier than those who were not.

Standards of weight gain vary among cultures, ethnic groups, and health care providers. Until recently, obstetricians severely restricted weight gain in pregnancy, and today it is not uncommon to hear of a physician who holds his or her pregnant women to a fixed number of pounds. Undiagnosed twins would clearly suffer malnutrition under such limits. In 1990 I visited a midwestern city where I learned that the common practice was to limit mothers of twins to a 35-pound weight gain. It is far better, when in doubt about twins, to err on the side of increased nutrition and growth so that the chance of low-birth-weight or premature offspring is reduced. (See Chapter 9 for a comprehensive discussion of dietary needs.) Mothers expecting multiples often show great weight gain in early and late pregnancy rather than in the middle, as is usually the case with singletons.

My midwife thought I was carrying twins the first time we met. She said I had that "look" about me — so large that my arms and legs looked like sticks.

I put on 60 pounds and I was absolutely huge — just like a ship in full sail.

My doctor said it couldn't be twins. I'd put on only 18 pounds and he said I wasn't large enough.

I was like a sow with suckers.

I lost sight of my feet at six months.

My belly button popped too early for one baby.

My weight gain was 55 pounds, but it was all out in front and I felt just great.

What a relief to learn it was twins. Imagine having a 16-pound baby.

My physician diagnosed twins at three months. I had gained 25 pounds.

I felt like I was carrying a 12-foot baby — there had to be two.

The doctor told me my abdominal muscles were "all shot," but I didn't know what he meant.

Sometimes it is easy to ignore the obvious. One mother of twins put on 80 pounds during her pregnancy, but neither she nor her doctor ever considered the possibility of twins — which she indeed produced.

At each prenatal visit the doctor or midwife measures the distance from the mother's pubic bone to the top of the uterus, known as the *fundal height*. Guidelines exist for normal distances at each stage of development. From about the third to the eighth month, a higher fundus than indicated in the guidelines suggests twins; it may reach the rib cage by thirty weeks. After the eighth month, growth is relative to the size of the baby, and measuring the circumference of the girth of the mother's abdomen may provide more clues about the pregnancy.

The extra stretching that occurs with a multiple pregnancy, in addition to higher levels of circulating hormones that soften the tissues, predisposes to separation of the abdominal muscles (*diastasis recti*). The woman may notice a peaking or bulging in the midline of the abdominal wall, which develops as the abdominal muscles and their central seam expand to accommodate the extra baby. If a woman's abdominal muscles are poorly supportive and she experiences

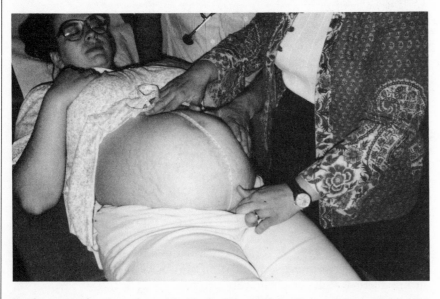

In the case of twins, the midwife finds a greater distance from the pubic bone to the top of the uterus (the fundal height) for the duration of the pregnancy.

severe backache, a corset such as the Baby Hugger (an all-cotton support designed by a physical therapist) may help. (See Resources.) However, early preventive exercise (discussed in Chapter 10) is much better.

Feeling the contours of the uterus through the abdominal wall, known as *palpation*, may reveal clues about a twin pregnancy. It is not just a simple matter of discerning two ''bumps''; usually the doctor or midwife feels three or more fetal parts, combinations of heads and breeches (buttocks and legs). Sometimes he or she may feel one fetal head that is very small in relation to the size of the uterus. If a fetal head can be felt low in the pelvis, yet the fundus seems too long for one baby, twins may be suspected.

Discomfort

Multiple pregnancy may cause mothers to experience more discomfort than they did in previous pregnancies, if this is not their first. The most common physical problems reported in the *Twins* magazine survey were inability to sleep, exhaustion, general discomfort and pain, water retention or swollen legs, nausea, and inability to walk more than a short distance. Mothers expecting twins may be more anemic because of the increased iron demand of two babies; anemia can cause or add to feelings of fatigue and irritability. Body size and lethargy may be problems for some only at the end of pregnancy. It appears, however, that some women are ''born to have twins.'' Contrary to most medical expectations, they feel wonderful and blossom through the pregnancy. These women may even experience more than one multiple pregnancy and enjoy each one with great enthusiasm. As with weight gain, some health care providers have a built-in bias that runs counter to women's intuition about their bodies. That is, feeling good discourages the suspicion of twins, whereas complaints of discomfort and pressure enhance the possibility.

Swelling of the hands and feet and dilation of veins are more pronounced with a multiple pregnancy, as the mother's blood volume is greatly increased to service the two placentas that are the babies' source of nourishment. Increased hormone levels in pregnancy also encourage fluid retention and relaxation of the walls of the blood vessels, perhaps leading to varicose veins.

Itching of the abdominal wall, a common irritation in pregnancy, is often worse with twins. The greatest itching, burning, and sometimes a sensation of numbness or even pain are localized around the

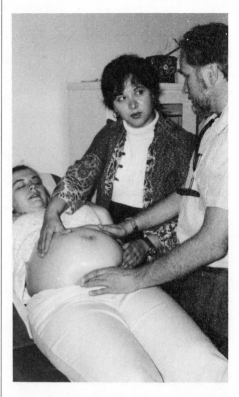

Sometimes an extra body can be felt. The midwife and obstetrician consult each other on the abdominal contours.

My three twin pregnancies were marvelous. I was sick the whole time with my only single pregnancy that came between.

I blew up like a balloon. My ankles were the same diameter as my thighs.

Typing became difficult because of fluid at my wrists and the stiffness in my fingers.

upper ribs and breastbone. (Friction massage can help.) The extra size of the abdomen in multiple pregnancy leads to generalized discomfort, awkwardness, and difficulty breathing and sleeping.

Fetal Movement

I was fortunate to have felt great throughout my entire pregnancy. I was thrilled in my last trimester when the babies were extremely active.

My doctor never believed I was having twins until they arrived. But Nick and I used to spend hours staring at the bumps. We were sure one baby could not move so much at once.

Multiples create more movement than singletons. Couples can sometimes diagnose twins by observing fetal movement, although they may have to watch the changing abdomen contours for quite a while. Only 9 percent of the respondents to the *Twins* survey suspected multiples because of an unusual amount of fetal movement. Awareness of the first fetal movements often occurs earlier in twin pregnancies. As with palpation, it is not just two moving parts, but several, that suggest twins. Mothers may feel the babies turning or kicking in all directions.Some mothers report activity levels within the uterus that are strong enough to interfere with sleep, while other women claim there was nothing unusual about the movements they felt during pregnancy.

Frequently a mother will notice different activity levels of the twins' movements. Many mothers notice exactly the same traits in their babies after birth as they displayed within the uterus. Toward the end of pregnancy there is little room for the babies to change position, and the mother can identify each twin by its position and become acquainted with each one's personality.

The parents' observations of their babies' characteristics during pregnancy may affect how they view the twins in infancy and thereafter. The child who is considered to have a certain trait will be expected to demonstrate certain behavior, which will be encouraged and reinforced. But perhaps it is the child who did not have as much room to move around in the uterus who becomes the active crawler, making up for lost time. Parents can encourage the less active baby before birth (see Chapter 6).

In the uterus Betsy preferred the left side. All I felt was a flutter from time to time. She is a flighty child, unlike her sister Barbara, who thudded hard and continuously in the uterus and is a more solid person.

While movement is obviously a sign of fetal well-being, the medical profession relies more on sophisticated tests, some of them potentially risky. Mothers themselves can feel and accurately record 90 percent of fetal movements and should be encouraged to be very aware of each baby. Relying on the pregnant woman for important observations about the progress of her pregnancy is something that many busy obstetricians may not be willing to do (although many are employing midwives, who are more apt to take the pregnant woman's observations seriously). In countless cases, however, the pregnant woman's feeling that something is "not right" about the pregnancy turns out to be a warning about a problem with the baby. Women must trust their intuition and demand medical intervention if they feel something has changed for the worse. This point was emphasized to me by mothers who had lost one twin or both during pregnancy.

Heartbeats

After the twelfth week of pregnancy it is possible to detect the fetal heartbeat with special equipment. The ultrasound Doptone is a more sensitive measuring device than the regular fetal stethoscope (fetoscope). Hearing two heartbeats confirms a twin pregnancy, but both may be difficult to detect if one twin's position muffles the sound of the other. If two heartbeats are suspected, the recommended procedure is for two examiners to listen and count the beats separately with two Doptones or one Doptone and one fetoscope (after the eighteenth week). It helps if there is a difference of eight to ten beats in the fetal heart rates, but often there is not. Couples can also try to

As a counselor for parents of children with special needs, I have been struck with the reliability of the mother's prediction during pregnancy that "something" was wrong.

Sure I felt a lot of movement. It was like having an octopus inside.

My midwife thought I was having twins when she found a heartbeat well away from where she expected.

My doctor said I was too small for twins, but I was always sure he was wrong. When I entered the hospital in early labor, I asked the nurse to see if she could pick up a second heartbeat. "You know, I think you are right," she said. Then the room filled with people.

My boyfriend was the one who was so sure. He came to one of my appointments and insisted that the doctor check for twins.

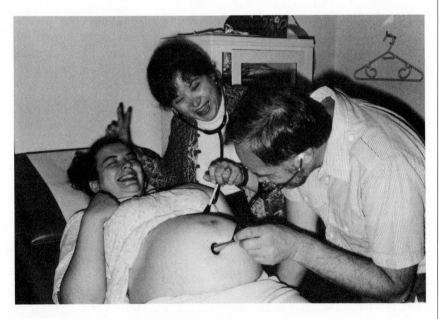

It takes two to hear the heartbeats of twins.

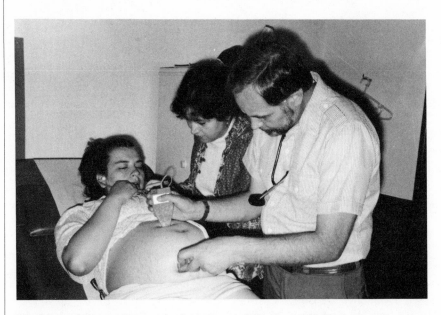

Mother and doctor listen to a heartbeat while the midwife looks on.

listen with a fetoscope or even an empty toilet roll cylinder or a plastic shot glass with a hole drilled through it. Parents or an examiner should be sure to take the mother's pulse at the same time to avoid mistaking the mother's aortic sound for a second fetal heartbeat. Identifying the heartbeat of each twin may help in determining their positions, although changes will occur, even as late as labor.

Hormones

Tests for hormone levels, which are increased in multiple pregnancy, may help in diagnosing twin pregnancy, but commonly a woman is sent for an ultrasound as soon as a multiple pregnancy is suspected. Human chorionic gonadotropin (HCG) is secreted by the chorion, the outer membrane that encloses the fetus. This hormone maintains the body of the fertilized egg in early pregnancy until it can develop sufficient hormones for its own survival. High levels of HCG, which can be measured in the mother's blood or urine, suggest multiple pregnancy. The hormone human placental lactogen (HPL) is a monitor of placental function and is associated with maternal weight. Low levels of this hormone during pregnancy have been linked to low birth weight and shorter newborns. The increased levels of this hormone from the two placentas in twin pregnancies provide guidelines for ruling out rather than confirming twins. In triplet pregnancies, levels of HPL are even higher. A new blood test to detect the rise of the hormone bHOG can predict a twin pregnancy as early as four to six weeks. Simple tests for these hormones could help to minimize the number of women who are required to have further screening, such as ultrasound.

X-Rays

X-rays have been available for decades, and the risks to the unborn child from exposure in early pregnancy are well documented. For this reason, x-rays have been replaced by ultrasound technology, which is considered safe, although the long-term side effects are unknown.

Ultrasound

Ultrasound technology uses sound waves that occur at a frequency beyond the range of human hearing to locate and identify hidden bodies of all types. The technology was first used to follow submarines, locate shipwrecks, and measure the depth of lakes and oceans. Also known as sonography, echography, B-scans, or Doppler, ultrasound procedures are now used in all fields of medicine, including obstetrics. Many obstetricians perform ultrasound in their offices, and in some states and other countries one or more ultrasound per pregnancy is mandatory.

Multiple pregnancy and the position of the placentas can be determined by ultrasound, along with the presentation of the babies. Ultrasound can also detect an ectopic pregnancy and twin transfusion syndrome (discussed in Chapter 7). Sound waves are passed through the twins' body surfaces at different angles and are deflected by different densities of body tissues. These echoes are amplified and displayed on a screen as white dots outlined against a black background. The resulting picture is called a *sonogram* (see page 49).

Persson in 1983 in Sweden found that 98 percent of twin pregnancies were detected by the seventh week with routine ultrasound scanning. Hugh and Oliver in 1985 diagnosed 94 percent of the twins in the group that underwent routine ultrasound scanning compared with 68 percent in the control group. Outcome was greatly improved with early diagnosis, and the incidence of unfavorable outcome was

My first scan showed twins, but in later pregnancy I had a follow-up scan that revealed triplets. People often ask me what my husband said when he heard the news and I tell them the truth — nothing!

The x-ray technician and my doctor told me I was having twins and showed me the two heads on the x-ray. But I saw a third head there and indeed I was right!

When we saw two little babies on the screen, we were awed by the miracle of their creation and humbled by our own inability to determine our lives.

My doctor wanted me to have an ultrasound because he suspected twins. I refused, right to the end. It wasn't the test itself, but I knew that I'd be rated as high risk. I wanted to feel in control of my own normal pregnancy.

My doctor did not agree that I was having twins and would not order an ultrasound. So I got an order from another physician, and there they were.

Because I had been taking both Clomid and Pergonal, as soon as I was pregnant my doctor suggested a scan to see if I was carrying twins. I was utterly stunned when I learned there were five! I found this out at twelve weeks, even though I had not gained a pound.

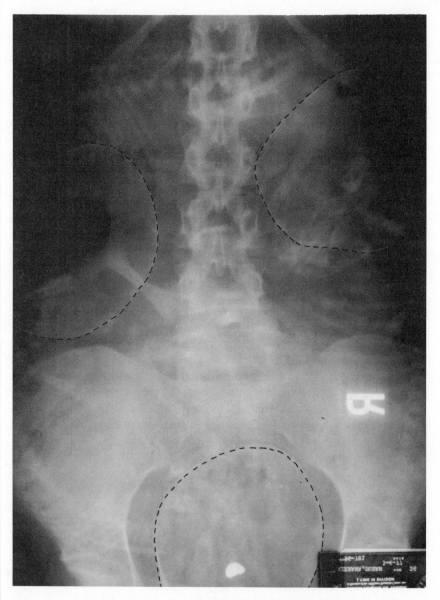

This x-ray shows that one triplet's head is in the pelvis, ready for labor.

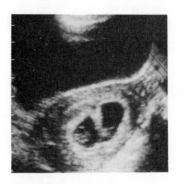

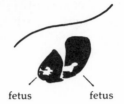

fetus   fetus

A.

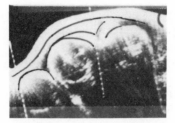

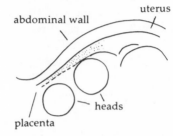

abdominal wall   uterus

placenta   heads

B.

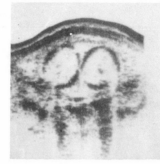

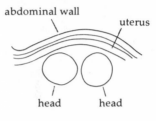

abdominal wall   uterus

head   head

C.

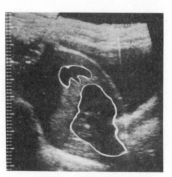

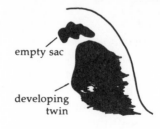

empty sac

developing
twin

D.

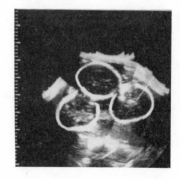

head

head

head

E.

Ultrasound is the most common way
to diagnose multiple pregnancy.
(A) Even as early as seven weeks,
twins can be seen in their developing
sacs. (B) Twins at twenty-three weeks.
(C) Twins showing the placental
plate. (D) The empty sac (a "vanished
twin"), right, shows that only one
twin is developing. (E) Triplets at
twenty-seven weeks.

I miscarried in my third month, but after a few weeks I was convinced I was still pregnant. My doctor was reluctant to believe me but sent me for a scan. You could still see the empty sac as well as the other twin growing healthily. As a twin myself, I did not particularly want twins and I also have another child. The miscarriage, then, was a relief more than a disappointment.

I was so angry when I had that second scan. They told me I was having twins at twelve weeks and now there is only one. I've been knitting two of everything, and my parents gave me two bassinets.

reduced from 60 percent to 25 percent: there were fewer occurrences of prematurity, low-birth-weight or growth-retarded babies, and stillbirths.

The actual ultrasound procedure is simple and takes only a few minutes. There may be some discomfort in early pregnancy when the mother's bladder has to be full to raise the uterus for a better view. Vaginal probes are now in use that do not require a full bladder and are more accurate in the first few weeks. Otherwise, the mother lies on her back, a gel is placed on her skin to transmit the sound waves, and an instrument called a transducer is moved over her abdomen. A picture is built up of the pelvic contents, and Polaroid photos are taken for the medical record. Often the couple may obtain one of the photos of their unborn twins. While ultrasound diagnosis is highly accurate, it is nevertheless not foolproof. Twin pregnancies have been identified where in fact there are triplets, the third baby being hidden by shadow or in the pelvis.

Detection of Vanishing Twin Syndrome

Sometimes twins are detected in early pregnancy but only one grows to term, a phenomenon called *vanishing twin* syndrome. With increasing use of ultrasound, it has been observed that more multiples are lost in the uterus than previously thought — some studies say as high as 80 percent of twin pregnancies. The reason that only one twin develops is not understood. In addition to errors in diagnosis, theories include malformations, which the body frequently rejects, and lack of oxygen for some reason within the uterine environment.

Symptoms of loss may include vaginal bleeding, cramps, or decreased hormone levels. More often there are no symptoms at all and the doomed twin is simply resorbed; rarely, remnants of the membranes and placenta may be delivered at birth. Thus, without ultrasound, women and their doctors would never know a twin had vanished.

One woman described losing a twin at fourteen weeks when she experienced bleeding. She felt sure she had been carrying twins, but her midwives, hearing a good fetal heartbeat with the Doptone, said she did not need to have an ultrasound. Subsequently, she delivered a healthy baby at home but did not pass all the membranes. Not wanting any intervention, she waited and a few days later delivered the rest of the membranes, which were torn at both ends. Ten days after that event, she delivered a small placenta, about three by four inches, with a torn outer sac and an intact inner sac.

Radiologist Jason Birnholz recommends that ultrasound scans be routinely performed in cases of bleeding during the first three months in case it is a twin pregnancy and there is a second, normal fetus. If not identified, this pregnancy could be lost through dilation and curettage (D&C), the typical procedure used to clear out the uterus after miscarriage. With recent improvements in diagnostic equipment, it can be expected that more twin sacs will be diagnosed in early pregnancy. The women in Birnholz's study who had one normal and one empty sac made up 5 percent of patients who received ultrasound examination in the first three months following bleeding.

Other Uses of Ultrasound

Ultrasound scans are also done to clarify the stage of the pregnancy and the development of the twins, if there is some doubt about the dates of conception and the size the fetuses should have attained. The information from the ultrasound is more accurate in early pregnancy; the pregnancy can be dated to the day up to about sixteen weeks.

Although I found out later that my insurance did not cover my scan, I was glad to pay for it to know for sure they were twins. The technician pointed out all the details.

Determining the progress of growth within the uterus has been considered a predictor of the outcome for twins. In early pregnancy the length from the crown to the rump of the fetus is measured. In later pregnancy the diameter between the skull bones is measured to assess the fetus's developmental age, although this is less helpful in twins because after the thirtieth week their growth rate may decline if the mother is not well nourished. Investigators have called for special scales for twin skull measurements, as singleton values do not apply. But standard measurements of the length of fetal thighbones or abdominal circumference growth charts can be used to predict the stage of growth for twins.

Sometimes ultrasound reveals the sex of the baby by the absence or presence of the male genitals. Not all couples want to know the sex; nor do all technicians tell them. I believe that it enhances bonding to know as much as you can about your babies. Babies have also been seen with their thumbs in their mouths and with erections in utero.

For decades physical therapists have made use of ultrasound in much higher dosages than those used for pregnancy. As a treatment it promotes healing and restores function following injuries to muscles, tendons, and ligaments. The long-term effects of exposing the fetus to diagnostic levels of ultrasound are not known. Some studies have shown changes in the amniotic fluid cells, and a study in Japan found that mice fetuses exposed to high doses of ultrasound developed more birth defects than fetuses unexposed.

In the case of multiple pregnancy, the risks of unknown long-term effects are outweighed by the benefits of a correct prenatal diagnosis and appropriate adjustments in care. Repeat scans at two-to-four-week intervals after the thirtieth week of pregnancy are recommended by some obstetricians. Others explain to the mother the (low) risk of twin transfusion syndrome, in which one twin develops at the expense of the other (discussed in Chapter 7), and let her decide how much ultrasound exposure she wants.

Besides detecting the presence of multiple fetuses and listening to the babies' heartbeats, ultrasound is used to monitor fetal hearts during labor. The type of ultrasound used during labor is continuous, unlike the pulsed Doptone, so a higher dosage is delivered. Further discussion of the use of ultrasound can be found in Chapters 8 and 12.

Awaiting Twins:

Parents' Feelings and Practical Considerations

PREGNANCY INCURS UNIQUE psychological states in both expectant mothers and fathers. The mood swings and emotional changes and dreams that are experienced form part of a normal and necessary process. Both parents are passing into a new developmental phase in their lives, with accompanying choices, anxieties, fears, and hopes. Fathers-to-be report more headaches and stomach upsets and have a higher incidence of absenteeism from work than at other times. Couples who make the best adjustment to parenthood are those who are aware and accepting of the fluctuating feelings in pregnancy and in fact explore and discuss them with each other.

Psychological Adaptation to Multiple Pregnancy

The adjustment to multiple pregnancy, of course, varies with each individual woman and depends on a multitude of factors including her partner's and family's support, marital status, age, economic situation, other children, fertility history, general health, acquaintance with multiples, and her own birth and upbringing.

The following chart describes two opposite poles of reaction to multiple pregnancy. Most women will fluctuate along the continuum between them, as ambivalence in pregnancy is common. It is important to recognize if you lean strongly toward the negative side so that you can seek counseling and support.

The Exciting News

The confirmation of a pregnancy may be good news or bad news, depending on whether the pregnancy was planned. Not all unplanned pregnancies are unwanted, and even those that have been anxiously awaited cause moments of ambivalence. If this is your first pregnancy, you will be adjusting to the idea that you will never be just a couple again. You can be an ex-wife or an ex-husband but never an ex-parent! A common concern of couples is the change in their relationship that the arrival of two babies will bring. The notion of

We both felt that planning to have a child is a serious life decision. People today make that choice responsibly. It is a shock, then, when you find that you are having twins. Suddenly you realize you had no control over this unplanned event. I'm getting used to the idea, but I need to have those babies in my arms. Then they'll be more personal and less amorphous.

When our twins are born, we will have four children under four. The difficulties of parenting are obvious; the nice aspects are not so easy to put into words. It is taking us a little while to get used to this pregnancy, although we know we'll love the babies when they arrive.

We had the perfect American family — a boy and a girl. I was so upset when I knew I was pregnant. I was one of a threesome and I hated it. Learning they were twins saved the day. I would have had to balance the numbers and now we are all square.

Twins run in my family, so I kind of expected it. I don't know why people make such a fuss about twins.

Reactions to Pregnancy

Negative	Positive
Insensitive disclosure of twin pregnancy by technician or doctor	Suspected twin pregnancy, confirmed with sensitivity and support
News experienced as a shock	News received as a wonderful surprise or dream come true
Unplanned pregnancy; unwilling to bear multiples	Planned pregnancy/conscious conception, optimistic about outcome of fertility treatments
Perceives large abdomen as "too fat"	Enjoys blossoming of her body
Feels like a sow, like she's having a litter	Grateful for abundance — "two babies for the price of one"
Resents size, appearance, social comments	Welcomes questions about large belly, due date
Anxious about high-risk pregnancy and going to term	Strongly motivated to learn about twin pregnancy and parenting
Irritated by bodily changes and discomforts of pregnancy	Views adaptation of body with sense of wonder and appreciation
Unaware of differences between babies; just feels kicks	Begins prenatal bonding with babies as unit and individually
Fears labor, sees Caesarean as an easy way out	Looks forward to labor, finds providers to support natural birth
Rejects idea of breast-feeding	Joyfully anticipates breast-feeding
Feels overwhelmed by the thought of having and caring for two or more babies	Sets up support systems for birth and postpartum

---

"double trouble" may raise doubts about their ability to handle the situation and become adequate parents.

With multiple births, the extra baby or babies are usually unplanned. Families are generally poorly prepared for news of a multiple pregnancy at the outset, let alone some of the prenatal restrictions and monitoring and the high possibility of a Caesarean. They greatly underestimate the workload involved in raising multiples in the first few years. The resulting stress contributes to increased incidence of postnatal depression, child abuse, and divorce. The situation is especially critical for poor, black, single, and teenage mothers. These are the ones who are often too busy or too tired to reach out for support, but of course they need it the most. Housing assistance, welfare, food supplements, extended leave from work (which is often used up prenatally), home care covered by insurance, and home visits for help with breast-feeding are all necessary. All multiple birth organizations are keenly aware of the information that a family with multiples — as well as their health care providers — needs to receive before, during, and after birth. Mothers of Twins Clubs need to take more initiative with outreach during pregnancy, and clinics can help by supplying names of expectant parents to such support groups.

Some mothers are intensely angry about being pregnant with twins. They don't want to face the physical, emotional, and financial burdens of the extra child. Almost 15,000 diaper changes are needed in the first year! Parents hear so often that they are lucky to have twins, and society doesn't support feelings of ambivalence about wanting two babies, especially if the mother had infertility problems. Other women may have used fertility drugs or have consciously conceived twins and feel wonderfully empowered to have exercised that choice. In cases where twins run in the family, the couple may have secretly hoped for twins.

A 1987 *Twins* magazine survey found that 61 percent of mothers suspected in the first or second trimester that they had a multiple pregnancy. Only 39 percent never suspected a multiple birth. Patricia Malmstrom of Twin Services in California found that 71 percent of 336 mothers she surveyed suspected that they were carrying multiples before it was confirmed medically. In the *Twins* magazine survey, 77 percent of the respondents were diagnosed with multiples during the first or second trimester. Sixteen percent found out in the third trimester, and 7 percent did not know of the multiples until labor or birth. If physicians had accepted their patients' intuition, they would have enormously improved their diagnostic rate. It is surprising in these litigious times, when many doctors perform extra and often unnecessary screening tests as a form of "defensive medicine," that women still have a problem convincing them to check for multiples. Seek a second opinion or consult a midwife if you suspect twins and your physician does not agree.

I was absolutely shattered. There I was on the doctor's couch, and he called out to his nurse, "I think I can hear a second heartbeat — come and listen," while I was supposed to lie there like a dead body.

We didn't really want any more kids after three girls, but when Sarah became pregnant we figured it'd be two boys or a boy and a girl. I nearly died when two more girls came out. "Who wants to tell him?" asked the doc as they were born.

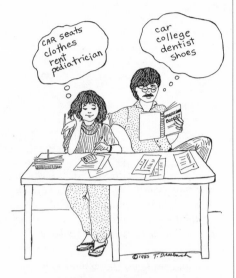

Line drawing by Terry Dresbach. Reprinted with permission from Twin Services, Inc.

When my husband heard I'd had twins, he forgot where he had parked the car. He even forgot where the elevator was.

I wasn't worried about paying for the birth. My thoughts raced ahead to two tennis rackets, two cars, and two kids in college together.

I nearly fainted when I heard the news. But what could I do? You can't send one of them back.

My husband and I were overjoyed. We think it is the most exciting thing that ever happened to us.

As with all important, and especially irreversible, events, the manner in which the news is broken plays a key role in the parents' reactions. Disbelief is usually the immediate response when twins are announced. "Get me a chair . . . ," "It must be a mistake," "Are you *sure*?" and "Why *me*?" are typical comments. Of course, if the midwife or doctor sends the mother for an ultrasound scan before making a diagnosis, perhaps merely hinting that her abdomen is rather large, the impact of the diagnosis is usually less marked. Because some women miscarry or go into premature labor following an unexpected diagnosis of multiple pregnancy, great sensitivity and support are required. The woman should sit down! The doctor should take time right then to answer her questions; at the same time, he or she should give the mother literature and the phone numbers of local Mothers of Twins Clubs and of Twin Services in Berkeley, California. Ideally a mother of twins (or higher-order multiples if that is the case) should call the expectant mother *that same day*, on the doctor's request.

The initial shock may pass quickly as a first-time mother realizes the advantage of having two children for the time and effort of one pregnancy — a ready-made family. If there are already other children at home, the news may bring genuine dismay, however. Two extra children may present a real burden on space, time, income, careers, and lifestyle. If twins complete the number of children planned, the parents are often thrilled. In cases where a fourth child was wanted but the twins make five, acceptance can be difficult, particularly if the parents are hoping for, say, a girl, and two boys are on the way.

Confirmation of triplets or quadruplets can be very threatening to the couple. In addition to the enormous changes that the care of higher-order multiples involves, the couple may be acutely aware of the hazards during pregnancy and birth. Guilt feelings are not uncommon as parents deal with the thought of such a large and sudden increase in family size and the attendant stresses.

Fathers, after the drama of discovery passes, usually become very excited by the prospect of twins. Two babies obviously involve the father more than just one, and participating husbands look forward to the birth of twins perhaps even more than the birth of singletons. Even when they have to take on an extra job to make ends meet, they may do so with great pride. Congratulations on their fertility, old wives' tales, and jokes about aphrodisiacs, sexual positions, and "help from the milkman" or the next-door neighbor can be expected. Finances usually come immediately to the father's mind — not just the expense of the doctor and hospital fees but long-term projections.

The attitudes of family members also influence the couple's reaction to the news of twins. One of the mothers interviewed for this book was separated, in school full time, and on welfare. With time marching on, she decided she wanted to have a child and was prepared to raise it responsibly on her own. She successfully selected a good genetic partner for the conception — but little did she expect that twins would result. However, the predicament of twins actually helped her family swallow their disapproval — they had ostracized her earlier in the pregnancy — and come to her assistance.

Time eases all adjustments. Parents with a few weeks or months to prepare for the birth of twins have a chance to gather enough supplies and make necessary changes in their self-image to prepare for their roles as parents of twins. Timely warning also aids a couple's expectations of the course of the pregnancy. Extra hunger, fatigue, weight gain, and swelling make more sense if there are two babies inside.

When twins are discovered for the first time in the delivery room, it is a shock for everyone — doctor and staff as well as parents. The couple may be so preoccupied with the birth of the first baby that they hardly hear the nurse remarking, "I think there is something else inside," or "Whoops, here comes another one!" Many a second twin has been named by the nurse or obstetrician while the parents look on bewildered. It is even more traumatic for the father who is killing time in the waiting room or the man at home who receives the announcement of twins by telephone. A California obstetrician relates a story about the birth of twins in which the father refused to accompany his wife through labor and delivery. The doctor felt annoyed at the husband for not supporting his wife, so he thought he would teach him a little lesson. The twins were swaddled and placed by the mother in such a way that only one baby was visible. After the father was called in and had spent some time admiring his single offspring, the second twin was produced.

Witnessing unanticipated happenings helps make them real. Mothers who have general rather than regional anesthesia for a Caesarean birth often wonder if the offspring are theirs, as they never see them actually delivered. The nurse tells them the news hours later or the next day and they learn from the medical chart which twin was born first.

Adoption

Adopting twins may sometimes be easier than adopting a singleton. Adoption agencies do not separate twins nowadays, and couples who want twins may have a shorter wait if prospective parents ahead

Even learning about the twins in labor is better than at delivery; at least you have an hour or so to adjust.

My family kept saying, "Oh, you're going to have twins." Then when I told them I really was going to have twins, the joke was on them — they didn't believe me.

I was walking down the hall when a nurse went by with two babies. "They're both yours, Mr. Lyons," she called cheerily.

My labor was long and exhausting. When the midwife announced there was a second baby I shouted, "I don't care — just hurry up."

When twins arrive unexpectedly, the hospital staff thinks it is either a great joke or a big thrill. Frankly, I was in such a state of shock, I didn't feel very positive at the time.

Because I was infertile, when my best friend had twins I really felt that one of those babies should have been mine. So when we went to the adoption agency, I put in my order for two.

After waiting eighteen months, we suddenly had thirty-six hours' notice that "something" was coming. We didn't know we would really get our twins until we went to the hospital. "Baby A" and "Baby B" were embroidered in a heart on each twin's jacket.

Depression was a major negative factor in my pregnancy. As a working professional, giving up my career to be on bed rest for twelve weeks and then to care for my sons was a forceful blow. The financial aspects were (and are) staggering. Child care and loss of income are difficult problems with no easy solutions.

of them on the list prefer to wait for a singleton. Not all adoptive parents are prepared to take on a twosome, but some parents have adopted a second pair of twins. One couple interviewed for this book decided from the beginning that they wanted to adopt twins. They wanted a ready-made family and a baby for each parent. When they mentioned this at an adoption group meeting, another couple also expressed a desire for twins. Of course, parents waiting to adopt cannot be promised twins, and if twins are available they are given a chance to change their minds. In 1990 a surrogate mother delivered twins, but the contracting family wanted only one child and chose the girl. The biological mother succeeded in getting the female twin back so that the twins could be raised together.*

Concern

The pregnant woman's moods closely follow certain phases. Before she sees actual physical changes and feels fetal movement, she may experience doubt and ambivalence. This is the beginning of becoming a mother — an endless growth process in which we come up against our supposed limits and learn to stretch beyond them. Knowing that these feelings are typical of pregnancy helps women cope. Feeling the babies move, however, is unmistakable evidence that the pregnancy is under way. Prenatal bonding is more of a challenge with multiples than with singletons because the mother has to integrate the extra baby or babies, relating to a pair or a group. (See Chapter 14 for a complete discussion of prenatal bonding.)

By the sixth month a mother of twins may be so large that she tires of friends and strangers asking if delivery is imminent. At thirty-two weeks the size of the uterus is the same as for a singleton at term (forty weeks). In the last trimester the mother may be overwhelmed by her huge body, aching legs, swollen ankles, itchy abdomen, heartburn, and constipation. The work of the lungs, kidneys, heart, and circulatory system is doubled and, unless she is very fit, fatigue sets in easily. Family and friends may treat her like a queen or like an invalid, forcing her to feel that her condition is abnormal rather than merely an unusual aspect of a physiological state. Pressure may be put on her to give up work earlier than she had planned and to curtail activities she enjoys. Couples soon hear all about the risks of multiple birth. Twins today are classified as high risk, although as one midwife

---

* Specify in your will that your twins will be raised together in the event of your death.

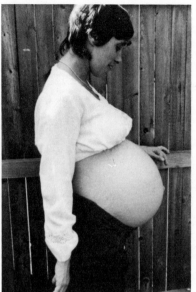

Seven months pregnant

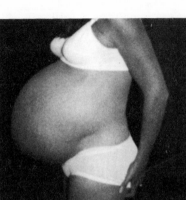

Nine months pregnant

Two babies take up a lot of room.

What I remember is pressure. Everywhere, from my bladder to my ribs. It was impossible to find a comfortable position.

One baby did somersaults to the left and the other one to the right. I was glad when things quieted down in the last two weeks.

People often said to me, "You're huge — you must be having twins," which only made me feel even more large and dependent.

I got so sick of strangers saying to me, "Tut, you shouldn't be out shopping when it's so close, dear." My husband told me to just lie about the due date when those busybodies asked.

My biggest fear during pregnancy was that the twins would be conjoined.

I was scared that something would happen to one of the twins.

put it, a better term is "special needs." If a home birth had been planned, the midwife or doctor will usually insist on a hospital delivery. Anxiety develops about difficulties that may arise during labor, such as the presentation of the babies and the possibility of anesthesia and Caesarean delivery. (See Chapter 7 for a discussion of the potential hazards of multiple pregnancy and ways to minimize them.)

The conduct of the latter part of pregnancy depends on the view of the physician. Progressive doctors counsel the pregnant woman on nutrition, sensible exercise, and rest and introduce no intervening measures. Other obstetricians may consider multiple pregnancy pathological and make recommendations ranging from a surgical corset and bed rest to surgery to close the cervix in the hope of preventing premature labor (see Chapter 11).

Choosing Your Health Care Provider

Find a doctor who has a midwife on his or her staff. Midwives typically spend more time with mothers, listening to their worries and offering advice. Check your obstetrician's Caesarean rate, ability to

Explanation of Abbreviations

Hct = hematocrit (iron test)
Hgb = hemoglobin (iron test)
G.C. = gonococcus (venereal disease)
G = gravida (number of pregnancies)
T = term (number of term infants born)
P = preterm (number of premature infants)
A = abortion (miscarriage)
L = living (number of living children)
LMP = last menstrual period (first day)
EDC = expected date of confinement
(due date)
Fe tabs = iron tablets
F.M. = fetal movement
F.H. = fetal heart
U.S. = ultrasound
P.T. = physical therapy
V.E. = vaginal examination
Dil. = dilation of cervix
Eff. = effacement of cervix
Vtx. = vertex (head) presentation
2X = twice
Abd. = abdominal
(L) = left.

Prenatal Flow Record

HOLLISTER maternal/newborn RECORD SYSTEM

PATIENT IDENTIFICATION

Patient's name: *Katie Finch*

Risk Guide for Pregnancy and Outcome

Preliminary Risk Assessment (detail risk factors from the HHS below)

- ☒ (0) No risk factors noted
- ☐ (1) At risk
- ☐ (2) High risk

Continuing Risk Guide (enter dates first noted and revise RISK STATUS)

Mo/day	Potential risk factors	Mo/day	High risk factors
/	3. Preg. without familial support	/	18. Diabetes mellitus
/	4. Second pregnancy in 12 months	/	19. Hypertension
/	5. Smoking (≥ 1 pack per day)	/	20. Thrombophlebitis
/	6. Rh negative (nonsensitized)	/	21. Herpes (type 2)
/	7. Uterine/cervical malformation	/	22. Rh sensitization
/	8. Inadequate pelvis	/	23. Uterine bleeding
/	9. Venereal disease	/	24. Hydramnios
/	10. Anemia (Hct < 30%:Hgb < 10%)	/	25. Severe preeclampsia
/	11. Acute pyelonephritis	/	26. Fetal growth retardation
/	12. Failure to gain weight	/	27. Premature rupt. membranes
/	13. Multiple pregnancy (term)	/	28. Multiple pregnancy (preterm)
/	14. Abnormal presentation	/	29. Low/falling estriols
/	15. Postterm pregnancy	/	30. Significant social problems
/	16.	/	31.
/	17.	/	32.

Initial Prenatal Screen

Mo/day	Test	Result
4/30	Hct/Hgb	34.5 11.7
4/30	Patient's Blood type and Rh	A+
4/30	Father's Blood type and Rh	O+
4/30	Antibody	Neg
4/30	Serology	Neg
4/30	Rubella titer	1:20
4/30	Urinalysis micro	Neg
4/30	Pap test	cl I
4/30	G.C.	Neg

Additional Lab Findings

Mo/day	Test	Result
6/19	Hct/Hgb	12.0
8/20	Hct/Hgb	12.5
9/8	Hgb	13.0
10/30	Hgb	12.5
11/30	Hgb	12.0
/		
/		
/		
/		

G 2 T 1 P 0 0 0 A L 1 LMP 3.2.79 EDC 12.7.79

- ☒ Attends prenatal classes
- ☐ Cesarean section
- ☐ For sterilization
- ☒ Breast ☐ Bottle feeding
- ☐ Circumcision

Anesthesia

Baby's physician *Rowe*

Flow Chart

Year 79 Pre-gravid 123

Date	Weight this visit	Blood pressure	Protein	Sugar	Est. weeks gestation (dates/size)	Fundal height	Fetal heart rate	Edema	RISK STATUS [0,1,2]	
4/30	125	110/70	N	N	7/10			–		Nutritional counselling – does not want
5/24	131	112/65	N	N	11/14	14		–		Fe tabs. For prenatal exercise program
6/19	136	109/70	N	N	14/20	20	144	–		FM reported. F.H. c̄ fetoscope
7/17	140	115/70	n	n	18/33	24	144	–		Large for dates? twins. Consider U.S.
8/20	146	106/60	Tr	n	24/24	28	140/150			Both F.H. audible. Pt refused Sonogram
9/18	150	95/65	N	N	28/28	33	145/150	+		Pelvic pressure, backache → PT
9/15	156	105/60	n	Tr	32/32	36	144/150	+		Active + well. V.E. 2 cm dil. 80% Eff.
10/30	161	100/65	N	N	34/34	38	140	+		1 vertex, ? 1 breech. Lots of FM
11/8	165	115/70	Tr	N	36	40	150/150	++		Fatigue – 2x daily rests
11/16	170	120/80	Tr	N	38	42	140/150	+		Finished work. Both vertex. Itch c/o abd.
11/23	174	118/75	n	n	38	44	145	++		Strong B-H Contractions. Doing well
11/30	178	125/80	n	n	39	45	140/148	++		Arrange for birthing room
12/8	181	120/70	N	N	40	46	140/150	++		4 cm dil. (L) head engaged

Physician's signature

Prenatal Care Chart: a case history of a healthy pregnancy. *(This record is copyrighted by Miller Communications, Inc., and may not be reproduced without permission of Hollister Incorporated, the exclusive licensee under said copyright.)*

perform version and breech deliveries (discussed in Chapters 7 and 12), and attitude toward natural birth and breast-feeding. Ask how many of the twin sets are normal weight at birth and what happens if a baby is sick or dies (see Appendix 3). Negotiate your birth plan ahead of time with the maternity nursing supervisor (see Appendix 2). You will need to remain flexible and to make decisions with your caregivers. Visit the neonatal intensive care unit at the hospital and take Caesarean classes to see what you hope to avoid. (Also see the Appendixes for guidance about ensuring your control over your birth experience.)

I usually wear size 12 maternity clothes but found that I needed a size 16 or 18 to go around my huge abdomen. I ate six small meals a day and paid special attention to my diet. One week, my doctor kindly announced that I had the biggest uterus in town.

Support

The pregnant woman's husband, relatives, or friends may give welcome support during the pregnancy or they may actually cause added stress. Much of the well-meant advice may focus heavily on the potential hazards of multiple birth or raise doubts about the mother's ability to care for two offspring at once. An expectant mother of twins may feel alone and isolated. There may be no history of twinning in her family and no multiples among her friends and neighbors. Some first-time mothers of twins feel that the situation is easier for them than for women who have had other pregnancies — they know nothing else. But experienced mothers, who remember the time it took to meet the needs of one baby, may be almost frightened at the thought of nurturing two. Although many more books and resources are available for parents awaiting multiples than a decade ago, most parents do not get enough information and support.

Parents expecting twins may find that while friends and neighbors share their excitement and enthusiasm, their experience with single children does not make them helpful resources. I strongly recommend that you seek out and visit at least two or three families with twins. Such visits can give you ideas about how you may want to organize your postpartum life. It is helpful to see a range of different situations. Compare a mother of twins who works with one who stays at home, perhaps with some help or even full-time help. Try to visit families who have other children too, if you already have children. Observing mothers of twins who nurse and those who bottle-feed should convince you that breast-feeding saves time, money, and energy as well as being an intimate and fulfilling experience.

Husbands were the most important support factor in helping women get through their pregnancies, according to respondents to

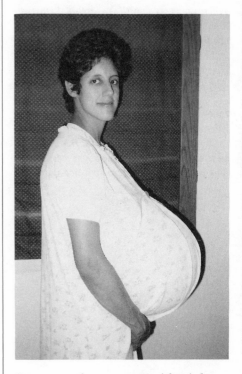

Seven months pregnant with triplets.

the *Twins* magazine survey. Some of the resource organizations available to mothers of multiples are discussed in Chapter 1 and listed in Resources. The Mothers of Twins Club is a great source of personal support and information. However, most mothers of twins get around to joining when their babies already are infants, unless the hospital has contacted a local chapter to arrange a postpartum visit or telephone call. I strongly recommend that you attend meetings and establish a relationship with members of the club nearest you *before* the birth so that you don't find yourself struggling through the early problems alone. Through these clubs it is possible to gather used supplies for multiple babies and thus save money for something like diaper service or home help. You can find out the address of your neighborhood chapter by writing to the national office of the Mothers of Twins Clubs listed in Resources.

The La Leche League (*leche* means "milk" in Spanish) is an organization concerned with the promotion and support of breast-feeding. You should be able to find a group leader in your area by checking the phone directory or a local maternity hospital. Otherwise you can write to the national office (see Resources). As with Mothers of Twins Clubs, I strongly advise that you contact a member of La Leche League prior to the birth. Then you will have someone to call when you are in the hospital or if you have problems in the first weeks at home. Thousands of mothers of twins have successfully nursed both babies and are happy to provide counseling and moral support. This is most essential because hospitals and many doctors tend to push bottle-feeding. Their attitude is that breast-feeding is a chore and nursing twins or other multiples is just about impossible. On the contrary, breast is best, and nursing is a joy. A double supply of formula costs more than $2,000 per year — money that could be spent on a washer, dryer, or household help. Unfortunately many mothers of twins who are told that twins "cannot" be breast-fed (some hear this from their doctors!) later regret having followed this wrong advice. Some people recommend bottle-feeding because it offers the advantage of the father's participation, but he can better share instead by changing diapers and doing other parts of the daily routine. (See Chapter 15 for specific advice about breast-feeding.)

Single mothers and others below a certain income level may be eligible for state assistance such as Medicaid, food stamps, and WIC (Women, Infants, and Children) nutritional assistance. These programs and their criteria for eligibility vary from state to state, so it is best to check with your state Department of Health. WIC is a federally administered program that provides vouchers for food and formula

When I was six months pregnant, I started to make extra soups, sauce, lasagna, pies, muffins, cookies, etc., and froze them. We had enough food to get us through the last month of my pregnancy and first few weeks after birth.

I was worried about the impact of four babies on a two-year-old. I mentioned my concern to my doctor who said that if the adults don't stress how unusual it is to have four babies it won't occur to a two-year-old.

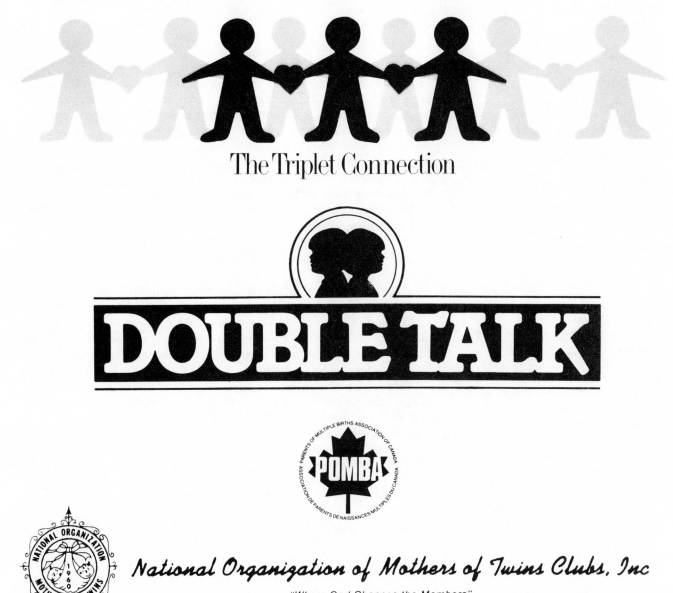

The Triplet Connection

DOUBLE TALK

POMBA

National Organization of Mothers of Twins Clubs, Inc

"Where God Chooses the Members"

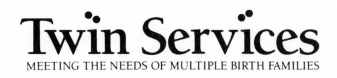

Twin Services

MEETING THE NEEDS OF MULTIPLE BIRTH FAMILIES

Turn anxiety into action: join the networks.

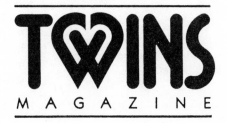

TWINS MAGAZINE

Breast-feeding was not discussed in detail in our childbirth education course. I was glad I had found support before the birth through La Leche League, as I was given tips on how to prepare my breasts — checking the nipples and exposing them to sunlight to toughen the skin.

My pediatrician did not charge the same for our triplets. We paid the full fee for the first, only half for the second, and the third child was free.

Haircuts were the only thing I ever recall where I got two for the price of one. And the barber made me promise not to tell any other mothers of twins.

I used a diaper service rather than disposable diapers for my twins because it was much cheaper, plus I didn't contribute to environmental problems.

A survey of the mothers in our club showed that a dryer was the most appreciated piece of household equipment.

as well as counseling and medical review of recipients who are at risk. State welfare benefits vary also but they increase for an extra child. In Massachusetts an expectant mother of twins on welfare would receive an extra allowance for a crib and layette. Parents of higher-order multiples, with persistence, may discover some state support. Organizations such as Twin Services are actively lobbying for the provision of a wide range of nonmedical services. A special project of the California Department of Health Services, Twin Services provides loans of infant equipment; education on nutrition, birth, breast-feeding, and parenting; counseling for prematurity and handicaps; and child care or homemaker services for single parents, teen parents, parents of supermultiples, and other families in crisis in the San Francisco Bay area.

Health insurance rarely pays more for twin births than for single births, although some physicians charge double. Check with your obstetrician, pediatrician, and hospital for their fees as well as with your insurance company for the reimbursements available. Hospital nurseries charge for both twin occupants, but perhaps the extra cost can be avoided if you keep the twins in your room (called *rooming-in*).

Some department stores give parents of twins a break. If you save all the receipts for baby clothing and equipment, the store may duplicate each item at no cost or at half price or some other discount. It never hurts to inquire about discounts for twins — store managers may never have given it a thought and may be happy to oblige. Usually twins create much attention from shoppers as well as from store clerks, and most businesses like to encourage good will.

Planning Ahead

Diaper service for twins is frequently provided for the price of one if you order it thirty days before delivery. While such service cuts down on laundry, twins use plenty of clothes, sheets, and towels that make a washer and dryer essential items. Even apartment dwellers can find portable washers to save them trips to the laundromat. All parents of multiples advise the purchase of laundry equipment even if it means that the father has to work a second job for a while or take out a loan. Many parents of multiples find they can afford such items from savings they realize on secondhand goods sold through Mothers of Twins Clubs and yard sales.

Try, if at all possible, to arrange household assistance for yourself when you return from the hospital. This basic need of all new mothers is much greater with twins or triplets, especially if they are delivered by Caesarean section. Some fortunate mothers of twins use household help for the entire first year; others engage a part-time nurse; others find a high school student or senior citizen to help for a few hours each day. Initially, fathers may take vacation time after the birth or make flex-time arrangements with employers. Relatives often rally round, but many couples no longer live near their relatives and have to rely on neighbors or hired help to clean, cook, and babysit.

Shopping is often a difficult prospect for a mother with twins. One woman solved the problem well ahead of time. Before the babies were born, she drew a detailed map of her local supermarket and made photocopies. Each week she had only to visually review the product aisles and check off the items she needed. This made it easy for her to remember everything while facilitating the shopping for visitors or neighbors who offered to help.

Many parents of twins find it simpler and less expensive to shop in bulk. Products are cheaper by the case, and three- or four-month supplies of nonperishables can be bought, leaving less shopping to be done weekly. Join a food cooperative that offers a wide range of organic products. I recommend that you make as many meals as possible and freeze them ahead of time.

Friends and family will want to bring useful gifts. Disposable diapers for travel or a few weeks of diaper service are obvious suggestions. Warn everyone before the birth that postpartum visitors will be welcome only if they bring a casserole or are prepared to help while visiting. Parents of twins appreciate practical baby clothes, not fancy matching outfits. There will be no time to iron frilly frocks with bows and lace. Stretch terry cloth and other easy-care fabrics are essential. Extra clothing is needed so the laundry does not have to be done daily. Large tote bags for outings with the twins are another gift idea. Infant car seats should be obtained beforehand. In most states and countries today it is against the law to drive the babies home from the hospital if they are not secured in the proper type of restraint. Some car seats can be used indoors as infant seats, and it is easier to pick up two handles than two babies. However, such dual-purpose car seats have to be detached and repositioned each time the family gets in and out of the car. A two-door car makes this even more of a struggle.

The following layette for twins has been adapted for a four-season climate from the book *The Care of Twin Children: A Common Sense Guide for Parents* by Rosemary Theroux and Josephine Tingley. The authors are both registered nurses and mothers of twins.

The quads had to be fed every three hours, as they were premature. This meant that every forty-five minutes, around the clock, another feeding would have to begin. We hired a night nurse for the first few weeks. Now we have a girl who comes to help during the worst hours of the day — four to six, Monday through Friday.

The biggest mistake made by mothers of twins is that we underestimate the amount of work and don't ask for enough help.

Looking after quintuplets meant nineteen hours of baby care a day. We had to prepare thirty-five bottles every day.

170–200 diapers per week* (from a diaper service) *or* 72 cloth diapers to allow for washing every other day

2 one-piece snowsuits, if applicable

6–10 fitted crib sheets (unless the babies join you in the "family bed")

2–4 heavy blankets or baby afghans

2–4 blanket sleepers

6 receiving blankets

2–4 machine-washable sweaters

8–10 plastic pants (Wool diaper covers are expensive but allow air circulation and are preferable to plastic pants.)

12 cotton undershirts

8–10 terry cloth stretch suits

12 cotton nightgowns

Bassinets are not considered essential items. Sleeping with your twins in the family bed (see "Sleeping" in Chapter 15) is the easiest solution, or the babies can be put down in padded drawers, laundry baskets, or even a large box. Twins shared the uterus for nine months and will prefer to stay together.

Many mothers of twins find a double baby carriage too cumbersome, particularly when negotiating doorways and using public transportation. Umbrella strollers that clip together or strollers in which the twins face each other are more manageable (see Chapter 15). The guide by Theroux and Tingley is highly recommended for advice about selecting equipment. The authors discuss the hazards of each item and considerations such as quality, price, and adaptability. Suggestions for safe use and maintenance are also included.

Because multiples often arrive early, it is a good idea to have everything ready and organized by the seventh month. Many parents of twins advise expectant mothers to consolidate all the baby clothing and equipment in one room, particularly if the house has more than one floor. It helps to have a spare bed, chaise longue, or even a large comfortable chair in the room so that the mother can rest and nap

* This would cost a tremendous amount of money per week if you used disposable diapers!

with the infants in the early weeks when the babies are fed so often. A basket on wheels is a very handy way to minimize bending and finding a place for all the odd items that accumulate during the day. A changing table of adequate height is essential, as mothers of twins bend over twice as often. Foot controls on diaper pails leave the parent's hands free.

Nursing mothers will need plenty of two-piece clothes. As with the infants' supplies, the greater the quantity you can afford, the less frequently you will have to launder.

Use the time before the birth to become acquainted with the special features and issues of twinship while you still have time to read! Also explore as a couple your philosophy about parenting in general and parenting multiples in particular. Discuss ways in which you can honor the special bonds of twinship while affirming each twin's individuality.

Although the idea of a pair, a unit, is foremost in your minds at the prebirth stage, select unalike clothes (don't buy very many as you will receive more gifts than you expect and most will be matching) and choose separate godparents for each child.

Other siblings in the family should be prepared for the twin birth. Some of the books for children listed under "Children's Books About Twins" in the References will help you explain what twins are and provide an opportunity for feelings to be aired. It is natural for children to feel displaced and jealous of any new arrival, especially if it is two or more. The advent of multiples has an enormous impact on the entire family, and siblings are pushed very much into the background. Parents, of course, are usually sensitive to these issues, but other people often are not. It is a good idea to arrange special treats and outings for the other children to look forward to when the babies come home.

We bought twin dolls for our daughter and she was very happy playing mother with her own pair.

Everyone told me that twins come early, so I packed one month ahead of time. All that happened was that dust collected on my bags. My twins were two weeks overdue.

Sharing Space: 6

Twinship Experiences in Utero

Developments in Prenatal Psychology

The exciting new field of prenatal and perinatal psychology offers a wide variety of accounts by children and adults of prenatal memories and preverbal experiences. Psychiatrists such as Graham Farrant, pioneer of the clinical study of such memories, and Stanislav Grof, author of many books including *Realms of the Human Unconscious*, have compiled impressive clinical evidence of organic memories going back to implantation and conception.

Neurologists, among others, have argued that memory capability depends on a myelin sheath around nerve fibers that does not develop until a child is learning to talk. However, Canadian psychiatrist Thomas Verny, author of *The Secret Life of the Unborn Child*, writes that from the sixth month of conception the fetus is sufficiently developed neurologically to receive, process, and encode information.

According to Massachusetts psychologist Arnold Buchheimer, memory storage is not an exclusive province of the brain — long-term learning is cellular. When we think of how much a one-celled creature like an amoeba can do, we realize that human memories can and do go back to the single egg and sperm cells.

It is beyond the scope of this book to explore in depth recent theories of mind and memory. However, ultrasound has shown just how sophisticated the activity and response of the embryo and fetus are. If all fetal organs and systems function well under the direction of the prenatal brain, why not the mind and memory as well? Why wouldn't the fetus remember events and emotions? Every mother who looks into the eyes of her newborn knows intuitively that her infant is already an individual with a personality and assumptions about the world. Every maternity nurse knows that each newborn is different.

Since cellular memories are behavioral rather than mental, they are held and expressed in specific parts of the body and may be accessed in later life through hypnosis, deep massage like rolfing, energy balancing techniques such as polarity or bioenergetics, craniosacral therapy, primal therapy, visualization, "rebirthing," evocative breathing, and other approaches.

David Chamberlain is a San Diego psychologist whose research into concordant birth memories of mother and child through hypnosis is presented in the 1988 book *Babies Remember Birth*. As the book jacket states, "Parents have always said so, but medical science is just coming to accept it: Newborns are far more conscious in the womb and at birth than they have been credited for. They arrive in the world not just feeling, sensing, and reacting, but thinking, communicating, and even remembering."

David Cheek is a retired obstetrician and hypnotist in San Francisco who has been documenting evidence of pre- and perinatal experiences for years. Cheek writes, "Prenatal memories have been presented to me often in workshops by patients and students who had only volunteered to explore their memories of birth. Initially, I was not looking for such memory because I was sure it did not exist. It seemed wise at least to listen to these reports."

While those who have not witnessed or personally experienced this kind of age regression are understandably skeptical, there is plenty of evidence supporting its validity. Recalled events can usually be verified by family members or medical records, and the patient frequently experiences a strong intuitive sense of resolution following regression. For the thousand plus members of the Pre and Perinatal Psychology Association of North America and the International Society of Prenatal and Perinatal Psychology and Medicine, the evidence of prenatal memory is indisputable.

Further investigation is needed to deepen our understanding of the physical and psychological dimensions of multiple pregnancy, but this chapter will present a few anecdotes and suggestions for expectant parents of twins based on the information now available.

Experience of Twinship in Utero

My interest in prenatal psychology arose from an understanding that many of us who work in maternity care are motivated by unresolved emotions about our own conception, pregnancy, and birth. Since writing the first edition of *Having Twins*, I have experienced many dimensions of my prenatal existence under the guidance of Graham Farrant and others, and I have concluded that my interest in twins stems from personal experiences of intrauterine loss.

My mother was six months pregnant with me when my five-year-old sister died, a fact that I did not realize until I relived my time in her grieving body during primal therapy in 1982. However, it took me some years to understand that the huge amount of grief I felt as an embryo was a result not just of my mother's emotions over that loss. I had other cellular memories from my period of gestation and to this day I hold a clear image and feeling of a disappearing embryo. This, coupled with my ever-present horror at any artistic rendering of a vortex, makes sense in the context of a vanishing twin (described in Chapter 4). Clinically, my mother, age thirty-nine and pregnant for the fifth time, was on bed rest to avoid threatened miscarriage, but in those days bleeding was not connected with the vanishing twin syndrome because it was unknown before the advent of ultrasound. After my personal experience of her bed rest was brought to my conscious mind, I understood my motivation for having always argued against the "therapy" of bed rest and my reasons for pioneering prenatal exercise in my professional work.

I have made many other connections with the loss of my twin, including feelings of being wrong, especially the wrong gender, which burdened me for years and led me to seek opposites in my relationships. Running a "kindergarten" for two sets of twins in my neighborhood when I was a preteen, writing *Having Twins* (especially my emphasis on healthy pregnancy), attracting and helping to heal another survivor whose story follows in this chapter are more examples. I have further explored my prenatal memories and those of others in a forthcoming book, *Inside Experiences: From Conception Through Birth.* Since delving into this field, I am prepared to suggest that anyone working with multiple pregnancy who is an apparent singleton and is not a parent of multiples probably shared the uterus with a twin at some stage.

Perhaps society's fascination with multiples stems not only from the fact that they were born together but that they shared conception and gestation. As a result of this unique experience, twins can serve in "nature's laboratory" by separately confirming prenatal events.

Sharing the uterus with one or more siblings is typically recalled as a struggle for space. Toward the end of pregnancy the uterus is experienced as a cramped environment even by most single babies. In an undisturbed intrauterine life, "good womb" experiences include feelings of cosmic unity and oceanic bliss, while pressure from the uterus provides important tactile stimulation. According to Esalen psychiatrist Stanislav Grof, the twin situation is a disturbance of this ideal intrauterine life and may give rise to "bad womb" experiences such as crowding and kicking. When two or more siblings compete for the same resources, there is the potential for a life-or-death struggle.

Generalizations are often made associating behavior with the type of twinning: same-sex twins are thought to be most competitive, for example. However, the dynamics of the intrauterine environment, the position of the babies, the tension or relaxation of the uterus and other muscles, and the birth experience play a role as great as, if not greater than, gender.

Jane Greer, a psychotherapist and twin expert in Douglaston, New York, frequently counsels twins who are experiencing conflicts between the bonds of twinship and the ties of marriage. One of her clients discovered through hypnotherapy that she felt kicked around in the uterus and pushed out during birth. Coincidentally, her twin phoned to say that she was undergoing primal therapy at the same time in another state. Her uterine experience was one of fighting for space and kicking out her sister in order to be born. Both twins confirmed that their prenatal situation was repeated in adult life. The twin who was pushed out at birth fell into relationships where she ultimately felt abused while the other felt she attracted people who wanted to be pushed around.

Such prenatal experiences form *engrams*, or changes in neural tissues to accommodate storage of experience. These engrams, also known as imprints, are registered in the body's cells prior to the advanced development of memory involving the cortex of the brain. They set up behavioral patterns in later life that can affect not only the twin relationship but interaction within the family and the choice of spouse.

Italian psychiatrists Bernabei and Levi describe a case of male dizygotic twins, one of whom was successfully treated for hydrocephalus, or excess cerebrospinal fluid, while in the womb. The condition was resolved by birth; there were no residual problems, and it was never discussed with the twins. However, by the age of seven, the nonaffected twin "assumed the role of doctor and leader," unnecessarily protecting and interpreting for his brother. The "protected" twin clearly resented the role forced on him and when asked to draw pictures of his family drew only his brother, with an enormous penis. After a series of discussions with the psychiatrists, the dominant twin explained that he had to protect his brother "because he had a sick head," a comment that clearly reflected memories of pre- and perinatal origin.

Graham Farrant was approached separately by monozygotic female twins seeking primal therapy. This procedure puts patients in touch with their physical and emotional feelings by causing them to regress to the earliest time at which they experienced those feelings. Both twins suffered from sexual confusion that had affected their marriages and subsequent separations. Extraordinarily, they began to experience similar problems independently and although they were not associating closely with each other, they would relive almost identical experiences. Most striking was their separate yet identical experience of conception. Both recalled two sperm entering one egg at the same time. Both experienced the first sperm pushing the competitor away from the egg, then fertilizing the egg, which split into twins. The brief presence of the second, Y sperm, which would have produced a male child, was sufficient to create their sexual confusion. After therapy, one of the women returned to her husband and the other entered a new and meaningful heterosexual relationship.

A participant at one of my workshops for regression experiences described the following experience of twin loss. (Her mother later went on to have two sets of twins). "I expected this to be another experiential process I would doze through. But midway through it, when we were those balls of cells fumbling slowly through the tube, I was *there* now. Feeling caressed by the tube, softly following toward something . . . a very secure feeling. Protected, safe, whole. But my serenity was to be short-lived. As soon as we entered the womb I split and became two. Shortly thereafter (it could have been weeks, the process was timeless), my "other" went away, forever. The vision that I have that goes with it is of a woman riding off into the darkness with her back to me, and all I see is the back wheel of a yellow bicycle, a sort of golden-yellow star rolling away into the darkness. From then on, my entire being, body and all, was bathed in sorrow — a deep, all-encompassing despair that permeated the whole universe for me. That was *all*, that was life. It was so *physical*. I was weakened by it."

She went on to describe her experiences of being born and giving birth and to discuss her lifelong aversion to golden yellow. However, as soon as she was pregnant and then postpartum, she found herself putting gold stars on everything — clothes, swing, birth announcements, toys. She concluded, "I do believe that my daughter is that spirit who has come back to me. Ninety percent of the time when people see her, here's what they say: 'You two must be *twins!*' "

Conception, implantation, and birth present survival issues that are more of a challenge to twins than to singletons. After the first twin implants in the uterine wall, the wall thickens, making it more difficult for the second to implant. Hanspeter Ruch is a twin and clinical psychologist in Winterthur, Switzerland, who as a research project for his higher degrees undertook primal therapy to journey back to life in the womb. He explains that as the second dizygotic twin he experienced implantation as one of "the most traumatic situations in my life," during which he felt, "I am not going to make it, I have to die — accompanied by strong physical feelings, wanting to scratch a hole into the wall with my hands."

Implantation tends to be overlooked in the literature of this new field. However, not only is it a powerful psychological dimension in twinning, but Ruch suggests that many second twins die because of physiological difficulties with implantation. Interestingly, geneticist Charles Boklage notes that the greatest loss of in vitro fertilized embryos, like naturally conceived ones, occurs in the uterus.

Once implanted, Ruch says that he experienced life in a soft, tender, warm ocean. This world began to change, however, as he sensed his "kingdom" becoming "limited, even constricted . . . with a sense of something outside of him, far away, yet bumping him . . . sometimes at random, sometimes like a response, a shadow, like two balloons slightly hitting one another." Initially, he felt playful and thought it would be fun to reach out to the shadow, but as he attempted to do so he simply spun around in the fluid. His impression at this stage was of "something in between with no end and no beginning." Later he describes "a kind of a wall . . . many times I touched it, crawled up and down, but I never found an opening." Wanting to reach out to feel "the shadow," he found that his skin and the other's could never touch; there was "always a skin in between" preventing contact.

Disturbances of Ruch's prior oceanic bliss became more frequent, intense, even violent, interrupting his sleep. He became progressively confined, and being kicked and hit in the back made him feel "unprotected and vulnerable." With no possibility of escape, he felt forced to struggle, becoming increasingly angry and frustrated.

"I became more scared and threatened by my brother's presence," he writes. "We started to fight much more, especially if one of us tried to turn. I felt pushed towards the walls, and furiously started kicking and striking out as hard as I possibly could. . . . My warm friend became an enemy and a threat. To survive I had to attack too, had to push him down."

As Ruch was powerless to resolve the situation, desensitization was his only option, and he became numb and less aware as a cover for his hurt and frustration.

"The time before birth was very scary to me. We were both like fragile flowers but already had a history of fights. The struggle between us became a question of survival. It felt as though one of us had to die."

As a result, Ruch always felt a tremendous pressure to compete with his brother in all areas of life. During therapy this competitive drive was associated to the primal struggle in the uterus. When Ruch relived and released the struggle, he felt free of this compulsion.

As a psychotherapist, Ruch emphasizes his belief that the way we are conceived determines the way we are born. For example, in his personal experience, the imprint of the struggle to survive, "to get in" at conception (entering the egg), was further strengthened by a subsequent struggle, to implant in the womb and to enter the world at birth. Such imprints lead to behavior patterns in later life that repeat the primal experience — in this case, one of struggle to enter.

Sharing the uterus with a mate/rival often leads to paradoxical feelings. Another twin said, "I can remember times when I would move my body in a way to get more room in the womb, but I would hold any joy about it inside. I couldn't let my body let Claire know about it because if I got more space, it meant that she got less."

Experiences of Twin Loss in Utero

Surviving twins have had the unique experience of both intrauterine sharing and intrauterine loss. Chapter 4 explained the vanishing twin syndrome, the incidence of which has been estimated to be as high as 80 percent of twin pregnancies. (Chapter 17 discusses the loss of one twin primarily from the viewpoint of the parents, with some exploration of the reactions of the surviving twin in infancy and childhood.) While much progress has been made recently toward understanding the grief process of adults and children, fetal grieving is not widely acknowledged. In this chapter I explore intrauterine bereavement and its potential long-term effects on the surviving twin.

Death of a twin during birth or shortly thereafter has a major impact on the survivor, who may carry an overwhelming burden of guilt. With intrauterine death or stillbirth, the survivor feels even more intimately involved and often feels directly responsible for the destruction of the twin. The earlier the loss, the more intense the imprint.

The conflict over space and survival in the uterus may manifest itself in later life as issues of identity and creativity. A twin who sought psychotherapy from Arnold Buchheimer for blocked creativity came to understand that as a surviving monozygotic twin he could not feel whole unless he gave up, or blocked, part of himself. After therapy, he was able to take possession of his self and his space in the world without fearing that harm would be done to another, and his professional work blossomed.

Christopher Millar is an Australian physician and family therapist who has concluded from his experience in primal therapy that he is a surviving twin. In his monograph *The Second Self*, he suggests that many famous writers and artists reveal their identity as a twin survivor through their work. Examples include Edgar Allan Poe's "The Oval Portrait," Dostoyevsky's novels, Lewis Carroll's *Through the Looking Glass*, Oscar Wilde's *The Picture of Dorian Gray*, Bob Dylan's song "Simple Twist of Fate," Paul McCartney's song "Yesterday," John Lennon's "#9 Dream," Leonardo da Vinci's *Mona Lisa*, Shakespeare's *Twelfth Night* and his "dark lady" of the sonnets, and Elvis Presley's song "I'm Left, You're Right, She's Gone."

Millar concludes that "such artists' creative drive results from experiencing loss of part of themselves. They are conscious of their immortality by being creative, an insurance that some part of them will exist after they are dead. Each creation is at once an attempt to regain their first creation, namely a copy of themselves, and an expression of their creative spirit which produced the copy in the first place."

In each of these examples, Millar believes that the dead twin was identical but female, a situation caused by a chromosomal abnormality called Turner's syndrome that could have been sufficient to cause the miscarriage. (Millar also suggests that a single pregnancy that results in the delivery of a baby with Turner's syndrome may have also started as a twin pregnancy.) Millar postulates that confusion about self following the death of a monozygotic twin in utero may result in autoimmune diseases. He also believes that the disordered gender identity of homosexuals and transsexuals may be a result of loss of one member of a mixed-sex monozygotic pair. That is, the loss of an identical self of the opposite sex results in sexual confusion. Another suggestion Millar makes is that a lost monozygotic twin may influence the development of schizophrenia, "loss of ego boundaries strongly suggesting some confusion about what is Self and what is not Self."

Physician George Engel, in describing his close bond with his monozygotic twin, reports a "diffuseness of ego boundaries, never feeling sure who was who," and says that he experienced a profound confusion between himself and his brother in dreams. He also was very aware of family anniversaries and dates of key events shared by himself and his twin. (See "Family Time" later in this chapter.)

Unaware Twin Survivors

Although children commonly fantasize about being a twin or being adopted, individuals who had no idea that they were a twin have discovered this fact in the course of therapy for various problems. (Many psychotherapists, however, are unaware of the impact of the twin bond and often never discover that a client may be a twin.)

Some singletons and mothers of singletons have a sense of incompleteness, feeling that a twin was lost. Kay Cassill quotes a woman who says, "Since childhood I've always felt very lonely. I couldn't overcome it and couldn't figure out why I felt that way. Even as an adult, I still felt this longing. It was when I was about to have my first child that my mother finally told me I was a twin and that my twin had died at birth."

Fascination with mirrors, reflections, and facial asymmetry, left-handedness, stuttering, and malformations have all been attributed more to twins than to singletons and may lead single adults to believe they once shared the uterus. However, Boklage's research showed that not only are twins more often left-handed than the rest of the population, but so are their siblings and parents. Therefore left-handedness and twinning have familial associations.

Twin survivors may be particularly sensitive and reluctant to make deep commitments to relationships for fear of sudden loss. And, like survivors of other tragedies, they often experience feelings of responsibility and guilt: "Why did I live and he/she/they didn't?" I contend that in the case of twins these feelings are special — primal and profound. First, unlike cases of survivor guilt from accidents, the experience of twin loss is not part of the conscious mind and therefore is unavailable for discussion, rationalization, and integration without assistance. Second, because of its deeply personal nature, the surviving twin may experience haunting feelings of being a parasite or destroyer. This is probably inevitable for survivors of the twin transfusion syndrome (explained in Chapter 7).

Graham Farrant believes that the vanishing twin syndrome is an emerging psychiatric condition. He describes one patient who, unaware of her twin history, always bought two items of clothing and another who bought a duplex house so the other side could be kept empty. Mothers of a surviving twin have reported various behavior such as the child talking to a make-believe companion, dreaming of a twin, or setting the dinner table for the nonexistent twin.

MaryEllen O'Hara, a psychotherapist and birth educator in San Diego, has no children yet but has suffered three miscarriages. All her life she experienced a feeling of "reaching toward someone" and had a recurrent dream that she was in a fog, with a piece of stretchy wall, "like plastic," between herself and the other person. She recalls trying to reach through it, wanting to grab and save the other. As a child, she often asked her mother if she had a brother; although she already had three brothers, she was always looking for a lost brother. Her mother suffered miscarriages six months before MaryEllen's conception and six months after her birth. During MaryEllen's gestation, her mother experienced bleeding and contractions between the fourth and fifth months. She had never discussed these episodes with MaryEllen who, much to her mother's astonishment, was able to describe exactly how her mother felt. Her mother remembers that MaryEllen reported her recurrent dream since the age of four and that as a child she often played with plastic, stretching it on her face and calling out. She was also fascinated with looking through glass, especially frosted glass or any silky, shimmery material.

During regression that she experienced as part of primal therapy, MaryEllen felt "weird sensations," and the right and left sides of her body felt different, lopsided, one side hot, the other cold. During one session she reexperienced the formation of her amniotic sac, " . . . watching a balloon inflate and feeling it coming out of the middle of me, and spreading all around me, with each breath . . . like a parachute or a sail. I was encased in it when done, like a larva in a cocoon." In both her recurrent dream and her regression she felt an "intense desire to unite with the other person." She sensed that he was a male, and her grief was profound when she experienced his demise. The experience of his leaving not only meant she had to be on her own but was "earth-shaking, the deepest connection to who I was — the male part of me." She subsequently realized how difficult it had been all her life to accept her "masculine" qualities, such as assertiveness and success at her career. She felt that her excess weight was where she stored her grief.

MaryEllen's connection with her uterine experiences allowed her to acknowledge her feeling of deep loss and realize that she could not "find" her twin. Gradually the dreams went away, as did her avoidance of her masculine qualities. She concludes, "It was a turning point for me no longer to search but to live my own life fully and to

have healthy, stable, male relationships without fear of abandon-
ment.''

Resolution of Repeated Miscarriage in the Survivor of a Vanishing Twin Pregnancy

A woman was referred to me recently by her obstetrician because of
her inability to achieve a successful pregnancy, having experienced
one ectopic pregnancy and three miscarriages by the age of thirty.
Her medical history included many diagnostic tests, some painfully
invasive and expensive, and she was understandably very depressed
and discouraged.

As I took a detailed history — including, as in the case of every
patient, information about her own conception, gestation, and birth
— I learned that her miscarriages always occurred between four and
six weeks of gestation. Her mother had also had three miscarriages.
My patient had conceived her first pregnancy at the same age at
which her mother conceived her. Her second conception occurred
around the time of her sister's birthday. (I am always on the lookout
for such anniversaries that may illustrate a family dynamic being unconsciously acted out in a generational pattern.)

Intuitively, I felt that something had happened to this patient
during her own fourth to sixth week of development and suggested
that she explore this possibility through regression.

In place of techniques such as hypnosis, controlled breathing,
and the like, I use a free, open-ended approach that I learned from
Graham Farrant. The patient simply lies on her back with arms and
legs uncrossed so she is safe from falling and is free to move. She is
gently encouraged to become aware of bodily sensations and underlying emotions and to allow herself to go back in time to the first
occurrence of those sensations, their primal origins.

During the first session, the patient felt disconnected from her
body, except for some nausea, and she expressed much victim language. Ultimately tears and anger poured forth over the myriad medical interventions to which she had been subjected. During the second session she went into deeper feelings and after a half hour of
inactivity she said that she was ''floating, dangling with a string
through my middle.'' (Such metaphors may be obvious to us, but the
patient may not realize that an image such as the string is the umbilical cord.) Then came grimacing and grief reactions. She said, ''It is
leaving, and I'm moving this way,'' as she slid slowly to the left. I

asked if it felt right to say "I'm leaving," wondering if perhaps her mother attempted to abort her. "No," she replied. "I'm staying, I'm hanging in here. But I'm so afraid and I don't want it to leave." I asked her if she was hanging on with her hands and feet and she said, "I don't have hands and feet yet." Thus I knew that her embryological development at the time of loss was prior to six weeks.

She had never heard of the vanishing twin syndrome, but when we discussed the possibility, she noted with amazement that (1) she had always wanted twins, (2) the child whom she had occasionally fostered was "coincidentally" a surviving twin, and (3) when she is pregnant, she feels she completes a part of herself that was missing. She later asked her mother about her gestation and discovered that her mother had experienced first-trimester bleeding.

In five more sessions, this patient reexperienced many prenatal events, including conception, which she described as a "splitting." I surmised from this description and her feeling that a part of herself was missing that she was a monozygotic twin. She often expressed her intrauterine existence with much grimacing of the left side of her face and body, which tied in with her feeling that her twin was to her left.

Over the four months that I saw this patient her demeanor improved markedly, her painful periods and headaches abated, and she became calm and cheerful, a "new person," as her referring physician observed.

In her seventh and final session, she seemed to complete a stage of bereavement for the lost twin and I closed with a guided visualization of her uterus as a nest, with affirmations of her ability to nurture a pregnancy to term. When she wrote to me about her subsequent pregnancy, conceived two menstrual cycles later, she said that she felt a turning point was her being able to regard herself as a nurturer, which suggests that she had imprints of being a destroyer from her own uterine experience. She had no more miscarriages and now has two healthy children.

It is important when a twin "vanishes" in the first trimester or dies in utero that the parents affirm the presence, right to life, and basic goodness of the intrauterine survivor. Joan Woodward, who conducted twin research in England, describes various degrees of rejection felt by surviving twins. Many report that their parents made cruel comments related to the uterine situation, such as "You took all the food" or "You crushed your twin" or "You dismembered him before birth." (One child, having been told such things by her parents, made a later suicide attempt.) While these were memories of actual remarks made to children, parental thoughts are always sensed by the child, even in the womb. I suggest that it is the parental consciousness that conveys negative messages to the fetus and causes a child to grow up thinking "I was a murderer in my mother's eyes." It is no wonder that such a child will feel undeserving, guilty, resentful, and alone and may develop a lifelong pattern of trying to please the mother to make up for the loss of the twin. When the lost twin is of the opposite and preferred gender, the surviving twin may experience further loss of self-esteem. Woodward found that female twins who lost brothers said they felt "useless as they were not the longed-for son." (I knew this feeling myself.) This is a common family dynamic, but it is intensified in the vanishing twin situation because death is involved.

"Family Time": The When and Why of Events Through Generations

An interesting monograph about the repetition of events from one generation to the next, called *Family Time: The Bridge Across the Generation Gap*, was written by an Australian psychiatrist, Avril Earnshaw. She suggests that the timing of family events is genetically encoded, that we inherit time-tagged messages precisely linked with emotional crises of our parents' lifetimes. These events shape our DNA and reverberate as anniversaries in our own adult lives and the lives of our children. She stresses that although the actual events may be different, related events occur at the same age. Maybe this explains simultaneous sudden infant death syndrome in twins and some of the amazing coincidences of twins reared apart documented by the Minnesota Center for Twin and Adoption Research.

Emanuel Lewis, psychiatrist at London's Tavistock Centre, describes a case of compulsive generational patterns. A woman's daughter, her stillborn twins, and her first grandchild were all born on February 1. The mother also had two sons, each from a twin pregnancy, and in each case the other twin died at the fifth month. Her last pregnancy was also twins, who were stillborn. The woman's two oldest daughters experienced unplanned pregnancies, which Lewis felt were unconscious replacements for the stillbirths.

Joan Woodward notes that twins who lose a twin in childhood tend to be fearful for their own children when they reach the same age. She describes one man in his forties who became ill when his daughter reached the same age as his monozygotic twin had been when he died in an accident.

Recommendations for Expectant Parents of Twins

All this fascinating material on prenatal and perinatal psychology can be used for the benefit of mother and babies, although some readers may perhaps feel that this is yet another avenue for parental guilt. I have counseled mothers, for example, who have made appointments for an abortion and then decided to go ahead with the pregnancy. They wonder what effect this will have on their baby or babies. (Incidentally, the discovery of a twin pregnancy in several cases personally known to me was the turning point. The mothers felt that two babies were too special and canceled their scheduled abortions.) As David Chamberlain points out, "Private truths are living history to your child . . . the honest revelation of your inner life is an alchemy that can turn negative feelings into positive ones." I suggest that such mothers explain to their babies, in utero, exactly how they feel and ask for time and patience as they adjust to the continuation of the pregnancy. Likewise, any negative situation should be explained to the babies, emphasizing that they are not the cause of the accident, divorce, job loss, family death, or whatever is the origin of the mother's anxiety. Every situation has the potential to be healed; the first step is acknowledgment.

Guidelines for Optimal Prenatal Conditions

1. Ideally, a baby, including twins, is wanted and planned. I have spoken with many mothers of twins who always wanted twins, who even willed their egg to split or prayed for double ovulation. Some mothers who have lost one or both twins have subsequently conceived another set. Parents ideally are equally aware of the desired conception during the sexual act. Consciously conceive your babies with meditation and visualization, especially if you are having an assisted conception (such as IVF, GIFT, or donor insemination).

2. Avail yourself of optimum nutrition, exercise, and family harmony. Aside from good nutrition and regular exercise, clear communication between the partners is important prior to conception as well as through the pregnancy and in the postpartum period.

3. Be aware of your family history, especially related to twins, and the age of your mother at the time of your conception.

Also significant is the time when a woman reaches the same age her mother was when she or her siblings were born. Avoid conceptions and births around anniversaries of miscarriages and stillbirths in the family.

4. Visualize your babies from the earliest time. If you did not consciously conceive them, begin communication with them as soon as you have a diagnosis of a twin pregnancy. Be open to any dreams, images, hunches, or other dimensions of intuition.

5. Entertain the idea of a soft, relaxed uterus that will yield so that each baby can stretch and turn comfortably. Place your hands on your belly as often as you can and reassure the babies inside that there is enough room, enough oxygen, enough nutrients, enough love and attention for each of them. Learn their various positions. Ask the midwife or doctor to draw each baby's position on your skin at each prenatal visit. Introduce the babies to the concepts of up, down, right, left, back and front, and body parts. When you feel one baby kicking, reassure the other that he or she is safe, keep breathing, and envisage your uterus softening with each exhalation. Use your hands to communicate with each baby. When the father and siblings do this, ask them to state their name each time, for example, "This is your brother Joe," so that the touch, voice, and family relationship are linked. Encourage activity in the quieter twin.

6. Affirm the individuality of each twin. Talk to the babies about sharing. Help them with their ego boundaries; refer to them by name. If you don't know the genders, make up some special pregnancy names. As psychiatrist Bernabei points out, "More than other people, twins must in each moment live with the problem and the question of identity of the 'I' and of the 'you' and their continuing relation." At no time is this situation more pronounced than during prenatal development. Increasingly routine use of prenatal screening means that more parents will know the sex, placental type, and perhaps zygosity of their babies before birth. Use this information to bond with each twin as an individual as well as to talk to them about their special bond of twinship.

7. Think positively about carrying the babies to term — however many there are. Take pride in the power and wisdom of

your body in responding to the challenge of multiples. Individuals create their own bodily realities; the life of a person is the life of the body. People can learn to voluntarily control blood flow, pulse rate, blood pressure, and other physiological functions. Visualize and verbalize optimal mental, physical, emotional, and spiritual development for your babies daily. Meditate on the babies' nutritional, emotional, and spatial needs. Emphasize the qualities you admire most in yourself and your partner as attributes for the twins to acquire.

8. Express anxieties, fears, and concerns. Worries and apprehensions may become self-fulfilling prophecies and lead to complications. Birth educators are continually challenged in their attempt to adequately inform parents of hazards and possible interventions while stressing the normalcy of birth. Each of us brings to pregnancy and birth our own agenda of unfinished psychological business, and this is where personal growth should be centered. Let yourself feel afraid and release the fear. Feelings need to be affirmed and explored, not rationalized. Pregnant mothers of twins who have been ordered to take bed rest, at home or in the hospital, for premature labor, high blood pressure, and other conditions can often resolve the complication if simply asked what their body is expressing (usually it is what they are repressing). Medical professionals often rush to treat symptoms without exploring causes, and the psychological dimension of complications is generally overlooked. (See Louise Hay's *You Can Heal Your Life* and Alice Steadman's *Who's the Matter with Me?*) If you cannot consciously connect with your fears, hypnosis, applied kinesiology, and dowsing are some techniques that can help.

9. Keep a journal. A written record of your thoughts and feelings will help you bond with the twins as a unit and as individuals as well as provide them with a wonderful record of their prenatal existence.

10. As your twins get older, listen to their memories about their birth and about the time before they began to talk. Many children spontaneously discuss such memories, but they are usually met with a skeptical reaction from adults and their expression of their memories is shut down once and for all.

A mother of twins recently told me that she overheard one twin say to the other, "You always kicked me when we were inside Mom," and the other twin admitted, "I remember kicking you a lot. I didn't have much room." Parents can best facilitate such conversations by acting calm and interested and asking open-ended questions such as "Tell me more . . . ," "When did you first feel that?," "How was that for you, Susie, when Tommy was born?," and so on. Let them say it was "warm, "dark," "tight" — whatever — spontaneously rather than using such terms yourself in questions. Be aware of birth symbols in speech, drawings, and play.

11. If you experience complications and have to undergo interventions, provide a running commentary for the unborn and newborn babies. They do understand: babies, years later, have been able to quote verbatim conversations in the delivery room! Caesarean babies need additional cuddling, body contact, and massage. (See the discussion of Caesarean section in Chapter 13.)

12. Honor your babies — they are your guides and teachers. Whether you consciously chose them or not, they chose you as parents!

7 Potential Hazards of Multiple Pregnancy

SOONER OR LATER expectant parents of multiples will hear stories of all the things that can go wrong. Although carrying and delivering two babies at once is more of a feat than producing merely one, the fact remains that pregnancy and birth are physiological states, not symptoms of a disease process. This is often forgotten in the increasingly technological approach to birth in the United States, where even low-risk pregnancies are often handled as potential pathology.

In recent years twin birth has come to be regarded as an abnormality with a gloomy outcome, although until about the 1950s good diet and common sense, with little medical intervention, were the only prescriptions given to women whose multiple pregnancies were anticipated. Every few years articles appear in the medical journals monotonously repeating unfavorable statistics of low birth weight, prematurity, and other complications and pleading for new methods of treatment. Few preventive measures — except bed rest and suturing the cervix to prevent premature labor — have been advocated, but the obvious importance of prenatal nutrition continues to be generally overlooked.

Mothers will hear — from well-meaning friends as well as from popular literature — that they have increased chances of anemia, high blood pressure, toxemia, placental problems, and postpartum hemorrhage. Complications predicted for their multiple offspring include congenital malformation, prematurity, low birth weight, and problems in presentation at birth. No wonder parents become anxious as delivery day approaches. Statistically it is true that the likelihood of some problems increases with twins, but not all the complications of singletons occur more frequently in a multiple pregnancy. Also, the samples of women used to generate the statistics are relevant. Research usually is conducted in large teaching hospitals, which tend to have more patients with complications than might be found in the general pregnant population. Twin births at small community hospitals or even at home are not included in such investiga-

Potential Hazards in Multiple Pregnancy

Fetal Complications

Prematurity
Low birth weight
Intrauterine growth retardation and growth discordance
Presentation
Cord problems (accidents, velamentous insertion)

Complications Unique to Multiples

Twin transfusion syndrome
Delivery of the second twin

Maternal Complications

Anemia
Pregnancy-induced hypertension (toxemia)
Antepartum hemorrhage and placental abruption
Maternal preexisting conditions (exacerbated by
    multiple pregnancy)

Maternal/Fetal Complications

Polyhydramnios

Fetal Disability: Congenital Anomalies, Defects, and Disease

Loss in the Childbearing Year

Loss in pregnancy (miscarriage)
Selective birth/reduction
Intrauterine death of one or more fetuses
Loss during labor (stillbirth)
Perinatal mortality among twins
Loss of a newborn (neonatal death)
SIDS: sudden infant death syndrome

tions. In one study, for instance, the problems associated with multiple pregnancy were not surprising considering that the mothers were poor minorities who had no prenatal care and whose twins in most cases were not diagnosed. Factors such as these inflate the reports of complications in multiple pregnancies.

Even today twins may not be diagnosed before birth, particularly in rural areas. Careful observation of the pregnancy and birth is the hallmark of good care. If multiple pregnancies are undetected and are treated as single pregnancies, poor outcome is not surprising. One study confirmed that if twins were discovered before the thirty-fourth week of pregnancy, the mortality rate was much lower than when the diagnosis was made only at the time of labor. Furthermore, early diagnosis correlates with higher birth weight; mothers carrying two fetuses are encouraged to eat more, as long as their physicians are enlightened about nutrition.

This chapter examines the complications that can occur in a multiple pregnancy as well as their medical management.

Fetal Complications

Prematurity

A birth after about twenty-six to twenty-eight weeks and up to thirty-seven weeks is termed *premature* or *preterm*. Birth at this time is by far the major cause of complications and infant death, whether the infants are twins or singletons. Prematurity accounts for two-thirds of the deaths of one twin and for 80 percent of cases in which both twins die. And prematurity is far more common in twin pregnancies than in singleton: 93 percent of singletons are born at term, but only 57 percent of white twins and 48 percent of black twins were carried to term in 1987 in the United States. Preterm delivery occurs in 35 percent of monozygotic twins but in 25 percent of dizygotic twins. O'Grady explains that the difference is due to a higher incidence of spontaneous rupture of the membranes in monozygotic pairs.

Preterm labor is associated with three-quarters of all the perinatal morbidity (illness) and mortality in the United States. Dr. Marsden Wagner of the World Health Organization stated in the *Birth Gazette* in 1989, "Infant mortality is not a health problem: it is a social problem with health consequences. The first priority for lowering infant mortality in the U.S. is not more obstetricians or pediatricians or hospitals, not even prenatal clinics or well-baby clinics, but rather to pro-

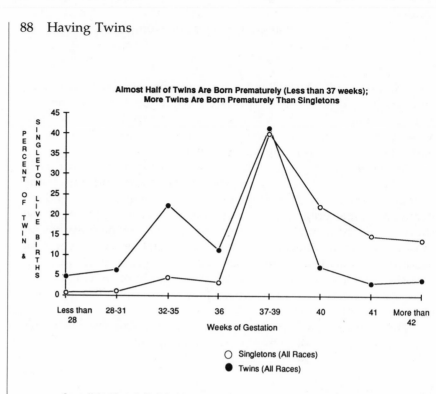

Almost Half of Twins Are Born Prematurely (Less than 37 weeks); More Twins Are Born Prematurely Than Singletons

○ Singletons (All Races)
● Twins (All Races)

Source: National Center for Health Statistics, 1987.

While multiple births often are premature, plenty go to term (thirty-seven weeks) and beyond.

vide more social and educational support to families with pregnant women and infants." Dr. Wagner recommended that the United States focus on problems of smoking, lack of social support, prenatal and postnatal paid maternity leave, other forms of maternity protection on the job, less obstetrical intervention, and increased use of midwives. Countries (such as Sweden and Holland) with some of the lowest perinatal mortality rates also have large numbers of midwives involved in maternity care and delivery and Caesarean rates less than 10 percent. In 1990, the United States ranked twenty-second in the world for perinatal mortality and had a 15 percent prematurity rate, which is not unexpected when one-third of all women in the country do not have prenatal care.

It has generally been accepted that the more babies there are, the earlier they will be born. The "crowding" theory is based on the idea that the uterus delivers the babies when there is no more room inside. In fact, most doctors and much of the public take for granted that twins "always come early." Along with the crowding theory, the general belief is that the uterus becomes overstretched, a theory not always based on fact. Often singletons weighing more than the combined weight of multiples are successfully carried to term.

Pre-eclampsia (a hypertensive condition occurring in late pregnancy), amniotic fluid infection with intact membranes (which predisposes them to rupture prematurely), polyhydramnios, and placental abruption increase the risk of preterm delivery. (All these conditions are discussed in this chapter.) Other theories on prematurity include psychological stress, differing maturation rates for babies within a set, and the concept that the fetuses themselves may initiate labor by secreting a hormone that stimulates contractions. Gail and Tom Brewer warn that falling blood volume from inadequate nutrition can trigger labor. When one baby is growing insufficiently or the babies have a blood group incompatibility, the life of one baby may have to be deliberately risked — an induced premature delivery, for example — to save the healthier one. (The prevention and treatment of prematurity are discussed in detail in Chapters 11 and 13.)

I was huge and very uncomfortable with my twins. When I went past my due date, I was really depressed. I called my obstetrician in tears and ultimately persuaded him to induce me. Each of the babies was over 8 pounds.

Low Birth Weight

The amount of weight the babies gain in the uterus is related to their rate of growth as well as the duration of the pregnancy. Both these aspects of fetal development are impaired if the mother is undernourished and if her weight gain is restricted. Most researchers agree that the birth weight of the offspring is related to the adequacy of the mother's diet and weight gain in pregnancy. Birth weight also is associated with the weight of the placenta — that crucial organ that supplies nutrients to the fetus.

Wide ranges of maternal weight gain have been observed in pregnancies with healthy outcomes. However, studies show that caloric intake in the presence of high protein, more than any other factor, helps avoid low-birth-weight babies and infant death. Older, heavier, and taller mothers do best with multiple pregnancy. Although empty calories of junk food are to be avoided, it was found that placental weight is consistently higher in groups of women who consumed supplemental calories, regardless of the actual type of food supplement.

Many women interviewed for this book delivered 8-to-9-pound twins. Larger babies have a better chance of survival as well as a better chance of later intellectual and physical development. Statistically, twins through age four weigh less than singletons of the same age. No subsequent treatment can make up for the lack of adequate nutrition and a healthy prenatal environment. MacGillivray observes in both his texts that the nutritional and metabolic requirements of a

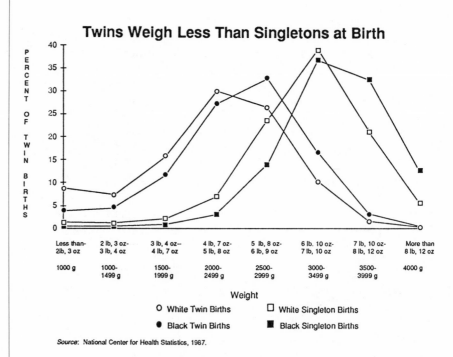

Twins Weigh Less Than Singletons at Birth

Source: National Center for Health Statistics, 1987.

Multiple births have low birth weight. (A weight of 1,000 grams is equal to 2 pounds, 3 ounces; 2,500 grams equals 5 pounds, 8 ounces; 5,000 grams equals 11 pounds.)

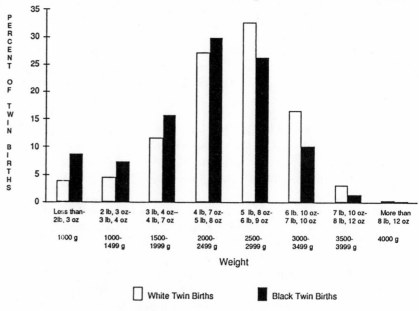

Black Twins Have Lower Birth Weight Than White Twins

Source: National Center for Health Statistics, 1987.

multiple pregnancy are not known and that increases over singleton requirements are not necessary. Yet more than thirty years ago the close relation between diet, fetal condition, and birth weight was discovered. An adequate diet reduced fetal death by one-third, according to Bourne and Williams in 1948.

Low birth weight is not the same as prematurity, although premature babies, especially multiples, usually weigh less than normal. Babies may also be "small for dates" or "small for gestational age." These definitions can be confusing as a baby may fall in one, two, or all three of these categories. About half of all twins weigh less than 5 pounds, 8 ounces (2,500 grams), which is the international standard definition of low birth weight. Birth weight is even lower for triplets, whose median weight is 4 pounds. Males usually weigh slightly more than females in twin births, and dizygotic pairs weigh more than monozygotic pairs. Monozygotic twins, despite the fact that they are "identical," often show the greatest disparity in birth weight because of inequalities in placental function. Discrepancies in growth between twin fetuses can also result from the competition for nutrients within the uterus, the most extreme cases occurring in the twin transfusion syndrome (discussed later in this chapter).

Among singleton births, only about 10 percent are low birth weight, whereas only about 10 percent of twins weigh more than 7 pounds, the average weight for a newborn singleton. In 1988, the incidence of low-birth-weight babies in the United States was 7 percent compared with 3 percent in Sweden.

Smoking, which diminishes appetite and depletes nutrients, is an even greater hazard if the maternal diet is inadequate. Smoking interferes with placental function, disturbs fetal respiration, and results in offspring that weigh less than babies of nonsmoking mothers. O'Grady states that women who have had fewer than three births, who weigh less than 95 pounds at the beginning of pregnancy, and who smoke during pregnancy are at "substantially increased risk for delivering low-weight twins." If an expectant mother simply cannot give up the habit, she should at least take in extra nutrients to compensate.

Intrauterine Growth Retardation and Growth Discordance

One twin may be discordant for growth (that is, may grow more slowly than the other twin) or may be growth retarded in comparison with normal rates. Differences in birth weight are usually expressed as a percentage of the weight of the larger twin. A difference of more

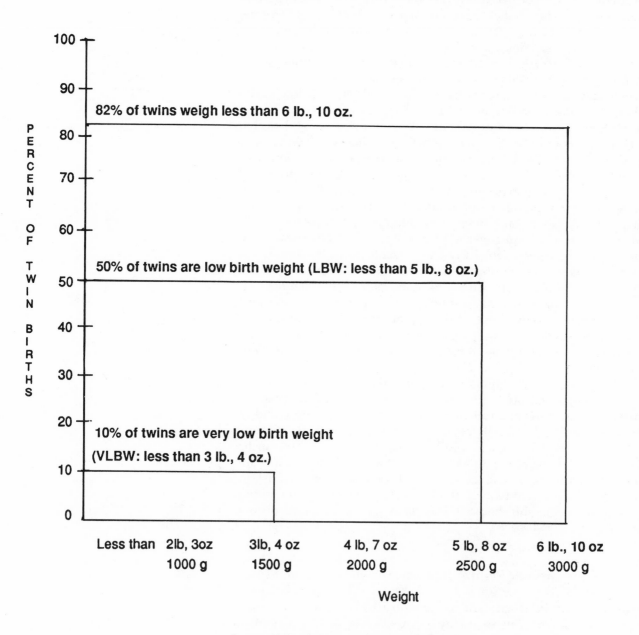

18% of Twins Weigh More Than 6 lb., 10 oz. at Birth

82% of twins weigh less than 6 lb., 10 oz.

50% of twins are low birth weight (LBW: less than 5 lb., 8 oz.)

**10% of twins are very low birth weight
(VLBW: less than 3 lb., 4 oz.)**

PERCENT OF TWIN BIRTHS

Less than	2lb, 3oz	3lb, 4 oz	4 lb, 7 oz	5 lb, 8 oz	6 lb., 10 oz
	1000 g	1500 g	2000 g	2500 g	3000 g

Weight

Source: National Center for Health Statistics, 1987.

than 15 percent is more likely to be associated with an infant who is considered "small for gestational age." Weight discordance most commonly occurs in monozygotic twins from twin transfusion syndrome (discussed later in this chapter). In dizygotic twins, discordance can be from polar body twinning or superfetation (discussed in Chapter 2) as well from expected differences from their different egg/sperm origins.

Evaluation of Low-Birth-Weight Babies (According to Blickstein and Lancet)

If a difference between the fetal head diameters of more than 5 mm is seen on ultrasound before the thirtieth week, head circumference or abdominal circumference measurements are made next. If the head circumference difference is greater than 5 percent or the abdominal difference is more than 20 mm, the next step is to estimate the weight of each twin. If a difference of 15 percent or more is found, the discordance is classified as grade I (this occurs in 20 to 25 percent of twin pregnancies). If the difference is greater than 25 percent, it is classified as grade II. This occurs in 4 to 9 percent of twin pregnancies, and those low-birth-weight infants have a perinatal mortality rate almost two and a half times that of infants with smaller differences. Intrauterine growth retardation is a major cause of stillbirth. Some researchers suggest that individual growth rather than differences between the twins is a better predictor of fetal problems because both twins may be affected by intrauterine growth retardation and the problem of low weight may go unnoticed.

Ultrasound scans are used to estimate the size of anatomical structures, and weight differences are more effectively diagnosed with Doppler ultrasound, which measures the blood flow in the fetus and umbilical cord.

Presentation

The parts of the babies in the uterus that present in the mother's pelvis may cause complications in a multiple pregnancy. Babies can change positions in the uterus at any time, even during labor, except when the presenting part is engaged in the mother's pelvis. Most single babies arrive headfirst, which is termed a *vertex* presentation. *Breech* presentation, in which a lower part of the body comes first, occurs in about 3 percent of singleton births. *Transverse lie*, in which the baby's body lies across the mother's pelvis, is very rare, as the uterus accommodates a baby better in the vertical than a horizontal

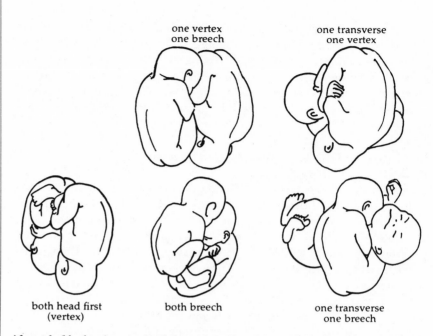

one vertex
one breech

one transverse
one vertex

both head first
(vertex)

both breech

one transverse
one breech

About half of twins are both born headfirst, but breech positions are more common than with singletons.

position. The presentation must be changed to vertex or breech for the baby to be delivered vaginally; otherwise a Caesarean section is necessary.

Twins are born both headfirst less than 50 percent of the time. The first twin is not in a vertex position 20 percent of the time. One is vertex and one breech in about 40 percent of twin births. More commonly, the second twin is breech. Both are born breech about 8 percent of the time, and other presentations account for the rest of twin births. In a small percentage of births, the second twin lies transverse or turns after the birth of the first to present with an arm or a leg or both (*compound* presentation), requiring either external or internal intervention by the obstetrician to turn that twin. Some researchers have found that the larger the difference in birth weight, the greater the likelihood that the heavier twin will be born first. Larger babies do well regardless of method of delivery, whereas low-birth-weight infants are much more vulnerable to trauma, even with a Caesarean delivery.

A breech birth is the most hazardous way for the baby to be born. Cord prolapse* occurs more often with breech presentation: there is

---

* A condition in which the umbilical cord, which is the baby's lifeline, drops out of the uterus into the vagina before the baby.

room for the cord to slip down because the baby's head is not against the cervical opening to seal it off. The feet or buttocks are delivered first with a breech and it may be difficult for the arms to be brought down and the head to follow. Sometimes the first twin is delivered vaginally, but a Caesarean section is done for the delivery of the second baby, especially if the obstetrician is not skilled in turning the baby (internal version) or in assisting a vaginal breech birth. (See Chapters 12 and 13.)

Cord Problems

Accidents with the cord, such as compression and trauma, are increased in multiple pregnancy, particularly in the rare situation where twins share one amnion and the cords can actually become entangled. Only 1 to 2 percent of twins share both chorion and amnion, and up to half of those do not survive, although this rate will improve with improved ultrasound detection. Several scans are often necessary to detect the condition. Careful surveillance of the pregnancy with ultrasound every two weeks and daily nonstress testing (see Chapter 8) for cord entanglement increase the chances of survival. Caesarean section prior to the onset of labor after thirty-five weeks makes sense for this type of high-risk pregnancy.

Another problem with the cord — velamentous insertion — occurs six times more often in multiple pregnancy than with singletons. In this condition, the cord is inserted into the membranes rather than directly into the placenta, and bleeding can occur when the membranes rupture if fetal blood vessels are torn. Vaginal bleeding and fluctuations in the fetal heart rate are symptoms of this rarely suspected condition.

Complications Unique to Multiples

Twin Transfusion Syndrome

When the placenta is shared by monozygotic twins, one baby may develop at the expense of the other, a condition known as *twin transfusion syndrome* or *feto-fetal transfusion syndrome*. Connections between blood vessels in placentas of monochorionic twins occur up to 15 percent of the time, and two-thirds of those twins die. (See the discussion of chorion and placenta formation in Chapter 2.)

Connections may be made from artery to artery, vein to vein, or artery to vein. Unequal distribution of blood and basic nutrients oc-

They had told me all along that my quads would be born by Caesarean. Their positions formed a perfect cloverleaf — all heads to the center.

curs when there is a one-way shunt from the high pressure in the artery to the lower pressure in the vein. This explains the difference in size, weight, and color at birth of twins who are genetically identical.

Doppler ultrasound techniques to measure blood flow in the umbilical cord and fetus may help detect twin transfusion syndrome during pregnancy if different growth rates arouse suspicion. In the absence of abnormalities, if there is a difference in the diameters of the fetal heads of more than 5 mm before the thirtieth week, the cause is probably twin transfusion syndrome. Ultrasound can also reveal discrepancies in the size of amniotic sacs, fetal movements, and size and number of umbilical vessels as well as other symptoms such as edema (swelling) or congestive heart failure. Lasers have been successfully to coagulate the shunts in the blood vessels.

Polyhydramnios (excess amniotic fluid) and oligohydramnios (depletion of amniotic fluid) coexist as a consequence of twin transfusion syndrome. (Polyhydramnios is discussed later in this chapter.) The donor twin is usually growth retarded with insufficient amniotic fluid. Sometimes the loss of this twin is accompanied by vaginal bleeding, sudden abdominal pain, and leakage of amniotic fluid without the onset of labor. In a pregnancy with polyhydramnios, such signs followed by diminution of girth and increased urine output of the mother strongly suggest the demise of one twin and the resolution of twin transfusion syndrome in the other. Ultrasound can confirm the situation.

Although twin transfusion syndrome has been reported in dichorionic twins and in twins with mixed blood groups (a condition called *chimerism*), it is generally associated with a monochorionic placenta, which always involves monozygotic twins. Thirty percent of fused dichorionic placentas are from monozygotic twins, and 1 percent of these show vascular connections, according to Dudley and D'Alton. If the third type of twinning (see Chapter 2) is more common than has been thought, twin transfusion syndrome could be explained by the genetic dissimilarity between the two fetuses and a possible reaction from their immune systems. The reported incidence of twin transfusion syndrome is variable, depending on the way in which the placentas and differences in hemoglobin and birth weight are analyzed and interpreted. Twin transfusion syndrome can occur in triplets, even trizygotic ones, as reported by Pons in France, where two such babies died in the uterus.

A Japanese study of 133 monozygotic twins found that in one-quarter of the pregnancies one twin died from twin transfusion syndrome. Eight of the surviving 33 babies had brain damage and other abnormalities. Machim in Canada gave a rate of 232 per 1,000 (23 percent) for monochorionic twins stillborn from twin transfusion syndrome. The prognosis is less favorable when a twin dies in the latter half of pregnancy; when death occurs in earlier stages, the surviving twin in most cases grows to term uneventfully.

Delivery of the Second Twin

Second twins are not invariably smaller, despite common belief, unless there are large discrepancies between the babies' weights. While many reports have suggested that death is more common in the second-born than the first-born (increasing with higher-order multiples), other researchers have not found this to be the case. Sometimes the difficulty results from the position of the second twin, but one ten-year study found that twins in the breech position (mostly second twins) had half the perinatal mortality rate.

If monozygotic twins share membranes and placental circulation, the risks at birth are greater and the second twin is delivered immediately if bleeding occurs. Another reason for haste in delivering the second twin is that if anesthesia is used for the birth, the second twin is exposed to it longer and may suffer more impairment. Anesthesia itself leads to complications, such as the need for forceps or vacuum assistance to replace uterine activity. The second twin may fall victim to such interventions when twins are not diagnosed. If the staff are unaware of a second baby, a uterine stimulant (oxytocin, ergometrine) may be given immediately after delivery of the first baby to inhibit postpartum bleeding. Such treatment can have the disastrous effect of shutting down the blood supply by augmenting uterine contractions. The second twin thus can become trapped inside the uterus as the oxygen supply is being cut off. Occasionally the second twin's cord can prolapse, appear as the cord of the first baby, and be cut mistakenly before birth. A prudent obstetrician does not cut any cords until all babies have been delivered.

Cases are reported in the literature in which intervals of days, weeks, and even months have occurred between the births of twins. Unpublished data from Northwestern Memorial Hospital in Chicago shows that intervals of up to 300 minutes are acceptable *if* the second twin is monitored and the vital signs are stable. Most obstetricians, however, including Dr. Leo Sorger, consultant for this book and an obstetrician in the Boston area known for his natural birth practice, prefer to deliver the second twin as soon as possible.

Maternal Complications

Anemia

Spellacy's 1990 study of 1,253 twin pregnancies showed that women pregnant with twins were 2.4 times more likely than women pregnant with singletons to develop anemia. Anemia is a condition in which the blood contains a reduced number or volume of red blood cells or insufficient hemoglobin (which carries oxygen to the tissues) within the red cells. Anemic persons suffer from fatigue, faintness, dizziness, and tingling of the extremities. Exertion increases these symptoms because the anemic blood cannot adequately oxygenate the tissues. Sufferers of anemia typically have pale skin and pale mucous membranes in the gums and inner eyelids and sometimes experience inflammation of the gums and tongue. Such persons may have disturbed digestion because of malnutrition and are often irritable. Many women are anemic before pregnancy, especially if they have had inadequate nutrition or heavy menstrual periods. Smoking also increases the effects of anemia.

Although anemia is commonly defined as an iron or folic acid deficiency, it is actually related to a lack of many nutrients in the diet. A balance of all essential vitamins and minerals must be present to facilitate absorption of the nutrients they contain. (For a complete discussion of nutrition, including vitamin and mineral requirements of pregnancy, see Chapter 9.)

Iron is essential for the formation of adequate hemoglobin. Blood tests measure the level of iron by determining the *hematocrit*, the percentage of red blood cells in the blood (the normal range is 36 to 47 percent) or the hemoglobin levels (the normal range for females is 12 to 16 gm per 100 ml). During pregnancy both the mother and offspring make greater than usual demands on the circulation for oxygen, which is transported by the hemoglobin. Decreased levels of hemoglobin in pregnancy can be caused by several different factors, however, so the hematocrit reading may be more reliable in some cases. In twin pregnancy, for instance, the mother's blood volume is greatly enlarged (by about 1,500 ml, about 3 pints) to flow through two placentas. An increase in the plasma component (which carries the red blood cells) in the mother's blood may appear to reduce the hemoglobin levels (a condition called *hemodilution*), when in fact the hemoglobin levels are adequate. In pregnancy, the increased work of the heart pumps the "thinner" blood faster in compensation.

Iron deficiency is the most common type of anemia in Western society. Most clinics feel it is cheaper to prescribe iron supplements than to determine whether women actually are anemic. Once the supplements are prescribed, a simple way to determine if a woman is taking the prescribed iron tablets is to ask her what color her stool is. Excreted iron turns the stool a blackish color.

Folic acid, like many other nutrients, is often insufficient in the average diet and, like iron, is depleted from maternal supplies during pregnancy. The protein construction of red blood cells depends on folic acid. Deficiency of this nutrient in animals has been associated with an increase in malformations of the skeletal, circulatory, and nervous systems.

A blood smear will reveal whether the blood cells are small and iron deficient or large and pale from insufficient folic acid in the diet, and appropriate treatment can be prescribed. Twin researchers Campbell and MacGillivray found a low occurrence of clinically significant anemia and do not recommend routine iron and folic acid supplements, which can have side effects.

Pregnancy-Induced Hypertension (Toxemia)

Consistent high blood pressure, known as *hypertension,* was found to be 2½ times more likely in twin pregnancies than in singleton pregnancies, according to Spellacy's 1990 study. In a blood pressure reading, the upper or first figure is systolic pressure, the highest pressure attained when the lower chambers of the heart contract to send blood out to the body. This pressure is lowest during sleep and varies in response to exercise, emotion, and anxiety. The lower or second value is diastolic pressure, the momentary resting pressure during the phase when the heart muscle relaxes. Since the heart actually rests more than it works, diastolic pressure is the more important value, although smaller changes are observed in it than in systolic pressure.

Hypertension in pregnancy is defined by obstetricians as a reading of 140/90 (measured in millimeters of mercury pressure), a rise of 30/15 over usual readings, taken on two separate occasions with at least one day's interval between the readings. (Internists diagnose hypertension if the readings are 160/100 on two occasions separated by six months.) Danger signs of hypertension include headache, visual disturbances, and vomiting. Modern obstetricians now feel that a rise in blood pressure in multiple pregnancy is to be expected. Such a rise is functionally associated with extra blood volume from the

When my doctor found out I was having quads, he wanted me to restrict salt and watch my weight. As a result I lived practically on just asparagus for the first three months. Then I transferred to a high-risk center, where they wanted me to gain as much weight as possible.

heart and the circulatory demands of extra placentas. The blood volume and nutritional status of a pregnant woman must be assessed before conclusions are made about hypertension. One study found that mothers of twins had a lower diastolic pressure in midpregnancy but that in the last three months pressure rose by 50 percent. The conclusion was that a diastolic pressure of 90 (accompanied by 20 percent protein in the urine) was probably not pathological in a multiple pregnancy. It has also been suggested that a rise in diastolic pressure (up to 95) serves to push the nutrients through the placenta. Bodies vary greatly in their response to physiological demand. One mother of quadruplets had no swelling, no proteinuria, and a consistent blood pressure of only 120/80.

Metabolic toxemia of late pregnancy, as pregnancy-induced hypertension formerly was called, occurs usually after the twentieth week and is defined as a combination of hypertension, protein in the urine (proteinuria), and swelling anywhere on the body. These three signs are checked at every prenatal visit because toxemia, untreated, can lead to eclampsia (convulsions from fluid retention in the brain), coma, and even death. (Women have had convulsions with normal pressures, however.) MacGillivray states in *Human Multiple Reproduction* that although the incidence of toxemia in multiple pregnancy is given as 20 to 30 percent, this condition is not a major contributor to fetal death as it is in the case of singletons.

In toxemia, blood pressure may be elevated in the last three months and may worsen with the progress of labor. In severe cases, immediate delivery is usual. If no protein is found in the urine along with the elevated blood pressure, the condition is classified as mild. Toxemia is considered more serious if proteinuria and hypertension are both present. Bed rest and sedatives are often prescribed but rarely succeed in controlling the condition.

Diuretics (water pills) and dietary restriction (typically low salt and low protein) have not been shown to improve toxemia. On the contrary, they may even cause or aggravate it. Swelling is the body's way of accommodating the increase in blood volume that is normal in pregnancy. A first-time mother expecting twins has 18 pints of fluid. This fluid is also related to fetal weight.

Theories about toxemia have ranged from autoimmune causes (in which the body attacks its components as if they were foreign elements) to problems of metabolism caused by poor nutrition. Most physicians declare that the cause is unknown and concentrate on the traditional yet ineffective therapy.

Since 1929 the nutritional theory has been advanced and toxemia of late pregnancy has been eradicated in some centers by aggressive prenatal nutritional counseling. But very few physicians examine the expectant mother's dietary intake or attempt to prevent or treat the symptoms with improved nutrition. Obstetrician Tom Brewer is convinced that the characteristic symptoms of toxemia arise from inadequate nutrition. Under ten years of his guidance, the prenatal clinics in Contra Costa County, California, saw a drop in the incidence of low-birth-weight babies from 13.7 percent of 2.8 percent and there was not a single case of toxemia. The only treatment was prevention: the clinics improved the diets of their low-income patients. Similarly, the late Agnes Higgins, a nutritionist at the Montreal Diet Dispensary, showed that for as little as $125 per pregnancy the Canadian government could supplement poor women's diets with adequate calories, protein, and other nutrients. Interestingly, the outcome of births at Higgins's hospital was the same as for private patients at the same hospital and significantly better than the Canadian average. Thus Higgins proved that it is possible to break some effects of the poverty cycle in pregnancy.

The counseling, support, and follow-up that are of paramount importance in such dietary programs pose a problem for most physicians, who have little training or interest in nutrition. The medical profession has traditionally focused on treating the symptoms and complications of malnutrition rather than understanding its nature and means of prevention. Inadequate nutrition is not a problem just of low-income groups. Unbalanced and unhealthy diets can be found in the wealthiest families. (See Chapter 9 for a complete discussion of optimal nutrition during the childbearing year.)

In the book *What Every Pregnant Woman Should Know: The Truth About Diet and Drugs in Pregnancy*, Gail and Tom Brewer explain that weight gain and swelling are normal, physiological adaptations of pregnancy. Treating these necessary changes with a no-salt, low-protein diet and prescribing diuretics to eliminate the body's fluids actually aggravate the symptoms. Low protein levels, caused by inadequate nutrition, cause water to leak out into the tissues from the blood circulation. This condition is worsened if salt is restricted and diuretics drive more fluid out. The result is an even more dangerously restricted blood volume. The woman continues to retain water, however, accompanied by a *sudden* increase in maternal weight and accompanying swelling and puffiness. Blood pressure rises markedly in an attempt to meet the demands that all the organs, particularly the placentas, place on the reduced circulation. Women who exhibit these symptoms may be further maltreated with amphetamines to

My doctor told me at six and a half months that I had gained all the weight allowed (20 pounds). I felt depressed and guilty as well as hungry much of the time. At childbirth classes I learned that other doctors don't restrict weight gain. It just doesn't make sense when you know the baby is still developing.

suppress appetite or antihypertensive and sedative drugs to lower their blood pressure. All this medication passes through the placenta to the babies, a risky and undesirable situation. If this course of events is allowed to continue, the woman's urinary output is reduced along with her blood volume, and kidney damage may result.

The most common cause of proteinuria in pregnancy, according to Gail and Tom Brewer, is simply urinary tract infections, which occur readily because of hormonal dilatation of the ureters (the tubes between the bladder and kidneys) in addition to pressure from the uterus. Even vaginal infections may give rise to a misleading diagnosis of proteinuria if a clean specimen is not obtained.

The "roll-over test" provides information on the blood volume during pregnancy. If an expectant mother's blood pressure is lowered when she rolls from her back to her side, the improved reading indicates that the blood volume is subnormal. This may be a warning sign of toxemia, although false signs can occur.

Gail and Tom Brewer cite many studies showing that adequate protein diets to meet the needs of pregnancy, with salt to taste, can prevent or reverse the toxemia syndrome. Sufficient calories must also be added in the diet; otherwise the body will burn the protein building blocks for fuel, wasting their nutrient value.

Antepartum Hemorrhage and Placental Abruption

Bleeding in pregnancy can result from the placenta lying partially or completely over the cervix or from its premature separation from the wall of the uterus (called *abruption*). Placental abruption is three times more likely to occur in multiple pregnancy than in singleton pregnancy, according to a 1990 study. Abruption has been linked to malnutrition and smoking and is rarely seen in well-nourished expectant mothers.

In vasa previa, the blood vessels of the cord present before the baby during labor and delivery, but the incidence of this condition is not increased in multiple pregnancy. Bleeding can also occur when the fetal blood vessels are torn or when the membranes rupture from velamentous insertion of the cord (see "Cord Problems" earlier in this chapter).

Maternal Preexisting Conditions

If the mother was suffering from certain disorders, such as heart or kidney disease, before conceiving multiples, she will definitely be considered high risk and will be very carefully monitored during the pregnancy. She will also experience an increased likelihood of Caesarean section.

Maternal/Fetal Complications

Polyhydramnios

The medical term for an excess of amniotic fluid within the uterus is *polyhydramnios* or simply *hydramnios*. Normally about two quarts of fluid develops within the amniotic sac in a singleton pregnancy, providing an environment in which the fetus is free to move and is buffered from bumps and jolts from the outside. More amniotic fluid is required for two babies. Although excess fluid can occur for no apparent reason, it is usually associated with fetal or maternal problems. A number of congenital abnormalities, such as vascular anomalies, cause this condition and it also often occurs when the mother develops gestational diabetes. Many researchers have claimed that hydramnios is more likely to occur in a multiple pregnancy and that the occurrence is equal in both monozygotic and dizygotic twinning. (One investigator, however, found that hydramnios was more common in singleton pregnancies.) The recipient fetus in twin transfusion syndrome (discussed later in this chapter), as a result of the increased blood flow, may produce large volumes of urine, leading to acute polyhydramnios. Hashimoto and his colleagues found that 10 of 75 twin pregnancies, analyzed retrospectively, had high levels of amniotic fluid. Nine of the 10 pregnancies were abnormal for other reasons too. The elevation of amniotic fluid volume alone, however, did not explain the high rate of prematurity.

Ultrasound-guided amniocentesis is sometimes performed to remove excess fluid (up to a quart or more) in a singleton pregnancy when the abdominal distention and chest restriction become too uncomfortable for the mother and to help prevent premature rupture of the membranes. With twins, the procedure can remove fluid from one or both sacs. One researcher describes two cases in Scandinavia in which a significant amount of amniotic fluid was drained from the amniotic sacs of twins. In one case both twins died prematurely, but in the other they were delivered in good condition at thirty-five weeks.

The criteria for defining excess fluid vary greatly, and making a diagnosis also is subjective. Reported incidences, therefore, may reflect difficulties in determining the condition. Twins confuse the matter of diagnosis because of the naturally increased uterine size, the extra placenta, and the doubling of blood volume over that of a singleton pregnancy.

Fetal Disability: Congenital Anomalies, Defects, and Disease

Many anomalies, defects, and diseases can be detected by prenatal tests, such as ultrasound, amniocentesis, and chorionic villus sampling (described in chapter 8) and fetal blood sampling (taking fetal blood using a fetoscope to view the babies).

Despite the difficulty in defining and collecting data, many researchers agree that the incidence of malformations is increased in twins, especially monozygotic twins and same-sex twins of both zygosities. The most recent report from the National Center for Health Statistics analyzed live births in 1973–1974 and reported that the incidence of congenital anomalies was 18 percent higher in multiple deliveries. Spellacy's 1990 study of 13 hospitals in the Chicago area found that malformations occurred three times more often among twins (especially monozygotic). It is not understood whether there is a common factor that predisposes to both monozygotic twinning and anomalies or whether anomalies result from some deviation during the splitting of the embryo that results in monozygotic twins. Strangely, anomalies in twins, even in monozygotic ones, are more commonly present in one twin only. Chromosomal events during fertilization can cause only one twin to have a particular disease such as muscular dystrophy or Down's syndrome.*

Some rare anomalies are unique to twins, such as conjoined twinning and acardia. Conjoined twins (sometimes referred to as Siamese twins) occur in about 1 in 200 monozygotic pregnancies. Division of the embyro that occurs later in the second week after fertilization may result in conjoined twins. The most recent study of conjoined twins, conducted in Japan, found an incidence of 10 per million births from 1979 to 1985. The rate was highest among mothers over forty who had several children. Conjoined twins are always joined at identical sites and are classified according to the site of the union. Seventy percent are attached at the chest, a condition often associated with congenital heart disease. Some twins live their lives

---

* Down's syndrome is a genetic disorder in which the child's mental and physical development are retarded. It is associated with congenital abnormalities, especially of the heart. Children affected by Down's syndrome may develop a characteristic mongoloid appearance.

joined together, as did the famous Cheng and Ang from Siam. Surgical division is attempted where possible. A set of twins born in Paris in 1974 were joined at the head. Fourteen years and twenty-six operations later, the girls were declared perfectly normal by their surgeon, Dr. Bernard Pertuiset.

Acardia is congenital absence of the heart, a condition that occurs in about 1 percent of monozygotic twins, either from failure of the heart to develop at all or from atrophy owing to circulation anomalies. The twin who pumps the blood in the latter situation often develops cardiac failure; this condition can now be seen with ultrasound and treated prenatally.

The largest category of congenital malformations comprises heart anomalies; according to Elizabeth Bryan, a cardiac malformation will affect one or both of the pair in about 1 in 50 of all twin pregnancies. Bryan pooled two studies and noted that both twins were affected in only 8 percent of monozygotic pairs and 4.4 percent of dizygotic pairs.

Pathological closure of the esophagus occurs up to five times more often in twins, but only 5 percent of the time both twins are affected. Many common anomalies, such as clubfoot and excess fingers or toes (polydactyly), are less serious. Twins actually had less incidence of congenital dislocation of the hip and Down's syndrome in the government's 1973–1974 report. The risk of lethal malformation in twins, according to Doherty, is 1.9, falling with increased maternal age. Lethal malformations cause about 8 percent of twin deaths but 18 percent of singleton deaths.

Most malformation occurs early in the pregnancy, although problems can develop in later pregnancy from the twin transfusion syndrome or compression of fetuses. Pressure on normal body parts from crowding can cause skull and facial asymmetry, torticollis (wry neck), and foot defects. However, since monozygotic twins have clubfoot and congenital dislocation of the hip 10 to 15 times more frequently than dizygotic twins, other factors are involved in the cause of these conditions.

The causes of birth defects not only are genetic but include malnutrition, smoking, alcohol and other substance abuse, infectious diseases, and environmental hazards. The same environmental influences may affect each twin differently because of gender, individual vulnerability, or slightly different age in a dizygotic pair.

Nutrition plays a role in birth defects. Multiple pregnancies make enormous nutritional demands on the mother, and if these are not met, physical and mental impairment of the babies is likely. Lower-birth-weight babies have more congenital abnormalities than normal-

Even though we already have a child with Down's syndrome, when the doctor explained the risks of checking both babies by amniocentesis, we decided not to have the test and to trust our luck.

birth-weight babies. In the 1973–1974 government study, babies weighing 5 pounds, 8 ounces, or less had about two and a half times as many birth defects as heavier babies. The lowest rate of anomalies was associated with birth weights over 7 pounds, 12 ounces. Birth defects were more common among the offspring of those who became pregnant within a year after giving birth and offspring of diabetic mothers. Male infants were found to have 41 percent more defects than females. Women with less income and education had a higher incidence of children with birth defects, which can be attributed to inadequate diet, poorer hygiene, greater occurrence of infectious disease, and less satisfactory prenatal care. The lowest incidence of infant congenital defects was found among women who had completed college or postgraduate education. A 1988 study by Khoury found almost 25 percent of malformed infants to have intrauterine growth retardation, compared with 10 percent of normal infants. The frequency of intrauterine growth retardation increased with increasing number of defects; for example, 20 percent of the infants with two defects had intrauterine growth retardation, compared with 60 percent of infants with nine or more defects.

Couples with a family history of anomalies or mothers over a certain age can seek genetic counseling (the age varies among counseling facilities but is usually late thirties to over forty). It is possible to detect many (but not all) anomalies prenatally by amniocentesis (discussed in Chapter 8). Availing yourself of genetic counseling or amniocentesis, however, may lead to another dilemma — the decision whether to have an abortion. For couples who would not undergo an abortion under any circumstances, an amniocentesis may still be helpful. If Down's syndrome is discovered, the parents can learn what type it is, which may influence their decisions about future childbearing. And prior knowledge of abnormalities gives the parents time to adjust to the news before the birth and to prepare for a handicapped child.

The risk of disability is also increased for multiples over that of singletons. Insufficient oxygen to the brain during pregnancy or birth can result in cerebral palsy, with varying degrees of physical and mental impairment. Brain damage that is observed in infancy may also be related to prenatal malnutrition. The March of Dimes estimates that one child in seventeen has a learning disability and one in twenty-four is mentally retarded.

Despite inconsistencies in evaluating and reporting complications, it is clear that women pregnant with multiples are at greater risk for complications. This is especially the case if their needs for early diagnosis, excellent nutrition, adequate rest, and good prenatal care are not met. It is important to keep in mind the many mothers of twins and triplets who carry healthy, normal-weight babies to term without any problems at all.

Loss in the Childbearing Year

Although the singleton perinatal mortality rate has improved in the United States — it was about 1.4 percent in 1979 and 1 percent in 1988 — the quality of the life that is saved must be considered. Physicians and medical scientists often claim that progress in technology has improved the mortality figures, but others feel that this is not the case. Instead, improvements in socioeconomic conditions for many people, smaller families, better nutrition and health care, and childbirth education have been cited as factors that are just as significant as technological tools such as ultrasound and fetal monitors.

Elizabeth Bryan reports that in at least 50 percent of twin pregnancies one baby is lost — most of those vanishing in the first trimester (see Chapter 4). Geneticist Charles Boklage claims that there is a greater prenatal loss of males than of females (although more males than females are born) and of same-sex dizygotic twins than mixed-sex dizygotic twins. Loss can happen in any trimester, during labor and delivery, and in the period after birth.

Loss in Pregnancy (Miscarriage)

Miscarriage is one of nature's ways of providing selection of the fittest pregnancies for survival. The body tends to reject a fertilized egg with any defect, which is why congenital abnormalities are infrequent in infants born alive. About one-sixth of all pregnancies miscarry, and this figure is much higher for multiple conceptions. Ian MacGillivray and his colleagues pooled data relating to first-trimester loss in pregnancies in which ovulation was not artificially stimulated and found that three times more twins than singletons spontaneously aborted. Miscarriage, like placental problems and prematurity, has been linked to malnutrition, smoking, and other substance abuse.

Death of a twin in the first trimester rarely leads to any complications. The earlier the loss, the more benign the effect on the pregnancy. The frequency of loss of one fetus of a multiple pregnancy ranges from .5 percent to nearly 7 percent (the majority of cases associated with monochorionic placentation, 70 to 80 percent of monozygotic twins). According to Enbom, the frequency of an antepartum death of one twin is 1 in 184 twin births. Eighty-two percent of remaining twins survive, but death or major morbidity affects almost half. If the death of one baby occurs at thirty-five weeks or more, immediate delivery is usually advised. The risks of prematurity from delivery need to be weighed against the potential hazards in the environment that contributed to the death of one twin.

Miscarriage may occur in the second trimester. Up to twenty-six weeks, the term *immature birth* is appropriate. The causes of second-trimester loss are similar to those in the third trimester — infection, placenta previa, and toxemia. Cocaine abuse may precipitate bleeding and cramping (the effect is not related to the strength of the dose). Some twins die in the second or third trimester and are compressed into the placenta (a condition called fetus papyraceus, discussed in Chapter 2).

Other losses occur in the last trimester from impaired function or placental abruption, cord accidents, toxemia, and twin transfusion syndrome (all these conditions are discussed earlier in this chapter).

Selective Birth/Reduction

When one fetus is found to be abnormal through ultrasound or amniocentesis and there are two chorionic sacs, parents have the option of "selective birth/fetocide." Prior to the advent of ultrasound, the mother would have had to terminate her pregnancy and sacrifice both the abnormal child and the healthy child or continue through the pregnancy and give birth to both babies. Often, parents who would accept a termination for a single abnormal fetus have much more difficulty with the idea of aborting a normal baby at the same time. The advisability of continuing the pregnancy depends on the severity of the baby's disease, the parents' reproductive history, and the estimated expectancy and quality of life for the abnormal twin. In some cases, either choice — to abort or to continue the pregnancy with both babies — may put the healthy baby at risk.

Selective reduction has been performed in cases where one twin but not both has a syndrome such as Down's, Hurler's, or Turner's, or Tay-Sachs disease, hemophilia, spina bifida, or Duchenne muscular dystrophy.

The reduction procedure usually involves cardiac puncture, but injecting air into the umbilical vein with a fetoscope has been performed. It is important not to inject any toxic substance into what may turn out to be a shared circulation. In early pregnancy the embryo can be extracted through the cervix. However, after the second trimester, the dead baby is carried along with the live one (the emotional consequences are discussed in Chapter 17).

Fetal Deaths per 1,000 Births

Year	Singletons	Twins	Higher-Order Multiples
1977	9.3	35.1	67.7
1985	7.9	27.9	76.3
1987	7.3	25.9	43.5

Source: Vital Statistics of the United States, vol. 2, Mortality, 1977, 1985, and 1987.

Every mother wants a healthy baby, of course, but such methods are not without risk to the healthy baby of the pair. Complications for the healthy baby include miscarriage, infection, premature labor and birth, and the need to terminate the entire pregnancy if a procedure fails. A rare possible complication for the mother is random clotting in the mother's fine blood vessels (disseminated intravascular coagulopathy, or DIC) as a response to the bleeding or resorption of the breakdown products of the lost fetus. A remote possibility is error in selecting the defective twin because of a change of position in the uterus. It helps if some dye injected at the time of the amniocentesis is still present in the amniotic fluid or if some distinguishing characteristic can be observed with ultrasound.

Intrauterine Death of One or More Fetuses

One of the less common complications is the natural death of one or more babies in utero, but it is ten times more likely than for a singleton. It is three times more common in monochorionic twins than in dichorionic. As the table shows, outcome improved between 1977 and 1985 except for higher-order multiples. This is because of the increased use of reproductive technology and the rescuing of ever-smaller babies.

Males are slightly more at risk than females. Monozygotic twins have a greater chance of intrauterine death than dizygotic twins, particularly if they share the chorion or, more hazardous, the amnion as well. Mixed-sex twins, followed by female twins, both monozygotic and dizygotic, fare best.

Intrauterine death carries the same risks as selective birth/reduction: premature delivery, infection, damage to the remaining baby or babies from the same ailment that caused the other death, and the clotting disorder of the mother's blood. A 1989 Israeli study examined two sets of twins (with second-trimester loss of one twin), one set of triplets (with second-trimester death of two), and one case of quadruplets (with third-trimester death of one) and found that no maternal complications developed and all fetuses found alive at the initial diagnosis were doing well after delivery.

There seems to be no problem retaining a dead fetus for up to four weeks, assuming close monitoring of the unborn baby and of clotting factors in the mother's blood. The first case of selective birth went nine weeks until the delivery of a healthy, normal baby.

Doppler ultrasound can detect abnormalities in fetal and umbilical blood flow and in the placenta that may lead to intrauterine death.

Loss During Labor (Stillbirth)

Stillbirth is defined as an infant born dead weighing at least 500 grams (about 1 pound, 1 ounce) or at a gestational age of at least twenty weeks. Although twins are more likely to die after birth than to be stillborn, about four times as many twins as singletons are stillborn. The triplet stillbirth rate ranges from four to six times that of singletons.

Some of these deaths may be preventable, as some twins are not diagnosed until labor. Some unforeseeable conditions that can cause death at term or during labor are prolapsed cord, velamentous insertion of the cord, or placental abruption (all discussed earlier in this chapter).

Perinatal Mortality Among Twins

Perinatal mortality refers to deaths within the first twenty-eight days after birth and fetal deaths of twenty weeks or more gestation (infant mortality, on the other hand, refers to deaths within the first year following a live birth). In all countries, the perinatal mortality rate for twins is higher than that for singletons. In the United States it ranges from three to five times greater. Ten percent of perinatal deaths in the United States are of multiple births. The rate is twice as high in monochorionic monozygotic twins as it is in dizygotic twins.

In 1988, the U.S. infant mortality rate was 9.9 per 1,000 live births. The perinatal mortality rate was 6.4 per 1,000. The post-perinatal rate (deaths between twenty-eight days and one year) was 3.5 per 1,000. The prematurity rate (babies born at less than thirty-seven weeks gestation) was 8.5 percent for whites and 18 percent for blacks. The overall incidence of low-birth-weight babies (less than 2,500 grams, or 5½ pounds) was almost 7 percent.

Louis Keith and his colleagues in 1980 observed that the pregnancy loss rate was highest among twin mothers in their first pregnancy, declined to a minimum among women with three or four children, and increased with subsequent births. The lowest loss, 3.5 percent, occurred for babies born at term. The overall mortality rate for second-born twins was 8.5 percent, for first-born twins 6.1 percent. As birth weight increased, mortality decreased, dropping dramatically when the first twin weighed 1,000 grams (2 pounds, 3 ounces) or more and the second weighed 1,250 grams (2 pounds, 12 ounces) or more.

The perinatal mortality rate has generally been greater for the second twin than the first twin, but this difference has been steadily decreasing. In fact, in one study in Scotland, all perinatal deaths in twins over 2,750 grams (6 pounds) occurred in the first-born twin. Twin boys used to fare worse than girls, but that too is changing. The perinatal mortality rate for twins is higher in young mothers having their first babies, the widowed, and the unmarried.

A 1980 study cited the perinatal mortality rate for twins as 11 percent, compared with 1.5 percent for singletons. Monozygotic twins had two and a half times the mortality rate of dizygotic twins in the study. But a Belgian study of more than 3,000 twin pairs showed that same-sex dizygotic twins suffer mortality at least as much as monozygotic twins. Monochorionic monozygotic twins had twice the perinatal mortality of dizygotic twins (9 versus 4.5 percent) as well as more congenital malformations and cardiac problems. Twins who share a single amnion have almost twice the mortality of twins with two amnions. Mixed-sex dizygotic twins with separate placentas have the lowest mortality.

Campbell and MacGillivray in their 1988 text *Twins and Twinning* came to the illogical conclusion that high maternal age, lower social class, short stature, and smoking do not have the significant influence on perinatal mortality or Apgar scores for twins as for singletons. They suggest that "other unknown factors which cause poor growth and preterm delivery are mainly responsible." They do not consider the importance of nutrition and psychological support.

Botting and her colleagues found that smaller multiples actually had a lower perinatal mortality rate than singletons but that the incidence was reversed for the largest multiples. A similar surprising finding was also reported in Spellacy's 1990 study in Chicago.

Loss of a Newborn (Neonatal Death)

Deaths in the first week of life are twice as frequent as fetal deaths. Prematurity is the most common problem among multiples, and the secondary complication of respiratory distress syndrome is the most common cause of death. Another frequent cause of death among premature infants is necrotizing enterocolitis (inflammation and death of tissues in intestines and colon), which is less likely to occur in babies receiving breast milk.

Neonatal deaths among twins born before thirty-six weeks can nearly all be related to respiratory failure, whereas complications with placental function were the cause of most deaths of babies born after thirty-six weeks. In 1986, the neonatal death rate in the United Kingdom was nearly six times that of singletons.

SIDS: Sudden Infant Death Syndrome

SIDS is the most common cause of death of infants between one month and one year of age, striking almost 8,000 infants per year in the United States, or 1 to 2 babies per 1,000 live births. The diagnosis is made by a process of elimination and includes those deaths in infancy for which no specific cause is found. SIDS is especially distressing for parents because of suspicions or accusations of wrongdoing or even criminal actions by police and medical examiners. With increased public and professional awareness of SIDS, it has become clearer that negligence by parents is not a cause of SIDS.

According to a 1986 article by Elizabeth Bryan, SIDS is at least twice as common among twins, both monozygotic and dizygotic, as among singletons. This is obviously because SIDS is highly correlated with prematurity and low birth weight, which occur so frequently among twins. While it is thought that the smaller twin is at greater risk, research in the United States has indicated that the risk is not higher when the statistics are adjusted for maternal age and number of children.

Some studies have found that the surviving twin in SIDS is at increased risk for up to one month after the death of the other twin. The risk is particularly high during the first three days. Families with infant deaths from SIDS or other causes had a 2 percent risk to subsequent children, according to one study. Of course, these are mere statistics; it is important to know the risk factors, which include race, birth order, birth weight, maternal age, marital status, socioeconomic status, and smoking.

Often a surviving twin is hospitalized for several days after a twin dies of SIDS, both to closely monitor him or her and to help the parents cope. Male babies tend to be more at risk. Some authors have suggested an abnormality of respiratory control, but the real cause of SIDS is far from known. Breast-feeding appears to be protective. Cigarette smoking near the infants, overdressing, and night sweats have been linked to SIDS.

Several cases of simultaneous SIDS in twins have been reported. Smialek reviewed nine cases of twins dying suddenly and simultaneously but could find no cause. He quotes a previous researcher who stated, "It is quite clear that it is the very quality of being a twin which somehow or other is combined with a predisposition to sudden unexplained death." Smialek suggests that something goes awry in the intrauterine environment of babies who later succumb to SIDS.

Because I have two friends who lost babies to SIDS, its occurrence has always been a fear of mine. Committed to the idea of a family bed for other reasons, I always felt reassured that my children as infants slept beside me. McKenna points out that in the infant the "social and physiological needs are inseparable, having coevolved over three to four million years in a caregiving microenvironment which, among other things, includes prolonged periods of parent-infant contact, one form of which is cosleeping." He suggests that the infant responds to the rhythmic auditory breathing cues and chest movements of the parents and that this is even more important for infants who are less healthy than the norm. (Even though SIDS deaths occur at any time of the day, the respiratory "fine tuning" at night protects an infant at risk.) McKenna's anthropological perspective has merit; it has been observed that the incidence of SIDS increases with the assimilation of immigrants. In particular, the rate of SIDS in Chinese infants in California was thirty-eight times higher than that of ethnic Asians living in Hong Kong, according to a 1990 study by Grether, where cosleeping occurs.

Chapter 17 explores the emotional reactions experienced by parents and siblings when twins die.

Prenatal Care and Screening Tests

8

IN THE PAST DECADE many new tests have been developed to screen the health of unborn babies. While helpful in certain circumstances, such as high-risk pregnancy, family history of disease, or previous problems with pregnancy outcome, these tests have drawbacks as well. The information they provide is not always clear-cut, there may be side effects to the tests themselves, and one test may lead to several more. I suggest Robin Blatt's book *Prenatal Tests* for more information and guidance on deciding whether to have certain tests. Genetic counseling can assess the risk of genetic disease within a family to aid in your decision.

Maternal Serum Alpha-fetoprotein Test (MSAFP)

The MSAFP is a blood test that measures a specific protein, alpha-fetoprotein (AFP), which is made by the baby and circulates in the mother's bloodstream and in the amniotic fluid. Elevated levels of the protein may indicate multiples because more babies manufacture more AFP. It can also mean a neural tube defect, such as spina bifida or anencephaly, in a singleton pregnancy, which is distressing to expectant parents. Low levels may indicate increased risk of Down's syndrome. According to O'Grady, virtually all uncomplicated twin pregnancies have an AFP level above the median for singletons. But because the normal range for singletons extends quite high, AFP screening fails to identify more than half the cases of multiple pregnancy. Also, there is a difference in the production of AFP between monozygotic and dizygotic pregnancies.

The MSAFP test is done between sixteen and eighteen weeks of pregnancy. Laboratories vary in their reliability with this test, largely owing to differences in classifying the length of pregnancy. One pregnant woman I knew submitted identical samples to three different laboratories and received three different results. Nevertheless this test is recommended by the American College of Obstetricians and

Gynecologists for all pregnant women. California was the first of several states to require physicians to offer the MSAFP test. Recently, MSAFP has been computed with HCG levels for greater accuracy. (HCG is human chorionic gonadotropin, a hormone secreted by the chorion in higher levels in multiple pregnancy. See Chapter 4.)

Follow-up diagnostic tests such as ultrasound and amniocentesis may put your mind at rest about the nature of your pregnancy if there is a query about your MSAFP test. Ultrasound for low levels of AFP may show that the dates are wrong or that the pregnancy is less than sixteen to eighteen weeks. Ultrasound for elevated levels may show that the pregnancy is past eighteen weeks. Level II ultrasound, which provides a more detailed picture, can study the babies for abnormalities.

Amniocentesis

This prenatal screening procedure involves withdrawing a sample of amniotic fluid, which contains the baby's cells, from the uterus. The purpose of this investigation varies with the stage of the pregnancy. When performed between the fourteenth and eighteenth weeks, it can uncover genetic defects or biochemical problems.

Amniocentesis can be more difficult with a twin pregnancy. Formerly, for a twin pregnancy with two amniotic sacs (see Chapter 2), dye was injected into the first sac after its fluid sample was removed so that the obstetrician would know if he or she tapped the same sac again. In 1990 Khalil Tabsh in Los Angeles recommended that some air be injected with the dye to form microbubbles that would be visible with ultrasound. This technique is also useful to determine if two amnions are present — the bubbles will remain on one side of the dividing membrane. With today's sophisticated ultrasound technology, however, the dividing membrane usually can be seen. If you decide on amniocentesis, search for a doctor who is experienced in performing the procedure with twins.

Amniocentesis may be recommended if AFP and HCG levels indicate that risk factors exist. Confirming the sex of each fetus is important because some genetic diseases, such as hemophilia and the Duchenne type of muscular dystrophy, are gender specific and may already be present in the family history.

Amniocentesis is most commonly used (between sixteen and eighteen weeks, although some doctors do it as early as thirteen weeks) to detect Down's syndrome if the mother is older than thirty-five. The recommended age has been continually lowered since amniocentesis was made available in the 1970s. Down's syndrome, also known as trisomy 21, occurs when three copies of the number 18 or 21 chromosome are made instead of two. This condition causes developmental disabilities including mental and physical retardation, and its occurrence has been linked to the mother's age, although other factors may also be involved. (See Chapter 7.)

Not all anomalies can be detected through amniocentesis. A normal amniocentesis does not guarantee a normal baby at birth; it simply indicates if the baby has the condition for which it was tested. The test usually costs about $1,000 and has some risks. The commonly cited statistic for singleton miscarriage rate after amniocentesis is ½ percent, but other studies have shown the rate to be as high as 1½ percent. Occasional orthopedic defects and injury to the offspring have been observed. A 1988 study in Holland described amniocentesis for 83 twin pregnancies. Seventy-seven taps were successful (in the others, there was insufficient fluid or only one sac could be tapped). Nine of the 166 babies were lost after the procedure, a rate of 5½ percent.

Amniocentesis can be used to detect autosomal recessive diseases such as Tay-Sachs, sickle-cell anemia, and cystic fibrosis. These diseases are caused by recessive genes, which means that both parents must carry the same recessive gene *and* pass it on to the same offspring. Because the twins of older women are more often dizygotic, the risk that both twins will have an autosomal recessive disease is only 6 percent. Couples in which both the man and the woman are carriers of the same recessive gene have a 25 percent chance of having a baby who receives both recessive genes and hence the condition. (Monozygotic twins, of course, would have the same disease.) They have a 25 percent chance of having a baby who is not affected and is not a carrier. They have a 50 percent chance of having a baby who is not affected but, like the parents, is a carrier. Certain recessive disorders occur more often among ethnic groups such as Ashkenazi Jews (Tay-Sachs disease), blacks (sickle-cell anemia), southern Mediterraneans (thalassemia), and Caucasians (cystic fibrosis).

Amniocentesis, like all genetic screening, is not without its emotional repercussions, especially if the results are not clear. Further testing understandably raises anxiety levels. Finding a serious problem with one or both babies leads to the dilemma of whether to abort both babies in the case of monozygotic twins or to choose "selective birth" in the case of one affected dizygotic twin. The first case of selective birth occurred in Sweden in 1978, when one member of a pair was diagnosed as suffering from Hurler's syndrome, an enzyme deficiency. (See Chapter 7 for a description of selective birth and Chapter 17 for a discussion of the emotional consequences.) Prenatal screening has thus thrust on parents an emotionally wrenching decision — whether one's child or children should live or die.

I believe that before a woman decides on amniocentesis for a twin pregnancy, she must have time to absorb the idea of twins and to reconsider her feelings about what now will be a double amniocentesis. Those who review the risks and doubt whether they have already bonded with their twins will discover plenty of evidence for the existence of prenatal bonding in Chapters 14 and 17.

Barbara Katz Rothman in *The Tentative Pregnancy* interviewed women who accepted the test and those who refused it. She found that amniocentesis delayed the mother's awareness of fetal movement, which may be a form of psychological protection until she is reassured by the results (which can take up to three weeks). Many obstetricians observe that babies become very quiet for as much as several days after the procedure, and this diminished activity also may account for mothers' delayed awareness.

Chorionic Villus Sampling

Chorionic villus sampling is a genetic test that can be performed earlier in the pregnancy than amniocentesis but requires much more skill. It is becoming available at several centers in the United States.

The chorions are located visually with ultrasound at their point of attachment to the placentas and are sampled there through the abdomen, cervix, or vagina, depending on their location. If the placentas appear to be fused, the sampling is done at opposite ends. The most recent data (unpublished in April 1990) was quoted to me by Dr. Pergament of Northwestern University. From a total of four centers, 174 twin pregnancies and 4 triplet pregnancies were sampled. In only one case was one placenta sampled twice, and the perinatal loss rate was about 1 percent.

The main advantage of the earlier chorionic villus sampling over amniocentesis is that termination of pregnancy, if necessary, is less traumatic in the first trimester than in the second, and selective embryo reduction can be performed instead of selective fetocide (see Chapter 7). The perinatal loss rate is also lower than with amniocentesis, especially for multiples.

Sometime in the future, pregnant women will probably be able to have a simple blood test to detect abnormalities rather than undergoing these invasive procedures.

Ultrasound

Ultrasound, which is fully described in Chapter 4, has many medical uses and is an especially effective technology for making diagnoses and detecting anomalies in pregnancy. It is used, for instance, as early as the first few weeks of a pregnancy to detect ectopic pregnancies and later to assess the relative sizes of multiple fetuses and to determine characteristics of the placentas and membranes.

Faced with increasing numbers of malpractice suits, obstetricians now recommend that multiple pregnancies be scanned frequently with ultrasound. This is done as often as once or twice a month to check for growth retardation, twin transfusion syndrome (see Chapter 7), and, in the case of monoamnionic twins, cord entanglement. If there is a discrepancy of one pound or more between the weight gains of the two fetuses together with edema (swelling) in the larger twin or different amounts of fluid in the sacs, all signs of twin transfusion syndrome, the pregnancy will be closely monitored in case a Caesarean section is required to save one or both babies.

Fetal Monitoring During Pregnancy

Fetal monitoring by machine was first invented for use in labor and is now done during a pregnancy if circumstances warrant. External monitors using ultrasound can be placed on the mother's abdomen and used any time during pregnancy and labor. During a high-risk labor, an internal monitor (ECG), which is more accurate, can be attached to the presenting baby's scalp (if dilation and descent in the birth canal permit).

Chapters 11 and 12 provide extensive details about the use of monitors, both at home and in the hospital, to record contractions and pick up any fetal distress before and during *labor*. The most common monitoring techniques during *pregnancy* are described in the following sections.

Nonstress Test (NST)

This test of fetal well-being is usually done in the last trimester, often when the birth is overdue or if there is a suspicion of premature labor. It may be done as early as the eighteenth week, although it is usually begun at thirty weeks and repeated in three to seven days. The test can also be used to determine whether a complaint of abdominal pain is caused by labor contractions (which will show up on the monitor) or by other problems unrelated to labor such as gas, intestinal problems, appendicitis, or kidney infections (which do not show up on the monitor).

Two external monitors (transducers of ultrasound) are strapped to the mother's abdomen to record the activity of fetal heart (one monitor per baby). The record is printed on paper so that any abnormalities can be observed and the data can be kept in the mother's file. If two machines are not available, each baby is monitored separately.

The babies' heart rates should maintain a healthy variability, changed only by sleep or drugs. This is known as a reactive NST and if observed twice a week indicates little probability of serious problems. In contrast, a nonreactive NST, which according to O'Grady occurs in about 20 percent of twins, is associated with problems such as cord entanglement, diabetes, oxygen deprivation, pregnancy-induced hypertension, intrauterine growth retardation, newborns with depressed vital signs, and death in the period shortly after birth. (Most of these problems are discussed in Chapter 7.) If the babies are sleeping, vibratory acoustic stimulation (VAS) may be applied to awaken them and stimulate heart rate and movement. This stimulation is also being used to study the development and maturity of the central nervous system of the fetus. Unborn babies respond to VAS with increased heart rate, movement, and startled responses, which vary with gestational age.

After activity, the heart rate should go up 15 beats per minute or more. If it does not reach this level, the test may have to be repeated soon. An absence of variation — low baseline and low spikes — is a bad sign. Deceleration (lowering of the heart rate) that is either late, early, or variable relative to a chance contraction can signify fetal distress. Late decelerations are the most ominous, indicating serious fetal distress. There are two kinds of variabilities. When the heart rate changes constantly within the normal range (an irregular saw-tooth pattern), it is a healthy sign. However, it is abnormal for the decelerations themselves to vary or to show inconsistent shape and timing. This may signify a problem with the umbilical cord. (For information on home monitoring, see Chapter 11.) Variable decelerations lead to the next test.

Contraction Stress Test (CST)

The contraction stress test is used to determine the babies' ability to withstand uterine contractions when the mother or physician have some cause for concern. The external fetal monitor is applied when the pregnant woman feels contractions at the rate of about three within ten minutes. The contractions may be spontaneous or the physician may have the woman stimulate contractions so the test can be performed. Contractions can be induced by breast and nipple stimulation or by use of an electric breast pump. If these techniques do not succeed in causing contractions, the oxytocin challenge test (described next) can be used.

If repeated late decelerations occur, it is likely that utero-placental insufficiency and chronic fetal distress exist. Delivery by Caesarean section is then done, whether one or both babies are distressed. While the NST and CST can be done in a doctor's office, the next test, the OCT, is almost always done in the hospital.

Both the NST and CST may give false positive results, which means that a healthy fetus may erroneously be judged to be at risk, leading to an unnecessary Caesarean section. A false negative result — an apparently normal test when the baby in fact is at risk — also can occur. Parents must know that no technology is perfect.

Oxytocin Challenge Test (OCT)

The OCT involves the intravenous administration of pitocin, a synthetic form of the hormone oxytocin, which the pituitary gland produces to cause contractions. Although the test induces uterine contractions, the possibility of the mother going into labor is slight unless it was imminent at the start of the test. The test is basically the same as the CST, but the OCT is used to make sure that each twin can take the stress of contractions without decelerations. A *positive* result on the OCT is *unfavorable*. Severe decelerations in one or both twins means that the twin or twins are in danger, and Caesarean section may be considered to save both of them.

Mothers should question their obstetrician about breast-nipple stimulation before going for an OCT.

While variability and accelerations of the fetal rate are important, with the two contraction tests it is more significant that no decelerations develop because slowing of the heart rate indicates fetal distress. The OCT may take hours to complete because it is started with a minimum dose of pitocin and the dose is increased only every half hour or so until three contractions occur in ten minutes. Many obstetricians allow their patients to sit, stand, and walk, which are much preferable to lying on the back. Other physicians feel that the OCT is too cumbersome and not appropriate for twins because of their high risk of premature delivery.

All these methods of monitoring are done with intact membranes. Internal monitoring, that is, with an ECG lead placed directly on the presenting twin's scalp, can be done only after rupture of the membranes.

Biophysical Profile (BPP)

When a fetus is not receiving enough oxygen, his or her respiration, heart rate reactivity, movement, and muscle tone will be affected.

The BPP assesses five variables of fetal health: heart rate activity, respiration, body movements, muscle tone, and amniotic fluid volume. Heart rate activity is monitored by the nonstress test (described earlier), and the rest of the parameters are assessed with ultrasound. A score of 4 or less on the tests is usually considered pathological and immediate delivery is indicated, except for babies less than twenty-eight weeks. A score of 2 indicates high risk and 0 indicates absent or abnormal activity. If the score is 6 or more, the test may be repeated the next day, which may be too late or too early, and thus some physicians have suggested immediate extended testing. A score of 8 or more is considered normal and indicates that the fetus is in good condition. False positives are possible, however, and they may lead to unnecessary interventions and maternal and fetal complications. Sometimes the placenta is graded as part of the BPP; grade 3 is mature (term).

Some investigators feel that decisions should be based on the individual components (amniotic fluid, fetal movement) rather than a profile or composite score. Controversy also exists over the normal amount of amniotic fluid and assessment of fetal movements such as trunk versus limb action. High-risk patients (including those who are postmature and insulin-dependent diabetics) are normally tested twice a week.

Mother's Assessment of Fetal Movement

Assessing fetal movement is part of the BPP, and many doctors consider the mother's assessment superior to the other single variables of the BPP. Counting fetal movements is based on the theory that if a fetus is in jeopardy, its movements will diminish before it dies. The mother checks for movement at a particular time every day or three times a week and, using a "kick chart," she can detect and report any change in activity level while there is still time to rescue the baby.

Sometimes the mother has to wait up to an hour to feel movement, but as long as fetal movement occurs within the first thirty minutes, further checking is not necessary at that time. Most fetuses don't sleep for more than an hour. (See "Fetal Movement" in Chapter 11.)

All of these screening tests, except ultrasound and amniocentesis, have been developed since I wrote the first edition of *Having Twins*. Prior to their development, mothers carried healthy, normal-birth-weight babies to term, as they do today without these tests. Keep in mind that procedures for investigating and monitoring high-risk patients tend to get used more and more for those women of lesser risk. It seems to be inherent that technology expands as far as the resources will stretch.

Making a decision about whether to have a test or about which test is appropriate may require a second or third opinion. Women expect a test to reassure them, but sometimes it provokes more anxiety if the outcome is not clear or further testing is necessary. It is much better to prevent complications by availing yourself of good health care and healthy nutrition, as emphasized throughout this book, and decrease your chances of needing these investigations.

9 How to Give Your Babies the Best Chance with Optimal Nutrition

IN MY RESEARCH for the first edition of *Having Twins*, it became clear that maternal nutrition and optimal weight gain were key factors for good outcome in multiple pregnancy, just as they are for singleton pregnancy. In the decade since then, the role of these factors has become more and more accepted, and it is rare today to hear of a physician who arbitrarily restricts weight gain and salt in pregnancy as in former years.

Much of this change is credited to obstetrician Thomas Brewer and Gail Sforza Brewer, who wrote, lectured, and campaigned tirelessly for improved nutrition in pregnancy, especially as a way to prevent toxemia and improve birth weight. Daily intake of 4,000 calories and 140–150 grams of protein for a twin pregnancy, recommended by the Brewers and other informed obstetricians, has generally resulted in term babies weighing at least 7 pounds. Gail Brewer had twins herself and they weighed 9 pounds, 3 ounces and 8 pounds, 9 ounces when they were born a few days past the due date.

The clinical work of Dr. Brewer in Contra Costa County, California, and the late Agnes Higgins of the Montreal Diet Dispensary has demonstrated the importance of good nutrition in pregnancy. In Dr. Brewer's ten-year nutrition project, there was not a single case of toxemia among several thousand mothers. Mothers ate for three and gained 50 to 60 pounds. Higgins found that adequate protein and calorie intakes were "markers" for the general level of a woman's nutrition. She recommended 1,000 extra calories and 50 extra grams of protein daily for mothers of twins.

Of the 125 medical schools in the United States, only 30 offer any instruction in nutrition. The average physician receives less than three hours exposure to the subject. Despite acceptance of the importance of nutrition in pregnancy by some clinicians — doctors and staff who treat pregnant women daily — the nutrition factor has not been embraced by doctors who research medical issues. There is a dearth of studies on nutrition in pregnancy, especially on the nutri-

Severe maternal nutritional deprivation has been associated with intrauterine growth retardation, premature labor, and increased perinatal mortality and morbidity. When total parental nutrition was provided to maintain adequate growth in four cases of fetuses small for gestation age because the mothers' nutrition was inadequate, there was no perinatal mortality or morbidity.
RIVERA-ALSINA ET AL., 1984

I am convinced that my girls' birth weights (7 pounds, 11 ounces and 7 pounds, 12 ounces) and good health were directly related to my early diagnosis of twins. I became fanatical about what I ate and how I took care of my unborn babies. My obstetrician, however, had to be convinced not only that I was carrying twins, which I knew intuitively from the beginning, but that I needed to manage my pregnancy in ways different from singleton pregnancies. I am grateful that I listened to my body and that my doctors ultimately did too.

tional demands of multiple pregnancy. A 1985 study found that in about two-thirds of premature and growth-retarded infants of multiple pregnancy the specific causes could not be identified. The researchers did suggest, however, that "preconceptual maternal malnutrition and poor diet in pregnancy might play a role." In contrast, a major medical text on twinning suggested that "most Western diets are quite sufficient in nutrients for increased fetal growth in twin pregnancies." That statement was based on the fact that in one survey mothers expecting twins consumed less protein and fewer calories than mothers of singletons. Despite a perinatal mortality rate for multiples that is four times that of singletons and a pre-eclampsia rate that is up to five times, the authors still claim that the cause of premature labor and pre-eclampsia are unknown.

In the ten years since I wrote the first edition of *Having Twins*, my own diet has changed considerably. I am more concerned today with quality, carbohydrate, fats, and the source of the protein I consume than I am with simply counting quantity. In my second pregnancy I ate much less animal protein than in the first and drank not one glass of milk — and had a baby two pounds larger! Nutrition is an immensely complex subject and it is a challenge, to say the least, to try to find "the truth," as philosophies are diverse and contradictory and eating habits die hard. Most of us know people who are overweight, eat junk food, or smoke and drink daily and who live to their nineties. And how can Zen monks live on brown rice and water for years and not suffer any vitamin deficiencies? But when it comes to eating for our preborn babies, we need to find out what is best, not just what we can get by on.

Eating is a life-sustaining activity that we engage in several times a day, so nutrition should be a relevant and fascinating topic of study. In this chapter I hope to whet your appetite to learn more rather than to provide rules and charts.

Some expectant mothers of twins have had difficulty eating the amount of food recommended by the Brewers' diet in the first edition of my book. The large quantities of eggs and dairy products make it economical but also high in fat and cholesterol. Mothers who pushed themselves to eat beyond their appetite for the sake of their babies' health were usually glad they did. But basic quality is more important than counting grams and micrograms. It is impossible to have a magic number to suit all mothers, and even then the value of a given food is influenced by soil quality, fertilizers, pesticides, harvesting, preparation, processing, shipping, storage, cooking, combining with other foods, and so on. On the other hand, the ideal "nutrition by intuition" is difficult in a society where, according to Christiane

Northrup, an obstetrician and nutritional expert in Portland, Maine, two-thirds of women have eating disorders to some degree. Anorexia and bulimia are very common in our culture and it's a challenge for women who find themselves pregnant to "switch gears" when it comes to food.

Mary Dillon and Stefan Semachyshyn cite in *Twins* magazine (1988) a Toronto study in which more than four hundred pregnant women were divided into three groups according to their diets. The mothers who received an average of 92 grams of protein daily fared best, with an average labor five hours shorter than the group that was given a poor diet. The less-nourished women had more cases of anemia, toxemia, and threatened abortions. That group also experienced 3.4 percent stillbirths and 6 percent miscarriages compared with zero in the better diet group. Almost four times as many babies were born prematurely to the mothers with a poor diet, and the babies were less healthy.

The Limitations of Numbers

People vary enormously in the way their bodies metabolize food, apart from all the lifestyle contributions, and routine meal plans therefore make little sense. While good intentions have produced diet sheets, RDAs (recommended dietary allowances, calculated and revised every five years or so by the Food and Nutrition Board of the National Research Council), and other guidelines, the fact remains that every person is an individual organism when it comes to nutritional requirements and all those guidelines are only rough estimates. The USRDAs on food labels are amounts established by the Food and Drug Administration as standards for nutritional labeling and do not include allowances for pregnancy and lactation. If an expectant mother of twins reads a percentage on a label, she needs to divide it by three: if, for instance, a cereal provides 45 percent of the RDA for iron, it provides only 15 percent of the RDA that the mother requires for herself and her unborn twins. If measured amounts are given on a label rather than percentages, the mother can add these amounts to her daily requirement, which should have been adjusted to account for her as well as her unborn twins. The US RDA values may err on the high side for nonpregnant adults, but they are low for a woman carrying twins.

The RDAs say nothing about individual requirements. They are based on amounts that will keep a population free from a deficiency of an essential vitamin, mineral, or other nutrient and were devel-

Most people don't need the full amount of the RDAs. They are "high" numbers, not minimal requirements to be met every day, which is why they're called Recommended Dietary Allowances, not Required Daily Allowances. They are general guidelines rather than a daily prescription.
ROBERT RUSSELL, M.D., associate director of the USDA Human Nutrition Research Center on Aging at Tufts University

oped only after widespread food processing caused deficiency dis-eases. What is optimal for each individual, with his or her individual metabolism and lifestyle, is not addressed at all by the RDAs. Despite the increasing loss of whole foods from the American diet, the RDAs for key nutrients such as iron and calcium were lowered in 1989.

It is not possible to calculate a person's exact nutritional require-ments except with the Vegatest. This method of testing for preclinical illness (that is, cellular changes that occur before a diagnosis is made), individual vitamin and mineral needs, food allergies, stressed inter-nal organs, toxins, and so on — anything can be tested if it can be produced in a vial — was developed by Helmut Schimmel, M.D., D.M.D., in Germany. It is a noninvasive biofeedback measurement and thus is ideal for pregnancy. After a specific deficiency has been determined, actual doses are prescribed using the same biofeedback system. This test is becoming more available in the United States, Australia, Great Britain, and Europe. I believe the Vegatest is a most important contribution to preventive medicine because it can detect disease in its preclinical stage, when its course can often be reversed by lifestyle changes. "Health insurance" should ideally be an annual Vegatest screening.

I explored my health profile with the Vegatest several years ago in Australia. Despite my habit of eating several times the RDA of vitamin C, I registered a deficiency for that vitamin as well as for some minerals I had hardly heard of, such as chromium and molyb-denum. The test also picked up a drug I had taken eight years earlier for a corneal abrasion that was still in my system. I was impressed! Seeing and hearing the results immediately (rather than sending blood away to a lab) convinced me to take supplements and homeo-pathic remedies. I normally eschew vitamin and mineral supplements because I simply have never known what I need and how much. Since the total amount of required vitamins and minerals add up to less than a teaspoon per day, I prefer to increase my intakes of appro-priate food rather than swallow a pill, which is not how nutrients normally arrive in the stomach anyway. The Vegatest can also find toxicities in the body that block absorption of iron or other nutrients. I am encouraging Stuart Zoll in Boca Raton (the nation's foremost Vegatest practitioner) to test women with premature labor contrac-tions, as the Vegatest explores emotional and environmental influ-ences as well as hormonal and nutritional ones.

The elements of good nutrition require deep understanding, and diet itself is more complicated than simply making the right food choices. The best foodstuffs may contain a certain amount of nutrients, but if the foods become stale or if overcooking destroys their nutritive value, dietary arithmetic does not reflect the true situation. The nutritive value of a food is also enhanced or diminished when the food is combined with other foods. Even more of a problem are animal products, which are heavily promoted by the meat and dairy industries but are grossly polluted.

I have observed an increasing awareness of nutrition among my clients; many of them choose more grains and vegetables in place of animal foods. The American Heart Association, the American Cancer Society, and the United States Surgeon General have warned the American public about the association of a poor diet with conditions such as heart disease, colon cancer, hypertension, diabetes, and obesity, to name just a few, and they recommend that dietary intake of red meats, sugar, and fried and processed foods be greatly reduced.

In May 1990, Jane Brody reported in the *New York Times* the early findings from the most comprehensive large study ever undertaken of the relationship between diet and the risk of developing disease. The study, begun in 1983 by Dr. T. Colin Campbell of Cornell University, examined the diet and health of 6,500 Chinese. Much lower occurrences of heart disease, cancer, and diabetes are seen among the Chinese, who consume only 7 percent of their protein from animal sources, compared with 70 percent for Americans. The plant-rich Chinese diet contains a third less protein than the American diet but three times more fiber. Fat intake is less than 20 percent among the Chinese.

Ideally an expectant mother has enjoyed good nutrition in her own developing years, particularly before she attempts conception. Her levels of weight and nourishment prior to pregnancy will determine the weight of her offspring (and, in some ethnic groups, the likelihood of twinning). Optimum prepregnancy and prenatal nutrition is the best safeguard against problems in pregnancy, birth, and postpartum, especially with multiples, and it is something you can take into your own hands. The mental and physical constitution of your offspring will also be influenced by your prenatal nutrition.

Toward Healthier Sources of Food

Now that it has been accepted that pregnant women need to eat extra for each baby, in this edition I want to recommend optimum sources of that extra food. Pregnancy is the ideal time to commit oneself, and the whole family, to a healthier lifestyle — changes that will last long after the delivery.

Food is man's [sic] most intimate contact, far more intimate than copulation. What you eat goes right inside you, is absorbed directly into the bloodstream and carried into every cell in the body, including, most importantly from the point of view of mental health and behavior, the brain cells.
RICHARD MACKARNESS, *Not All in the Mind*

Nutrition is more controversial and more complex the further one delves. A trip to any bookstore will show how many different diets have been devised. There are various types of vegetarian diets (vegan, no animal products; "lacto," in which dairy products are consumed; "ova," in which eggs are eaten). Some schools of thought push raw fruit and vegetables; others feel strongly that both these foodstuffs should be cooked, as in macrobiotic food preparation.

The sanest and most interesting discussions of nutrition are those written not by dieticians or academics, but by cooks. Among the best I have found are *Food and Healing* by Annemarie Colbin, *The New Laurel's Kitchen* by Laurel Robertson, books by Carol Flinders and Brian Ruppenthal, and *The Complete Guide to Macrobiotic Cooking* by Aveline Kushi. These are just a few of the abundant titles that can be found in health food stores, and the ever-increasing number of these cookbooks shows the changing dietary habits of the American population.

Macrobiotics is based on the traditional diet in Japan, before it was contaminated by Western products like white rice, white flour, sugar, and so on. First popularized in the United States by George Oshawa and further developed in Boston by the Kushi Institute, macrobiotics is also the subject of a worldwide movement. Concerned with more than just nutrition, it is a philosophy of balance — yin and yang — and includes a medicinal or therapeutic use of food. Macrobiotic diets have been somewhat successful in reversing all kinds of cancer (see *Recalled to Life* by physician Anthony Sattilaro). However, I don't care for their prohibition of fresh fruits, juices, raw vegetables, salads, and nightshades (tomatoes, potatoes, peppers).

In this chapter I give a few tables of measurements to demonstrate the nutritive value of certain foods in the macrobiotic diet that are not commonly used in American diets (for example, sea vegetables). I believe it is better to spend your time shopping for healthier ingredients and learning how to prepare them than weighing and measuring serving sizes. If you choose only high-quality foods and get the majority of your calories from complex carbohydrates rather than fats and sugars, you will be in good shape.

Calories and Weight Gain

How much weight should a woman expecting multiples gain? Fifty to 60 pounds seems to be an average healthy figure for mothers of twins, but what about the woman who is carrying an unsuspected

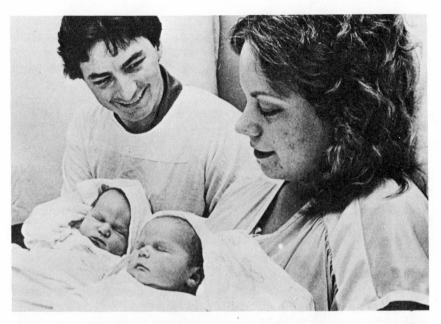

Maternal weight gain must be encouraged for optimal outcome. This mother of twins gained more than 90 pounds. The babies weighed 8 pounds, 9¼ ounces, and 9 pounds, 8½ ounces. This was the mother's first pregnancy.

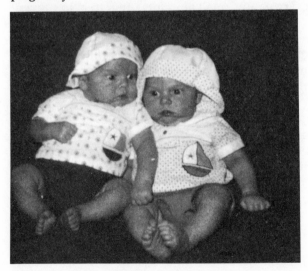

The size and maturity of these one-month-old twins pay tribute to the mother's high prenatal weight gain.

I gained 75 pounds with my triplets. One was stillborn but the others weighed almost 7 pounds.

My twins weighed 7½ pounds and 8½ pounds although I gained only 28 pounds. We live on a farm and I was as plump before the pregnancy as I am now.

The heaviest surviving twins were born in Arkansas in 1924. They weighed 14 pounds and 13 pounds, 12 ounces.
Guinness Book of World Records

I ate good food all through my pregnancy. Boy, was I hungry! I used to wake before six A.M. and have to get something to eat. Then I would go back to sleep. I couldn't keep my eyes open — just like a newborn babe after he eats.

triplet? Arbitrary numbers have no place here — these are only target numbers to reach because optimal weight gain is essential. In addition to the weight of an additional baby, there is increased weight from the placenta and increased amniotic fluid, maternal stores, and blood volume.

Prepregnancy weight is significant. Women who are overweight may have normal to large babies even if they gain little weight during the pregnancy. But overweight women are often the most malnourished, and they must take care to eat well during pregnancy. If a woman's prepregnancy weight is less than 115 pounds, she needs to gain more weight than an overweight woman might need. *Never* diet to lose weight during pregnancy and nursing. It is strange that in a society where obesity is so common, women in the childbearing year feel concerned about temporary weight gain.

Some maternity care providers are concerned about the rate of weight gain (which in multiple pregnancy is going to be faster than usual). Rate of weight gain is highly variable, so listen to your body! Although the babies grow more slowly in the first few months than later in pregnancy, many mothers find a tremendous need for energy in the first trimester to fuel the transition from the nonpregnant state. Major hormonal changes affecting the respiratory and cardiovascular systems contribute to the fatigue they commonly experience. While some women are ravenous in the first trimester, others feel nauseous and may vomit a lot. Try eating small amounts often to help prevent "morning sickness," which may occur at any time of the day when blood sugar levels are low. Fresh grated ginger added to food or made into a tea can relieve nausea, as can tiny amounts of umeboshi plum (a macrobiotic diet ingredient available from health food stores). It is also easier to eat more small meals through the day, especially toward the end of pregnancy when the stomach is crowded into a smaller space above the vastly expanded uterus. Mothers of multiples do have to take care that they are eating enough. If you have difficulty consuming an adequate amount of food or have nausea or obsessive cravings, consult the recommended nutrition books in Suggested Reading.

Basic Nutrients

Carbohydrates

Extra calories are required for your body's increased workload in a multiple pregnancy. If you do not consume sufficient high-energy foods, your body will burn protein for fuel rather than using it as the essential body-building material it is for the babies, placentas, and uterus.

Carbohydrate is the most abundant foodstuff in the diet, and the two forms that supply fuel to the body are sugars and starches. Sugars are generally present in fruits, while starches are found in vegetables and grains and their products.

Sugars found naturally in fruits, vegetables, grains, and beans are simple carbohydrates. In contrast, whole grains, such as brown rice, oats, buckwheat, barley, millet, and corn, are complex carbohydrates and provide for the slow release of energy in the body. Grains also contain protein, B vitamins, iron, and other minerals.

The maintenance of blood sugar levels is very important, especially for the function of the brain. The type of carbohydrate eaten is significant for maintaining blood sugar levels. Complex carbohydrates are digested slowly and maintain more even levels of blood sugar. Although fruit, which contains fructose, a simple carbohydrate, takes time for digestion, the other simple sugars, such as table sugar (sucrose), are absorbed immediately. This quick digestion explains the rush of energy that follows eating candy, pastry, syrups, honey, or other "pick-up" foods. Unfortunately, this high-energy state soon passes and is replaced by a low-energy state as the blood sugar levels drop. Although people vary in their resistance to these hypoglycemic attacks, weakness, irritability, and anxiety are commonly associated with the vicious cycle that results from eating too many simple sugars. The vicious cycle also strains the liver, which stores sugar as glycogen and releases it in emergencies to try to maintain equilibrium.

Metabolism of sugar drains the body of nutrients, vitamins, and minerals. Like salt, sugar is often added to canned and processed foods. Sodas and various juice "drinks" are loaded with sugar. For example, one can of Pepsi contains 10 teaspoons of sugar. Sugar contributes about 25 percent of the calories in the typical American diet, and most Americans eat their weight in sugar each year.

Your dietary goal, especially in pregnancy, is to eat more complex carbohydrates in their less processed, more natural form. Whole grains should compose about half of your diet.

Protein

Protein forms the basis of the body's structure, and because it is not stored by the body it must be obtained from food every day. Utilization of protein becomes very efficient even when its intake is limited, and it is rare in the United States to see a protein deficiency.

Protein is broken down by the body into amino acids. There are twenty-two amino acids, ten of which are considered essential amino acids because, unlike the others, the body cannot manufacture or convert them. They must be obtained from the diet. Animal protein contains all the essentials, which is why meat, fish, fowl, milk, and eggs are considered classic protein sources.

The RDA of protein for a woman pregnant with one baby is 60 grams. A woman pregnant with twins needs about 100 to 110 grams, with triplets 135–145 grams. Protein is also available from many other sources (see the chart on the following pages) that do not have the liabilities, such as high fat and toxin content, that animal protein has. While certain grains and legumes (beans, lentils, peas) may be incomplete in their amino acid content, in combination with other protein sources they form the necessary complete protein.

One of the first nutrition writers to carefully consider these combinations was Frances Moore Lappe, who wrote *Diet for a Small Planet* in 1971. In her 1982 revision of the book she said that combinations of protein could be more flexible and that the balance did not have to be achieved at each meal, but could occur over a few days.

The major consideration with animal protein is its source. The meat of diseased animals that are bred with sex hormones to stimulate growth and that consume antibiotics, pesticides, and herbicides is frankly unhealthy. Also, livestock are generally slaughtered under unsanitary conditions that detrimentally affect the quality of the food.

Poultry has less fat content than meat, but if it is commercially raised it has many of the same problems regarding wholesomeness. The spread of feces during slaughter and processing contributes to the high content of salmonella (which can cause food poisoning) in chicken. Although food poisoning is rarely lethal, up to one-third of the U.S. population suffers from it each year.

While fish are usually free from many of these hazards, they may come from polluted waters, and labeling is not required. Eggs are a whole food, but the hens who hatch them generally are dosed with antibiotics and hormones, are kept in tiny cages, and are debeaked because they find their environment so stressful that otherwise they would kill each other. The eggs such chickens lay are higher in cholesterol than those of free-range chickens, lack the essential fatty acids, and taste very inferior to natural eggs.

Health food stores carry meat and poultry products that are raised naturally and eggs from free-range chickens. Kosher poultry

How many people consider when they sit down to eat their steak that they are getting a dose of penicillin? Fifty percent of the antibiotics manufactured in this country are fed to livestock.
Christiane Northrup, M.D.

Protein Content
in grams per 100 grams
(3½ oz. or ½ cup)

Meat

Beef	14–22
Pork	9–22
Chicken	15–23
Eggs	12–14
Fish	16–25
Cheese	14–28

Beans

Azuki beans	22
Kidney beans	20.2
Soybeans	34
Mung beans	23–24
Lima beans	20
Tofu	1
Lentils	7
Seeds/nuts	11–30

Grains

Brown rice	7
Wheat	9–14
Oats	13
Buckwheat	11–15
Millet	10–13
Barley	8–9
Rye	12–13

Source: U.S. Department of Agriculture, Japan Nutrition Association, and *Aveline Kushi's Complete Guide to Macrobiotic Cooking* (1985).

(such as the Empire brand) is also raised free from drugs. Such products are worth paying the extra price.

Whole grains and beans are excellent sources of protein without the disadvantages of meat and poultry. However, most of us were not raised on such foods and we need to learn how to cook them so they are digestible and appetizing. They are very easy to store because they do not require refrigeration, and they can be bought in bulk, which is a big consideration for the busy postpartum mother of multiples. They can be cooked ahead and stored in the refrigerator (rice can be kept for five days, legumes for about three).

Fats and Oils

Fats supply more than twice the energy (calories) per gram than do carbohydrates and protein. Fat-soluble vitamins A, D, E, and K and fatty acids for cell metabolism are also carried in fats and oils. Fats digest slowly, give a more "filling" feeling, and are (unfortunately) well absorbed by the body. Cooking and salad oils, butter, margarine, shortening, and mayonnaise contain fat, and these items are used to add variety and flavor to the preparation of many foods.

Nuts and seeds contain oils and should be kept fresh and stored in the refrigerator because they can turn rancid. Often rancidity can be disguised with salting and roasting, oiling, and flavorings. Peanuts (actually a legume, a pea) often harbor a carcinogenic mold; Valencia peanuts are more resistant to the mold than other types. Fat is also present in animal flesh, where environmental poisons may be concentrated, making it wise to take even more care in the use of animal products. Meat contains approximately 14 times more pesticides than do plant foods and dairy products 5 times as much.

It is recommended that fats should be no more than a quarter of a person's total calorie intake. Outside of pregnancy and lactation, this is about two tablespoons of oil or butter, including that used for cooking and salad dressing, and a handful of nuts or seeds or a serving of nut butters. Two to three times these amounts are recommended for expectant mothers of multiples.

Housewives used to obtain fresh oil frequently, but today storage and handling requirements have changed this pattern. Raw, natural oils readily become rancid because they are unsaturated; that is, gaps exist in the molecular chain (which in saturated or hydrogenated fats would be filled with hydrogen molecules, making them solid, like butter and lard). Oxygen fills these gaps and the subsequent changes in the molecular structure cause the oil to smell and taste bad as well as impairing its biological usefulness. Free radicals form when the fatty acids become oxidized and smell rancid. These substances have been associated with cardiovascular disease, cancer, arthritis, and premature aging. Antioxidants are added to prevent these problems, and refining is done before commercial sale, so that the product is no longer natural.

"Polyunsaturated" tends to be equated by consumer with "healthy." Udo Erasmus, a Canadian researcher in dietary fats writes in *Fats and Oils* that in addition to the two essential fatty acids* and about eight other valuable polyunsaturates, there are "literally hundreds of polyunsaturates possible, many of them unnatural, some harmful, and many of them present in refined and hydrogenated oils."

Light, oxygen, and heat destroy the essential fatty acids in oils, yet oil, even if cold-pressed and unrefined, is generally sold in transparent bottles. Heating oils for cooking alters their chemical composition and turns the fatty acids into poisonous breakdown products that interfere with essential fatty acid functions in the body. Erasmus recommends flax (linseed, which he regrets is not available in North America in a fresh and pure form), pumpkin, soy, and walnut oils for nutrition because they contain both essential fatty acids, and coconut and palm kernel oils or butter for cooking. I prefer to use unsalted butter from an organic farm, sparingly — at least I know what I am getting, unlike with margarine, although neither contains the essential fatty acids. Butter adds flavor and is often less heavy than oil in cooking. Olive oil is low in essential fatty acids and thus there is minimal change during cooking. Make sure that the olive oil you use is extra-virgin, unrefined, and cold-pressed. Toasted sesame seed oil adds delicious flavor to noodles and Oriental stir-fried dishes. Sesame seed oil is partially unsaturated, and it is easy to press without using heat, so it does not have to be refined.

It is clear that the typical American diet, with about 40 percent fat, not only lacks adequate essential fatty acids but is loaded with undesirable forms of fat as well. The problem is cutting down the amount of unhealthy saturated and unsaturated fats as well as choosing sources of LNA and LA such as mackerel (see Odent's comment on fish oil and the prevention of preterm labor in Chapter 11). While fish and chips may taste great, fried foods may increase heartburn in pregnancy and should be avoided as much as possible. Eating leaner cuts of meat, avoiding the skin of chicken and fish, and limiting the intake of cheese, sour cream, and other rich dairy products will lower

---

* Essential fatty acids LNA (linolenic acid) and LA (linoleic acid) must be obtained from food sources. They govern every life process in the body, including oxygen transport and formation of prostaglandins to regulate tension in the arteries and thus blood pressure. Both are involved in the secretion of all glands and in the formation of the brain during fetal development.

the fat intake. Chewing pumpkin seeds, walnuts, soybeans — even grape seeds — is the easiest and freshest way to obtain the essential fatty acids.

High blood pressure, abnormal elevation of cholesterol, and obesity are not just diseases of middle age but can occur in young children. Greasy plates mean greasy arteries. Fatty streaks believed to be the precursors of atherosclerosis have been found in the aortas of young children, according to Dr. Christiane Northrup. The changes that you make in your diet during pregnancy will benefit your twins in the short and long term.

Minerals

In addition to protein, carbohydrates, and fats, the body requires vitamins and minerals. Minerals include, in decreasing order of amount required, potassium, chloride, sodium, calcium, phosphorus, iron, zinc, iodine, magnesium and traces of copper, manganese, fluoride, molybdenum, selenium, chromium, and cobalt. RDAs are given for calcium, phosphorus, iodine, iron, magnesium, and zinc, but for the rest only "safe and adequate daily intakes" are proposed as there is insufficient information on which to base allowances. I concentrate here on calcium, iron, and sodium because opinions regarding their roles in health and disease vary widely.

Calcium
Calcium is the most abundant mineral in the body and is the main component of bones and teeth. It helps the functioning of the heart, muscles, and nerves and plays a major role in blood clotting after bleeding. Inactivity tends to deplete the skeleton of calcium, which is why old or bedridden people incur fractures easily and why bed rest may be undesirable in multiple pregnancy. Pregnant and lactating women require 1,200 mg of calcium per day, an increase of 400 mg over normal daily needs for an adult female. For a woman pregnant with twins the requirement is increased to about 1,800 mg per day. Calcium intake must be adequate, particularly during the last two months of pregnancy, because more than half the calcium required will be deposited in the fetal bones at that time.

Milk, cheese, yogurt, and other dairy products immediately spring to mind when calcium is mentioned. But while the average American eats more than 350 pounds of dairy produce a year, milk is not part of the Eastern diet, except in India. Most Asians, blacks, certain ethnic groups such as Ashkenazi Jews and Mediterraneans, and about a quarter of whites suffer from lactose intolerance, which interferes with the digestion of milk. After the age of about four, people lose the ability to secrete the enzymes lactase and rennin. The milk combines poorly with other foods and forms curds in the stomach. Some authorities believe that if your ancestors are, say, Dutch, German, or British, then the familial line has become accustomed to dairy products and for you the food is satisfactory. Others, particularly macrobiotics, believe that milk is mucus-forming and clogs up the body, often causing pimples, acne, phlegm, and allergies (to name a few of more than forty symptoms). Many also feel that milk is a growth food only for the young and that an adult who still drinks milk is not fully weaned!

Some physicians question the safety of synthetic vitamin D, which is added to milk. Other additives include iodine (from disinfectants used in cleaning cows' udders, milking machines, and storage tanks) and dioxins if the milk comes in a chlorine-bleached carton. (The common use of corn as a filler in beverage cartons is leading to increased cases of allergies.) Christiane Northrup has observed that many cases of female diseases such as breast cysts, endometriosis, uterine fibroids, and vaginal discharges can be reversed or substantially improved by eliminating dairy products. Breast cancer incidence (and twinning) are highest in Holland and Denmark and very low in Japan. The National Women's Health Network in the United States has long been advocating research into the role of dietary fat in breast cancer. I wonder if dairy products are a major culprit: Holland and Denmark are major dairy-producing countries, and dairy products are not part of the Japanese diet. Vegetarian physicians bemoan the fact that parents of children with chronic ear infections would rather see their children go through multiple hospital admissions, with tubes placed in the ears, than eliminate their daily glasses of milk, which will often clear up the problem.

Every schoolchild knows that "milk is one of the four food groups and the major source of calcium." However, the amount of phosphorus in milk impairs the body's absorption of calcium. Colbin points out that animals much larger than humans maintain their bone structure not from drinking the milk of another species but from eating a vegetarian diet — leaves, grass, and vegetables. Furthermore, calcium drain may occur from dietary imbalance such as excessive protein and phosphorus in animal foods, which make the body acidic and cause calcium to be released from bones to alkalize the effect. This is the major cause of osteoporosis, a disease that is increasing

You can be absolutely certain of one thing: milk is the most political food in America. According to the Los Angeles Times, *the dairy industry is subsidized (meaning the taxpayers foot the bill) to the tune of almost three billion dollars a year! That's 342,000 dollars every hour to buy hundreds of millions of dollars' worth of dairy products that will in all likelihood never be eaten. The storage bill alone for the surplus that will never be used is forty-seven million dollars annually. The demand for dairy products has declined substantially, as it is becoming more apparent that they are not the perfect foods they were once touted to be.*

But production is continuous. Be assured that much of the publicity referring to the health benefits of dairy products is commercially motivated. . . . Although the real reason for the advertising campaign is to reduce the surplus, the ads attempt to convince you to buy milk for its many so-called health benefits.

HARVEY DIAMOND, *Fit for Life*

Calcium Content
in mg per 100 grams
(3½ oz. or ½ cup)

Dairy Foods

Goat's milk	120
Cow's milk	118
Cheese	50–850

Vegetables

Parsley	200
Turnip greens	130
Broccoli	130
Collards	188
Kale	187
Watercress	90–151

Legumes

Kidney beans	130
Soybeans	190
Tofu	590

Nuts and Seeds

Sesame seeds	630
Almonds	282
Brazil nuts	169
Hazelnuts	186

Fish

Canned salmon (with bones)	200–250
Canned sardines (with bones)	300–400

Sea Vegetables

Agar	400
Wakame	1,170
Kombu	800
Hijiki	1,400

Source: Michio Kushi and Aveline Kushi, *Macrobiotic Pregnancy and Care of the Newborn*.

with modern civilization. Ironically, older women, who have trouble digesting milk, are consuming large quantities for its calcium, but the protein in the milk leaches the calcium out of their bones. Because osteoporosis is a disease that begins slowly in the childbearing years, pregnancy is a good time to become aware of the paradox of milk as the ideal source of calcium. Dr. Campbell states that the Chinese study showed that no animal products are needed to prevent osteoporosis. Ironically, osteoporosis tends to occur in countries where calcium intake is highest, and most of it comes from dairy-rich products.

Unfortunately, we are so accustomed to the media barrage that promotes dairy products as healthful that it seems like heresy to point a finger at them. Pregnant women and nursing mothers in particular are usually exhorted to drink pints of milk a day for both the protein and calcium content. It has not always been understood that a lactating woman does not need to drink milk to make milk, although fluid intake is essential. Individuals who substitute increasing amounts of dairy products as they give up red meat must be particularly careful. Modest amounts of dairy products in cooking or as garnishes are less of a problem than when they are regarded as a dietary staple.

I am fond of cheese, although I never drank milk, but during my pregnancies I experienced uncomfortable levels of mucus production after I ate dairy products, at times affecting my breathing and hearing. My last child developed the same symptoms, plus gastric distress, when he nursed after I had consumed dairy products, especially ice cream. Many pregnant women (and nonpregnant as well) react in this way to dairy products. Goat's and soy milk may be more digestible than cow's milk for both mothers and infants, and feta cheese, which is made from sheep's or goat's milk, can be substituted for other cheeses.

Some substitutes for dairy products are amasake, a sweet liquid made from brown rice that can be eaten with cereals such as granola, and Rice Dream, an ice cream substitute also made from brown rice. Whole wheat pancakes and sauces can be made with soy milk, and soups can be "creamed" without milk or yogurt by blending in some tofu or rolled oats.

Pregnant women must decide for themselves whether they consume dairy products for their taste or for their protein or calcium content. Taste preferences are, of course, personal, and should be indulged only in moderation if you have any signs of intolerance, but for protein and calcium consumption, many other foods are better sources, as the adjacent chart demonstrates.

Sea vegetables contain the highest calcium levels of all foods and abundant minerals, trace elements, and vitamins. Hijiki, for example,

Mineral Content of Sea Vegetables, in mg per 100 grams

Sea Vegetable	Calcium	Iron	Iodine	Potassium
Agar-agar	567	6.3	0.2	0
Dulse	296	150.0	8.0	8,060
Hijiki	1,400	30.0	0	0
Irish moss	885	8.9	0	0
Kelp	1,093	100.00	150.0	5,273
Nori (green and red)	470	23.0	0	0

Source: Sara Shannon, *Diet for an Atomic Age.*

contains ten times more calcium than a comparable volume of cheese, milk, or other dairy food. It is also high in iron, protein, and vitamins A, B_1 and B_{12}. Seaweed comes from Maine and Japan and can be found, dried, in health food stores. Agar functions like gelatin and is easy to use in desserts. Wakame and dulse can be added to soups. Strips of kombu placed on the bottom of a pan of beans will prevent them from sticking as they cook and will add minerals and nutrients to the meal. Seaweed granules are available with other spices (garlic, ginger, or cayenne) to season food as a salt substitute. Vitamins D and B_{12} are also contained in sea vegetables, which is important for diets without milk or other animal protein. Sea vegetables, after soaking to soften and remove excess salt, can be sautéed with other vegetables (and some grated ginger and soy sauce), baked, stir-fried, steamed, and eaten with salads — they are a most versatile and delicious food.

Individuals with thyroid dysfunction should consult their physicians before adding sea vegetables to their diet because some sea vegetables have a high iodine content. (The mineral content of sea vegetables varies widely, as the table illustrates.) Lawrence Wood, M.D., author of *Your Thyroid*, considers the basic American diet already too high in iodine. Excess iodine results from milk consumption, use of iodates as dough oxidizers in making bread, and the (often excessive) use of iodized table salt rather than sea salt. In contrast, the U.S. Food and Drug Administration has found a tendency toward steadily declining iodine levels; it recommends that no additional sources of iodine be introduced into the "U.S. diet." The RDA for iodine is 150 micrograms (one gram of iodized salt contains half that amount), 175 micrograms during pregnancy, and an additional 50 micrograms during lactation for the nursing infant.

Urinary iodine excretion is a reliable indicator of a person's iodine status. Although one researcher in Japan has documented effects from excess iodine consumption in Japan, this is not the case with the small daily amounts added to the typical Japanese diet. I have asked several Japanese physicians about their traditional seaweed consumption during pregnancy and they reassured me that there have never been any known complications. Japanese women crave sea vegetables if they live abroad, especially during pregnancy.

I suggest omitting the foods with excess added iodine to enjoy the natural source in sea vegetables. For those who eat primarily natural, whole foods, sea vegetables are a safe and healthy addition to the diet and a better source of many essential micronutrients than land-grown foods. With knowledge and practice they become a delicious addition to your diet. Further information about sea vegetables can be found in Evelyn McConnaughey's *Sea Vegetables: Harvesting Guide and Cookbook* and in any macrobiotic cookbook.

One of the bonuses of our starting to eat sea vegetables is that our two older children, who never liked milk, just relish them.

Iron

Although the iron needs of the body are comparatively small, most people are aware that adequate amounts are vital and that anemia is relatively common in women and men, despite the amount of meat consumed by the average American. The most important function of iron is its involvement in the transport of oxygen to the tissues. Together with protein, iron forms hemoglobin in the red blood cells to bind with oxygen. Hemoglobin gives the blood in arteries a bright red color; the blood in the veins is darker because its oxygen has been given up. Protein, folic acid, vitamins B_{12} and C, plus trace elements such as copper and cobalt are also required for the production of red blood cells.

Menstruation is usually blamed for iron deficiencies in women, but more typically the cause is the modern diet. Iron deficiency may manifest itself in loss of appetite (which hinders the cure), fatigue, and hair loss, even in early pregnancy.

In multiple pregnancy, the maternal and fetal demands of iron and other substances necessary for red blood cell formation are elevated. Not only is additional iron needed for both the mother's and the babies' circulations, but a store of iron for the babies' postpartum life must be laid down as well. With two or more babies the requirements are increased proportionately. Furthermore, in the last weeks of pregnancy, each fetus doubles its own iron requirements; babies born prematurely are often anemic because their liver is immature and they have not stored sufficient iron.

What seems to be anemia in pregnancy may only be the result of the increased plasma volume in the circulation, which has the effect of diluting the quantity of red blood cells. A simple check is to stretch open your hands and look at the color of the lines — they should be deep pink to reddish, as should the mucous membranes of your lower eyelid. A physician should do further tests before prescribing iron supplements.

Getting enough iron is not simply a matter of dietary intake — the way it is absorbed by your body is important too. Foods containing vitamin C and protein aid absorption of iron when they are eaten at the same meal. Some iron is even added to your food if you cook with iron pots and pans. Liver and meat supply heme iron (both protein and iron) directly, which is more easily absorbed by the body and has long been advised as a remedy for anemia. However, liver and meat are high in toxic components such as hormones, pesticides, and antibiotics.

The U.S. Food and Drug Administration and the Food and Nutrition Boards of the National Research Council state that dietary intake of iron cannot meet the demands of pregnancy and recommend a supplement of 30–60 mg for a singleton pregnancy. The daily iron requirement of an adult woman is given as 15 mg, and estimates for a twin pregnancy begin at 50 mg. The average American diet, according to Ballentine, contains 14–20 mg a day, of which only 10 to 20 percent is actually absorbed, depending on the rest of the diet. Excess iron from supplements is excreted from the body and turns the stool black. Iron capsules may cause constipation and occasionally vomiting, so women often take less than the prescribed dose. Also, routine prescriptions of iron and other supplements may mask more complex and serious dietary deficiency, so the use of supplements needs to be monitored carefully. The average Chinese adult, who shows no evidence of anemia, consumes twice the iron that the average American does, but the vast majority of it comes from vegetables.

Vitamin B_{12} and folic acid (found in bright green foliage, among other foods; hence its name) are also important in the prevention of anemia. Both play a role in the development of new tissue, and in pregnancy the production of cells is greatly accelerated, particularly

Iron Content in Various Foods
in mg per 100 grams
(3½ oz. or ½ cup)

Whole Cereal Grains

Millet	6.8
Buckwheat	3.1
Soba (buckwheat noodle)	5
Oats	4.6
Brown rice	1.6

Beans

Azuki	4.8
Chickpea	6.9
Lentils	6.8
Soybeans	8.4

Vegetables (raw)

Dandelion greens	3.1
Kale	2.2
Swiss chard	3.2

Sea Vegetables

Arame	12
Dulse	6.3
Hijiki	29
Nori	12
Wakame	13

Seeds and Nuts

Pumpkin seeds	11.2
Sesame seeds	10.5
Sunflower seeds	7.1
Walnuts	3.1

Meat and Poultry

Beef	2.5–2.7
Chicken	1.6
Eggs	1.3

Dairy Foods

Cheddar cheese	1
Whole milk	Trace

Source: U.S. Department of Agriculture and Michio Kushi and Aveline Kushi, *Macrobiotic Pregnancy and Care of the Newborn.*

for twins. Brown skin pigmentation, especially on the faces of women who take oral contraceptives or who are pregnant, may be related to folic acid deficiency, according to Ballentine.

Vitamin B_{12} is needed only in minute amounts (4 micrograms in a singleton pregnancy), and it is supplied by oatmeal, whole grains, sea vegetables, eggs, and fish. Tempeh, made from fermented soybeans, provides 1.5–3.6 micrograms per 100 grams. If small amounts of animal food are included in the diet occasionally, vitamin B_{12} deficiency is almost nonexistent (a deficiency can result, however, after many years of strict vegan diets).

Sodium (Salt)

There is no RDA range for sodium, but recommended amounts range from 500 mg to 2,400 mg (about a teaspoonful), according to the Food and Nutrition Board.

In contrast, the typical American diet has 1 to 3 teaspoons a day, and those who eat many canned and processed foods and drink artificially softened water are taking in about 4 teaspoons daily. Salt appetite is determined by habits, especially those formed in early childhood, so the effects of excess salt may take years to show up. In *Diet and Nutrition*, Ballentine explains that *preventing* high blood pressure requires much less salt restriction than treating it. Thus, keeping salt intake at a reasonable level from infancy through adult life pays off more than trying to eliminate salt completely after one's blood pressure has started to climb.

Sodium is an essential nutrient that is required not only for the fetus but for the amniotic fluid as well. Sodium requirements increase with the demands made by maternal tissue, muscle function, digestive system, and blood circulation. Cravings for salty foods such as olives and pickles, the subject of many pregnancy jokes, are often a response to a biological need and point to a dietary imbalance.

During pregnancy, the blood volume increases, in the case of multiples on the order of 100 percent or more. Adequate fluid levels must be maintained so that sufficient blood volume can permeate each placenta. (A helpful guide is that the woman's urine should be pale yellow, excluding vitamin tints.) That means that expectant mothers of twins should consume more than ten glasses of fluid a day, including teas, soups, and other liquids. According to Dr. Tom and Gail Brewer, when the level of circulating blood does not meet the demands of pregnancy, particularly in multiple pregnancy, a serious state of inadequate blood volume (hypovolemia) results. In addition to interfering with the function of the placentas, low blood volume predisposes the mother to dehydration.

Cardiac patients and patients with kidney disease may need to restrict salt intake, as kidney and heart disease give rise to essential hypertension. Many such patients can maintain their health with less than ⅛ teaspoon of salt per day. But, as the Brewers emphasize, in pregnancy more salt helps build up the blood volume to transport nutrients. For this reason, salt should not be decreased in cases of toxemia (which are more common in multiple pregnancy).

Commercial salt has several additives, including iodine, whereas evaporated sea salt (usually from France) does not and contains other natural minerals as well. Use sea salt to taste and realize that there is plenty of sodium in milk, cheese, processed meats, canned vegetables, snack foods like potato chips and nuts (unless unsalted), and many baked goods if you eat such foods.

Vitamin and Mineral Supplements

Eastern cultures have always understood both the nutritive and the medicinal properties of food that Western societies are only just beginning to understand. People who swallow large doses of megavitamins and other supplements from health food stores are actually moving into the realm of pharmacology. They risk overdose, secondary depletion of other nutrients, and potential interaction with medications they might be taking.

Vitamins and mineral supplements are often prescribed to provide insurance for the mother and fetus. They are a cheap form of preventive medicine, especially for low-income mothers. But they cannot supply all the nutrients and enzymes that your body needs during pregnancy, and they often contain additives, preservatives, and artificial colors. Rarely is the diet lacking in just one particular nutrient. Good health demands a holistic approach and not token remedies.

Our approach to iron and other deficiencies is usually medical rather than nutritional, and the wider perspective of dieticians is underutilized. The routine prescription of iron and vitamins is much simpler and quicker for the busy doctor than arranging an in-depth session of nutritional history and counseling. Supplements are also convenient for the busy or lazy person who does not want to evaluate and improve his or her eating habits or does not trust food to provide enough nutrients. However, patients may consider the supplement a treatment, and many people erroneously believe that the more vitamins one takes, the better one's health will be. Some vitamins, such as A and D, if taken in excess can be stored in the body and actually

If we took all the vitamins recommended, a whole year's supply would not fill a thimble.
Dr. David Reuben, *Everything You Wanted to Know About Nutrition*

As well as improving my diet with more whole grains and green leafy vegetables, I started cooking with iron pans when I was pregnant. My hemoglobin increased so I didn't need any iron supplements.

reach toxic levels; they also can be teratogenic (likely to cause birth defects). Other vitamins, such as C, are water soluble, and any excesses are usually excreted, although aggravated cases of scurvy caused by sudden withdrawal of large doses of vitamin C have been documented. If you are going to take supplements, make sure they are free from additives, sugar, and artificial color, and take only what is prescribed by your doctor.

Some midwives and doctors ask expectant mothers to keep a record of their food intake for several days, with detailed descriptions of each food, including brand names. Similarly, it is an interesting exercise once in a pregnancy to analyze your diet using the *Nutritive Value of Foods* guide, which is also published in *The New Laurel's Kitchen* by Laurel Robertson. This cookbook provides RDAs for all of its recipes, many good transition dishes, and good advice on food and nutrition in general.

The Loss of Whole Foods

The typical American diet derives its balance from various components, such as meat, which is all protein and no carbohydrate, and refined starches, which are all carbohydrate and no protein. Many conventional eating habits thus seem to make sense as combinations of such components — the rich dessert after the steak dinner, for instance. However, certain natural foods are themselves whole, and a mixed diet based on such foodstuffs provides a great variety of nutrients without the disadvantages, such as high cholesterol and additives, of the conventional American diet.

Processing and refining of many food products enables them to remain longer on the store shelf without spoiling, but the processes also remove valuable nutrients. Refining separates the protein, fiber, minerals, and vitamins from the whole food. Grains are stripped of the bran and germ (which are sold to health food stores), and now even wheat flour must be enriched to compensate for the loss of nutrients during processing. Small amounts of processed and refined foods are not a problem if the diet is generally otherwise balanced. However, excessive intake of refined starches and sugars can be harmful. The average American receives 25 percent of his or her calories from refined sugar and 45 percent from fat. These refined substances become a double liability because the body must release stored nutrients to metabolize them.

It is unfortunate that whole foods that contain all their original nutrients normally are sold only at "health food" stores or the "nu-

We can achieve most, if not all, of our essential nutrient intake from a mixed diet of different sources. The vast majority of people who are eating highly fortified products don't need vitamin fortification in the first place, just like most people don't need vitamin supplements.
Irwin Rosenberg, former member of the National Academy of Science's Food and Nutrition Board, director of the USDA Human Nutrition Research Center on Aging at Tufts University

I ate a tremendous amount of good food during my pregnancy and I felt great. My appetite was just unbelievable, which is actually what led my doctor to suspect twins.

tritional foods'' aisle of the supermarket. These names alone suggest that anything else is less healthy and less nutritional. Similarly, nutritious whole foods are almost impossible to find at fast-food outlets and school cafeterias. For these reasons, cook carefully at home and enjoy only the best choices available at parties and restaurants.

Recommended Diet

A diet consisting of the following foods will be balanced and healthy at all times. Pregnant and lactating mothers of multiples should eat as much as they can, choosing whole grains and vegetables as staples, with legumes or animal protein at each meal. Fruit, nuts, and seeds can be eaten between meals as snacks.

Whole Grains. Whole grains include brown rice, corn, barley, millet, oats, buckwheat, bulgur, quinoa, and rye. These grains come in many forms such as corn grits, pasta, and flour and can be used in many foods such as bread, cereals, and couscous. These complex carbohydrates, together with starchy vegetables and potatoes, should provide half to two-thirds of the calories in the diet.

Vegetables. Choose a mixture of surface, leafy, and root vegetables each day. Surface vegetables include squash, pumpkin, cucumber, peas, beans, zucchini, cauliflower, and celery. Leafy vegetables are bok choy, collard greens, kale, Swiss chard, parsley, watercress, lettuce, endive, escarole, and broccoli. Root vegetables include carrots, onions, radishes, parsnips, turnips, daikon (long white radish), and potatoes.

Fruits. Fruits make ideal snacks between meals as they tend to cause fermentation in the stomach (particularly melons) when eaten with grains and starchy vegetables. Fruits can be eaten fresh, stewed, or dried. Prunes and dried apricots are a good source of iron. Too many dried fruits, however, will cause water from your body to be reabsorbed.

Legumes. Legumes include soybeans, chickpeas (garbanzos), lentils, azuki beans, tofu, tempeh, kidney beans, split peas, pinto beans, lima beans, navy beans, and black-eyed peas.

Animal Protein. Fresh fish from a fish market is best. It is worth a special trip as supermarket fish is usually older and often smells (fresh fish is odorless). Search for poultry, meat, and eggs that are naturally grown. Sardines are very high in clacium.

Fats, Oils, and Butter. Eat 4–5 tablespoons per day of the best quality.

Desserts. Eat fruits, cooked or fresh, depending on what is in sea-

Is it really worthwhile to alter lifelong eating habits and adopt the view that steak and other meats do not need to fill up a third of the plate for a meal to be nutritious and satisfying? That is, can the new approach really make a difference? The answer is an unequivocal "yes."
Tufts University Diet and Nutrition Letter

Toward the end of my pregnancy when my twins were huge, I used to blend the high-protein powder sold in health food stores into a shake with fruit and low-fat yogurt. It was quick to prepare and delicious.

As my pregnancy advanced, there seemed to be less and less room for my stomach. I found that six small meals a day rather than three large ones were a better idea.

I found carrying triplets that I would have double meals, like one dinner at six o'clock and another one at nine.

son. If you must use sweeteners, try rice syrup, barley malt, amazake, and pure maple syrup instead of white sugar. Try agar instead of gelatin and kudzu to thicken sweet sauces to obtain the mineral benefits of seaweed.

Seeds. Seeds include sesame seeds (which are high in calcium and can be roasted with sea salt to make a delicious condiment called Gomasio, to be sparingly used over grains), sunflower seeds (which in a spinach salad help counteract the oxalic acid, which makes the calcium less absorbable), and pumpkin seeds (which supply the essential fatty acids). Keep jars of these seeds handy to use as garnishes.

Nuts. Choose less fatty kinds such as almonds and walnuts.

Snacks. Try to snack on fruit, raw vegetables, rice cakes, whole grain crackers, unsalted popcorn, trail mix, and, occasionally, fermented cheese if it does not disagree with you.

Beverages. Choose from spring water, herbal tea, bancha or twig tea (noncaffeine teas, available from health food stores), fruit and vegetable juice, and natural nonalcoholic beer.

General Principles

Eat seasonal foods as much as possible. Select organic produce that is locally grown. For example, baked turnip and squash is a most delicious dish, satisfying and warming in winter. These vegetables cost less than fifty cents a pound. Contrast this with a winter salad of expensive imported lettuce and hothouse tomatoes.

Mix the colors in your food. Use yellow and green vegetables every day, especially cooked leafy green vegetables. Choose foods that will offer a variety of tastes — sweet, bitter, and so on. Every day eat some raw as well as cooked vegetables.

Cooking Hints

Shop for the best-quality food and cook it as skillfully as possible. Avoid aluminum pots because aluminum is a toxic metal that has been linked to Alzheimer's and Parkinson's diseases. Use cast iron, glass, or earthenware for cooking. Steam vegetables, and bake and broil rather than fry other foods.

Wash fruits, vegetables, and raw poultry very carefully to get rid of bacteria and harmful microorganisms. Some people recommend a few drops of chlorine bleach or organic detergents when washing foodstuffs (make sure to rinse them well).

Cook animal flesh thoroughly to destroy bacteria.

Save vegetable stock for soups because the cooking water contains many nutrients. Miso (fermented rice, barley, and so on), which is high in protein and even more delectable in pregnancy, can be kept for a long time in the refrigerator and used very simply for soup with added sea vegetables. Soups can be eaten every day — even twice or more a day. Soups are ideal for mothers of multiples with diminishing stomach space and high fluid requirements.

Soak grains and legumes in water overnight to improve cooking and digestibility. Beans in particular need to be well cooked (a pressure cooker helps) and well chewed. Adding herbs such as coriander and cumin improves digestibility and protein content. Growing sprouts on your windowsill guarantees some fresh green vegetables in the winter.

Tofu can be found in the produce section of most supermarkets in various consistencies. Made from soybean curd, this traditional Asian food can be made into dressings, omelets, or dips, and it can be served cubed in soups and vegetable dishes, stir-fries, and spaghetti sauce. Silken tofu can be blended into a shake or "smoothie" with fruit, wheat germ, and vegetable protein powder, making an ideal snack for expectant mothers of multiples with restricted stomachs. Tempeh is another soybean product that lends itself to cubes, slices, and "soyburgers."

Food combinations need consideration. Unfortunately the standard American breakfast — orange juice and cereal or toast — is a bad mix, the citrus causing the grain to ferment in the stomach. It's better to eat the citrus on arising and wait a half hour or so before consuming grains. Don't eat in haste or anger. Food is to be appreciated and enjoyed.

Meal Suggestions

The following meals are an example of what foodstuffs can be eaten when animal products are reduced. An expectant mother of multiples should eat as much as she can in each category. A wonderful book of natural food recipes, divided into the four seasons and with helpful instructions to minimize time and maximize efficiency, is *The Book of Whole Meals* by Annemarie Colbin. Additional cookbooks are given in

Suggested Reading, and mail-order whole food wholesalers are listed in Resources.

Breakfast

Fruit. Orange juice or grapefruit. Eat it a half hour before eating cereals or toast.

Cereal. I make my own completely organic granola: rolled oats, wheat germ, pumpkin seeds, sesame seeds, sunflower seeds, lecithin, raisins, sliced almonds, and crushed walnuts. Amasake, or low-fat yogurt for dairy eaters, plus more fruit, such as berries, stewed apples, stewed prunes, banana, peaches, apricots.

Toast/Muffins. Whole grain, very lightly toasted. Use naturally sweetened jam without added sugar or a small amount of butter or tahini (sesame seed butter, which is very high in calcium).

Beverage. Cereal grain coffee, bancha or herbal teas.

For variety and extra nutrients: Whole wheat pancakes with barley malt, maple syrup or berry toppings sweetened only with fruit juices. Eggs several times a week.

Morning Snack

Sourdough bread with tahini or nut butter.
Rice cakes or fruit.
Celery and carrot sticks.

Lunch

Soup. Vegetable or lentil soup or miso soup, with tofu cubes for added protein and seaweed for calcium.

Grains. Bread or pita pockets or barley.

Vegetables. Kale, butternut squash.

Salad in warm weather. Mix many different ingredients — two or three kinds of lettuce, sprouts, carrot, cucumber, beets, red and green pepper, mushroom, radish, tomato (vine-ripened and locally grown).

Humus (made from chickpeas and tahini) or whole wheat soy pizza.

Beverages. Nonalcoholic beer, juice, or mineral water in warmer weather. Spring water, herbal tea, or hot cider in colder months.

Afternoon Snack

> Whole wheat crackers, soy or cottage cheese, sardines.
> Dried fruit and nuts.
> Herbal tea or grain "coffee."

Dinner

> *Soup.* Potato or pumpkin in winter, tomato or asparagus in summer.
>
> Mackerel, corn, beans, carrots, swiss chard *or* lentil loaf, millet, broccoli, zucchini, parsnips with hijiki seaweed *or* udon (whole wheat) or soba (buckwheat noodles) and stir-fried tofu or tempeh with mixed vegetables: endive, onion, garlic, carrots, mushrooms, scallions, beans, broccoli, red pepper, snowpeas, bean sprouts.
>
> Azuki beans and brown rice *or* whole wheat or Jerusalem artichoke spaghetti with (preferably homemade) tomato sauce and tofu cubes *or* roast chicken with potatoes, squash, turnip, parsnip, and whole wheat stuffing, collard greens.
>
> *Dessert.* Apple crisp with whole grains *or* couscous cake with agar-jelled fruit *or* stewed apricots and Rice Dream (nondairy "ice cream") *or* fresh fruit.
>
> *Beverages.* Nonalcoholic beer, juice, or mineral water in warmer weather. Spring water, herbal tea, or hot cider in colder months.

Substances to Avoid

Substances that most commonly deplete the body of vitamins and minerals are alcohol, coffee, sugar, drugs (antibiotics, sleeping pills, street drugs), birth control pills, laxatives, and tobacco. Luckily, many pregnant women often develop a strong aversion to many of these harmful substances.

Cigarettes

The harmful effects of cigarette smoking on general health are well known, and the Surgeon General has warned against the impairment of protein and carbohydrate metabolism. Smokers are advised to take in extra vitamin B_6, B_{12}, and C and bone minerals. Nicotine has a harmful effect on fetal respiration and metabolism; smoking increases

I had smoked two packs a day for ten years, but the day I found out I was having twins, I stopped completely.

the chance of fetal death by 50 percent. Smoking also reduces the mother's appetite, which discourages the weight gain that is so important for a healthy pregnancy outcome, especially with multiples, and has been shown to reduce the length of pregnancy. While only a little more than a quarter of the U.S. population smokes today, women smokers are on the increase. Tobacco is also associated with osteoporosis. Avoid being a passive smoker and inhaling from others' cigarettes. If you have trouble quitting smoking, ask your doctor to refer you to a program to help you.

Caffeine and Additives in Beverages

Coffee, black teas, colas, sodas, and other beverages containing caffeine should be eliminated from a prenatal diet or reduced as much as possible. High intakes of caffeine (about eight cups a day) have been linked with complications in pregnancy.

From the minute I was pregnant, I suddenly could not stand even the smell of coffee. I guess your body tells you what you don't need.

Sodas also contain many additives, especially sugar (as much as ten teaspoons in a ten-ounce can of Pepsi). In hot weather, drinking such sweet soda leads to dehydration as the sugar pulls fluid out of the circulation. Soft drinks also weaken the bones because they contain phosphoric acid, which impairs the absorption of calcium. A 1989 study at the Harvard School of Public Health found that women who were athletes in college and who also drank sodas had twice the chance of their female teammates who did not drink sodas of breaking their first bone after age forty.

The long-term effects of sugar substitutes in pregnancy are not known. When in doubt, leave them out. Try mixing fruit juice in equal amounts with bottled water. If you do not have a good source of drinking water, bottled water with a slice of lime or lemon is quite delicious and doesn't leave the aftertaste of drinks with artificial sweeteners.

Alcohol

Consumption of alcohol by expectant mothers, according to the March of Dimes, is the third most common cause of mental retardation in newborns in some areas of the United States. It has not been established how little is safe, but the amounts are reduced as more studies are done. It is known that as little as 10 grams of alcohol (one drink) per day leads to a small but significant decrease in birth weight. Too much alcohol during pregnancy can cause serious, long-lasting effects on the child. Typical symptoms of the fetal alcohol syndrome include physical and mental defects, such as a small body and brain, poor coordination, and deficient attention span. The appearance of such a child may be characteristic — narrow eyes and a short nose with a low bridge. Heart defects and behavioral problems have also been observed. Nonalcoholic beer may be a substitute for some women.

Drugs

Any kind of drugs — street narcotics, over-the-counter medications, prescription drugs (check carefully for risk during pregnancy) — put your babies at risk. Before you take nasal sprays, cough medicine, antihistamines, sedatives, painkillers, sleeping pills, salves, ointments, and so on, ask to see the package insert, which usually contains information about the drug's actions, side effects, and contraindications. If you do not have access to the insert, consult the *Physicians' Desk Reference* at the pharmacy counter or your local library. *Peace of Mind During Pregnancy: An A–Z Guide to the Substance That Could Affect Your Unborn Baby* by Christine Kelley-Buchanan provides information on nearly two hundred substances.

If you have a special condition for which your doctor prescribes a drug, the dosage may be critical in pregnancy. Follow the instructions carefully. It may be possible to do without the medication or to try an alternative therapy such as homeopathy, meditation, or visualization. Just because a drug has been approved by the Food and Drug Administration and prescribed by your physician does not mean it is safe for your unborn babies. Mothers found out many years later that DES (a drug used in the 1950s to prevent miscarriage) caused vaginal abnormalities in their female offspring. Tetracycline (which causes staining of the offspring's permanent teeth) was another medication that was once thought harmless during pregnancy.

Radiation

Avoid unnecessary dental or other x-rays. Sit at least twenty feet from color television sets and don't linger in front of a microwave oven. Other household appliances that produce low levels of radiation include alarm systems, paging devices, remote-control garage door openers, and cellular phones. Do not sleep with electric blankets or water bed heaters — they have been associated with miscarriages. Decrease or eliminate the amount of time you sit in front of a computer with a cathode ray tube video display terminal. If you live near high-voltage power lines, a nuclear power plant, or nuclear waste disposal site, increase your intake of sea vegetables and miso. The calcium, iodine, and sodium alginate in sea vegetables help remove radioactive substances from the body. Shannon in *Diet for an Atomic Age* cites evidence that the Japanese who consumed miso and brown rice were protected from radiation sickness after the bombing of Hiroshima.

Further information on the increasing amounts of radiation in the world can be found in Paul Brodeur's landmark work *The Zapping of America* and orthopedic surgeon Robert Becker's *The Body Electric*.

Household Products and Environmental Toxins

Avoid contact with paint, solvents, glues, stains, pesticides, herbicides, and harsh cleaning compounds. Nontoxic detergents are available in health food stores. Avoid inhaling car exhaust, gasoline fumes, or chemical fumes.

The success of the fast-food industry has shown how difficult it is for busy working people to take the time to study nutrition, shop for the most healthful foods, and prepare them in the most nutritious way. Yet the growth of health foods stores and the proliferation of health food books and magazines shows that an increasing number of people are cultivating the art of cooking nutritious meals. It takes time and commitment to change one's diet, and each individual will go at her own pace. Since we are what we eat (and so will your babies be), it is certainly worth the effort. Eating should be an avenue for creativity, growth, change, and increased body awareness. Exercise, rest, and relaxation are also important for physiological and psychological well-being. Physical activity allows nutrients to be more efficiently digested and circulated, which alleviates many of the discomforts of pregnancy. The next chapter examines the significance of exercise and relaxation in a healthy pregnancy and as preparation for birth.

10 | How to Prepare Yourself for a Multiple Birth

EXERCISE AND NUTRITION are the most significant factors in preparing your body for the demands of a multiple pregnancy and birth and for ensuring the health of your babies. Rest and relaxation are also integral components of a healthy lifestyle. Both exercise and relaxation aid the distribution of nutrients within your body's systems and alleviate symptoms of physical discomfort as well as mental stress.

Exercises

Ideally, you have been exercising regularly long before your pregnancy. If not, you may be at a loss about what kinds of exercise you should do and when you should begin. It is never too late to start. Women want advice and guidance in early pregnancy, and classes for the first trimester are offered in some of the more progressive hospitals. It is during the early months that you need to learn correct posture to prevent backache and to discuss your emotional changes in a support group. It is important to share the pregnancy experience within a learning environment as well as to look ahead to what may happen at the birth. Some twins come early, so it is a good idea to get into the earliest classes you can. Special classes for expectant parents of multiples are ideal, if you can find them.

Private childbirth educators, clinics, as well as hospitals may offer an "early bird" series or ongoing classes for all stages of pregnancy. They may be exclusively lecture and discussion or may be balanced with exercises, relaxation, and comfort measures. Fitness classes for early pregnancy may be offered through the physical therapy department of your local hospital. The district or state chapter of the American Physical Therapy Association should also be able to recommend an obstetric physical therapist. Some YWCAs offer classes in movement and exercise for prenatal and postpartum women, as do some yoga studios. It may be difficult to evaluate the qualifications and ability of some of these instructors. However, a good guiding principle is that if you are taught to do something that hurts, your body is telling you that it is wrong. Your instructor should have specialized training in prenatal and postpartum exercise, and ideally everyone in the class should be pregnant. (Regular exercise classes will be too vigorous for most expectant mothers of twins.)

In addition to calisthenics and stretching, low-impact aerobic activity can be done recreationally. Such activity is important to improve two vital body systems, blood circulation and respiration. The earlier you start gentle aerobic exercise, the better you will feel, particularly as you may find even walking difficult toward the end. Dancing, swimming, walking, and cycling are examples of this kind of exercise and are easily done in early pregnancy. Health clubs, Y's, and some hotels or motels offer membership with access to a pool. Swimming is ideal for expectant mothers, especially with multiples, since the buoyancy of water lightens your body weight, which greatly facilitates movement, and there is no stress on joints or pelvic floor muscles. Some women continue to pursue fairly vigorous activity throughout the pregnancy, which is fine if they feel comfortable, but make sure you have plenty of rest too. Jogging with the extra weight of twins puts too much strain on the pelvic floor. There is no point pushing yourself to run a mile while you suffer "falling-out" feelings in your undercarriage. As we will see in Chapter 11, however, some women are going to have a hard time persuading their doctors even to let them get out of bed!

Carrying twins means carrying twice the load, so clearly you have to make a double effort to stay in shape. Extra-strong abdominal muscles are needed to protect your back as you move about through pregnancy. The pelvic floor muscles, which support the uterus from below, also have to be in optimum condition so that problems with urinary control do not develop. A complete description of the structure and function of these vulnerable muscle groups can be found in my book *Essential Exercises for the Childbearing Year*. You will not be doing the Jane Fonda Workout! Although the American College of Obstetricians considers multiple pregnancy to be a contraindication to exercise, the standard prenatal exercise program at my former

I swim sixty laps every day. Of course, I don't know if I'll keep it up to the very end — carrying quintuplets. But right now I feel great.

I knew I was having twins by the fourth month. That didn't stop me from doing anything. I felt great doing regular exercise and had an easy pregnancy. In the eighth month I learned that the twins were going to be triplets.

My doctor felt that it was my regular exercise sessions at the spa that helped me to carry my babies to term.

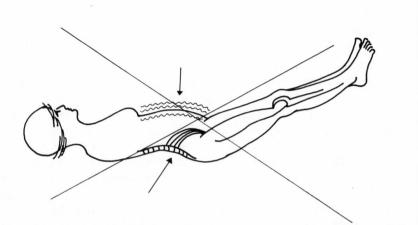

Never raise both legs because this can strain the back.

clinic, the Maternal and Child Health Center in Cambridge, Massachusetts, is safe and necessary for any woman expecting multiples. I do not advocate vigorous exercise in pregnancy for anyone. Instead I emphasize body awareness — with particular attention to the essential muscles affected by childbearing such as the pelvic floor and abdominals.

Moderation is the key to any program. You cannot force your body to move quicker than its own pace, so you have to become acquainted with what you can comfortably achieve and to distinguish this from difficult movements that require you to jerk, strain, or hold your breath. Harmful exercises and bouncing must be avoided. Double-leg raising and full sit-ups with outstretched legs are still being taught in many places to both males and females. These movements are not recommended at any time and are definitely contraindicated during the childbearing year, when muscles are stretched, ligaments are softened, and injury is thus more likely to occur. These strenuous trunk and leg motions put a dangerous strain on the lower back while they supposedly strengthen the abdominal muscles. Paradoxically, such exercises can be performed by substitute muscles so that you are not rewarded with improved abdominals for all your effort and agony.

All exercises and other forms of exertion should be performed on *outward* breath. Perform all movements slowly and rest between them with a couple of deep breaths. Deep breathing is particularly important for mothers of multiples. The pressure from the large uterus restricts the diaphragm above and impedes venous return from the legs and pelvis. Conscious deep breathing alleviates these problems.

A few exercises done properly and regularly serve you better than a mixed bag repeated quickly many times. Beware of programs that require that an exercise be done a fixed number of times (the "magic" number is usually fifteen or twenty, which leads rapidly to fatigue and boredom) without explaining the rationale and benefits of the repetition. Such regimens also fail to arrange the exercises in a logical sequence of difficulty. Exercises must always be progressive if there is to be constant challenge and improvement. That is, rather than simply increasing the number of repetitions of the original exercise, the starting position or movement maneuver should be modified. It is even more important to evaluate your "entry level" so that you begin with the appropriate movement for your individual condition. Usually exercise programs claim to be designed for the "average person" when, especially during pregnancy, everyone is different and needs to exercise at her own pace.

The Abdominal Wall

It is quite common for a pregnant woman to develop a "separation" of the abdominal muscles at the midline,* particularly if she is undergoing the extra stretching required for twins. Sometimes this gap is picked up at a second pregnancy, but it may have occurred in the first. Examination of the central seam of the abdominal wall should be done prior to starting any exercises involving trunk movements. It is also a good idea to check the gap frequently throughout the pregnancy as the muscles can part at any time.

To check the gap, lie down on your back with bent knees. Feel up and down the midline of the abdominal wall for a gap between the two vertical bands of muscles on the sides. Check as you exhale and put your chin on your chest (which contracts the recti muscles so you can tell if they are parallel or not). In pregnancy you may see a bulging that looks like a sausage. Postpartum, you should feel for a gap after the third day.

If you can fit three or more fingers, placing them horizontally between the muscles, don't bother to do the curl-ups described next. If your recti muscles cannot stay together when the weight of your head is raised, it makes no sense to overload them by bringing the shoulders off the floor as well. Instead, continue with head raises,

* The medical term for this condition is *diastasis recti*. The vertical fibrous band connecting the abdominals at the midline stretches.

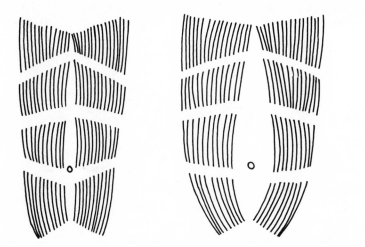

The abdominal muscles can separate in the same way that a zipper parts under stress.

chin to chest, while you cross your hands over the gap and give support to the muscles on each side. After the babies are born you will need to continue this exercise until you can raise your head, then later your shoulders, with the muscles parallel without your hands to help. Then the gap is closed. (If you require more details, consult my book *Essential Exercises for the Childbearing Year*, 3rd edition.)

The chart of essential exercises on page 160 summarizes the basic essential exercises to be done in the childbearing year. You can do additional ones, but if you perform these diligently, each one just a few times twice a day rather than during one long session, you will be well ahead. These are the same exercises you will need to begin within a day after the babies are delivered. The muscles you prepare are, logically, the ones you will also restore, so there is only one simple program to be learned. Mothers of twins often find it takes much longer than they expected to get their waistlines back to normal. Getting the muscles into good condition prior to the birth makes this job much easier.

You will notice from the illustrations that, apart from the all-over stretching exercise, the knees are always bent. This helps to tilt the pelvis so the lower back can stay protected on the floor. For the same reason, the trunk is curled only halfway, rather than in a full sit-up position. Because the waist never leaves the floor, the lower spinal area is never at risk. If you are not accustomed to doing abdominal

Essential Prenatal Exercise Chart

Do each exercise twice at first, progressing at your own pace to five times. The sequence can be repeated in reverse order. Relax and breathe deeply between each exercise.

1. Deep breathing with abdominal wall tightening on outward breath.

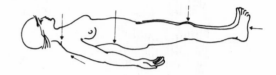

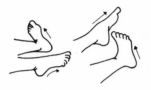

2. Foot exercises: stretch, bend, and rotate.

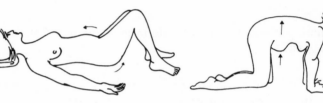

3. Stretch out the kinks: on the bed, against wall.

4. Pelvic floor exercises.

5. Pelvic tilting: various positions.

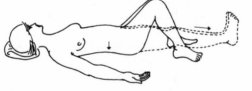

6. Leg sliding.

7. Straight curl-up.

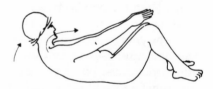

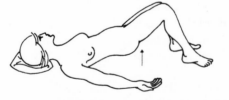

8. Bridging.

9. Diagonal curl-up.

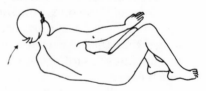

When standing up, roll over onto the knees and push arm with the arms. When rising from the floor, go on to one knee and straighten legs to stand.

10. Posture check.

Relaxation session: Twenty minutes in any position of comfort twice daily.

muscle exercises, your front neck muscles may protest a little at first. Remember to tuck your chin in first and then curl up.

Although the abdominal muscles are placed in front of the spine, they are nevertheless the muscles (rather than those in the back) that support the spinal column. The various muscles of the abdominal corset work together in curl-ups. Straight curl-ups involve a forward movement of the trunk, and diagonal curl-ups bring one shoulder toward the opposite hip.

If you are a beginner, try these curl-ups first with outstretched arms (but do not hang on to your knees at any point). Some women are able to come forward only a few inches, and it makes no sense to force or strain the movement any further. With time and practice, strength will improve. Sometimes the upper back is stiff and cannot readily curl forward. You can check this by sitting cross-legged and seeing if your forehead reaches to the floor in front of you. After the outward physical signs of the pregnancy have started to occur, which can happen as early as three to four months in a multiple pregnancy, just do what you can do. Muscles that have already started to stretch can be maintained in good condition, but further strengthening cannot be expected.

Pregnant women who are in good shape or in early pregnancy can perhaps achieve one of the progressions of the curl-up exercises. It is harder to raise your head and shoulders off the floor with your arms folded across your chest, and the 100 percent test is to clasp your hands behind your head. As your pregnancy progresses, the size of your abdomen will interfere, so you can return to an easier arm position or change to all fours. Raising the pelvis and lower back on hands and knees is another way to work the abdominals against the force of gravity, which may be more comfortable.

When you do curl-ups, your pelvis is held stable while your trunk moves. With pelvic tilting the reverse occurs, which focuses the effort on the lower abdominals. The trunk stays on the floor while the pelvis is tilted back to align with the spine, flattening the hollow in the lower back. Bending the knees makes this easier, so the first progression is to maintain the backward tilt of the pelvis while your heels slide slowly forward. Extend your legs only as far as you can without letting your pelvis tilt forward. When your abdominals are strong enough to keep the pelvis down while both legs are extended (heels in contact with the floor), you are ready for the final progression.

For the starting position, bring both knees over your waist so your back is rounded. Very slowly, allow your legs to move down and out — a coordination of both lowering and straightening. The

Posture Checklist

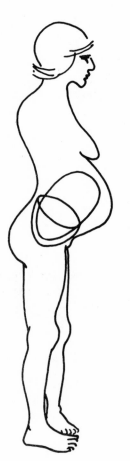

Incorrect Posture

To correct posture:

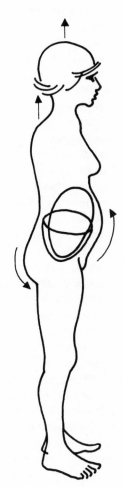

HEAD

If neck sags,
chin pokes forward, and
whole body slumps.

Straighten neck,
tuck chin in, so
body lines up.

SHOULDERS AND CHEST

Slouching cramps
the rib cage and
makes breathing
difficult.
Arms turn in.

Lift up through
rib cage and
pull back
shoulder girdle.
Roll arms out.

ABDOMEN AND BUTTOCKS

Slack muscles
= hollow-back.
Pelvis tilts
forward.

Contract abdominals
to flatten back.
Tuck buttocks under and
tilt pelvis back.

KNEES

Pressed back
strains joints,
pushes pelvis forward.

Bend to ease body
weight over feet

FEET

Weight on inner
borders strains
arches

Distribute body
weight through center
of each foot.

100 percent test is to keep the pelvic tilt under control, with both legs straight at an angle of 45 degrees. However, you must move only as far as you can in this direction *without your pelvis leaving the floor*. It is not necessary to go any lower than halfway or you become involved in the leverage problems that characterize the reverse of this exercise (double-leg raising, the hazards of which have been explained). The analogy of a seesaw may make this clearer. Obviously the small pelvis is going to be raised from the floor before the long heavy legs. Any movement with the most difficult phase at the onset does not deserve to be called an exercise. With double-leg lowering, you start from the easiest position. You have total control and progress only as far as you feel you can. In all these abdominal exercises, your awareness and commitment are to the lower back. Anyone can sit up or straighten her legs — the point here is to control the pelvic tilt at the same time.

Pelvic tilting can be done in a back-lying, all-fours, side-lying, kneeling, sitting, or standing position. It is important to learn how to do tilting in the last two positions because we mostly sit or stand. In squatting, the pelvis is tilted back as far as it can go, so further active movement is not possible. This, along with the enlargement of the pelvic outlet, is probably why squatting is a commonly chosen position for birth in many societies. Pelvic tilting movements in all positions help relieve stiffness and aching in the lower back.

The position of the pelvis and its two or more passengers is the keystone to good posture. As your pregnancy advances, your body weight moves forward, increasing the pull on the lower back. It becomes more difficult for the abdominal muscles to hold the bony basin in a good position. The buttocks contribute by pulling the pelvis down from behind. High-heeled shoes add to the problem, as they tip the body and pelvis even further forward. A checklist to help you attain a comfortable and attractive stature is included on page 162.

I found sandals to be the most comfortable footwear, and I could let out the straps as my feet got more swollen.

The Pelvic Floor

Another muscle group that is particularly vulnerable during the childbearing year is the pelvic floor. Like a hammock slung within the pelvis, pelvic floor muscles must support the weight of the uterus and other organs such as the bladder and bowel. Because we mostly sit and stand, it is rarely relieved from its load or the force of gravity. Sudden increases in intra-abdominal pressure such as a laugh, cough, or sneeze strain these muscles. If they are weak, these activities result

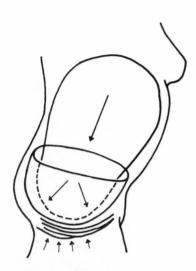

Multiple pregnancy puts a greater strain on the pelvic supports.

Some of my friends used to wet their pants when they coughed, so I just thought it was normal in pregnancy.

I gave up jogging at three months, as the pressure on the pelvic floor was too uncomfortable.

in leakage of urine — one of the classic signs of pelvic floor dysfunction. Other symptoms include "falling-out" feelings, lack of sexual satisfaction for one or both partners, and inability to void completely. Smokers and other people who cough frequently have increased likelihood of pelvic floor problems. Constipation and straining must be avoided at all times. Exercise and diets with plenty of fluids and high fiber, rather than processed foods, will help prevent constipation.

The pelvic floor muscles run from front to back and are also wrapped around the three openings. These circular muscle fibers are known as sphincters and form a figure eight. The front half of the figure is shared by both vagina and urethra (the passage from the bladder). This is why exercises that interrupt the flow of urine strengthen the birth canal. Urinary control is improved and the muscles are more supple and able to withstand the stretching during delivery by the fetal head. Hormonal changes during pregnancy soften and prepare the tissues for such distention, which is achieved by the first twin so the second usually follows easily through this area.

There are no short cuts to developing pelvic floor strength; you need to do at least fifty exercises a day. Contract the muscles only two or three times before resting as the muscles fatigue easily. Awareness of these muscles may be slow to develop because you cannot witness the muscle contractions (which occur at the middle of the vagina) and no bones move. Closing an eye is similar to contracting the sphincter muscles. Just as you can close your eye tightly or make a very hard fist, so you should try to do a strong, slow, uplifting pelvic floor contraction. It is the same action as interrupting the urine flow. Avoid contracting the pelvic floor in positions where your legs are crossed, as these lead to substitute activity in other muscle groups such as your thighs and buttocks. Sexual intercourse offers the best opportunities for practice. Your legs are apart and your partner can provide feedback about the quality of your vaginal sphincter. These muscles are important for the sexual response of both partners. There are two types of nerve supply to the vagina, and the upper areas are more effectively stimulated if the vaginal canal is snug. Take care that you perform a drawing-up movement, not bearing down. Do only the number of pelvic floor contractions that your partner can clearly feel and rest a minute or so before continuing. You should feel them yourself, with your finger, and also ask your midwife or doctor to evaluate the muscles.

Many expectant mothers are concerned that they have little interest in sexual gratification during pregnancy, especially toward the end when their body seems to have grown out of bounds. Other couples find that freedom from contraceptive measures and from fear of pregnancy affords them greater spontaneity, relaxation, and reassurance than before. Most doctors have little time or interest in discussing basic concerns like sexuality. Some still use blanket prohibitions such as "no sex for six weeks before and six weeks after." This philosophy is considered old-fashioned and is not based on any medical evidence. Any restriction that is placed on sexual activity for medical reasons should be thoroughly explained to both partners to avoid misunderstandings and resentment. Some physicians are very cautious in the case of twins because they fear that orgasm — from any means — may cause premature labor. Occasionally a woman will go into labor following orgasm, usually when the pregnancy is at term. Premature labor has never been proved to result from a couple's sexual activity; understanding this should spare couples from suffering feelings of guilt. It would be a great breakthrough if sex could be successfully used to induce labor instead of hospital admission, intravenous oxytocin, and fetal monitoring!

Many mothers of twins are too large and uncomfortable in the latter months of pregnancy to have any interest in sexual relations. You should not, therefore, feel that the following suggestions are yet another "how to" list of things that pregnant women are supposed to be wanting and achieving.

Although I spent the last few weeks in bed — too huge to move — sex was the last thing on my mind. Imagine trying to make love over a couple of active puppies.

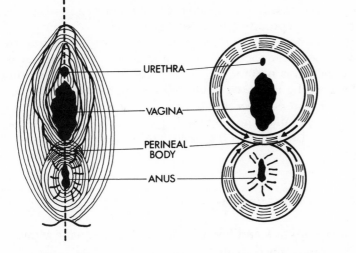

The muscles that circle the birth canal also function in bladder control.

Some Suggested Positions for Sexual Intercourse in Pregnancy
Lovemaking can be difficult with a huge abdomen, but try some of the following positions to find one that is comfortable for you.

Man Kneeling. The woman lies on her back on the edge of the bed. Her feet are supported on one or more chairs at a distance so that the man is able to kneel between her legs. Pillows may be needed to bring the woman's pelvis to a higher level.

Side-lying, Approach from the Rear. The woman lies on her side with knees partially drawn up. The man lies on the same side, just behind her, with his chest a reasonable distance away to bring the genital organs into alignment. This position permits fondling and extra stimulation of the woman.

Right Angles. The woman lies or sits on the bed with her knees drawn up. The man lies on his side at a right angle so her legs can rest across his body.

Squatting. The woman squats with her knees bent or sits with legs extended. The man kneels and rests on his heels. (Some women have difficulty balancing in the squatting position or find that their legs go to sleep.)

Both Kneeling. The woman rests in a forward position with her shoulders on pillows and her knees bent. The man kneels behind or sits with outstretched legs.

Frequently sexual interest increases in pregnancy, particularly in the middle months, which may bewilder some husbands who anticipate that pregnancy will be a low point in their marriage and sex life. Some men are very proud of the growing evidence of their contribution; others are concerned that the mother or babies will be hurt by sexual activity. Sensitive communication and good humor are real assets.

Infection is no more a risk in pregnancy than at any other time as long as the twins are protected by unbroken membranes. Intercourse should never occur after the bag of waters has ruptured. Another contraindication is vaginal spotting of blood. This may occur after a head engages in the pelvis and the cervix sinks low into the vagina.

Physical Considerations

The awkwardness and loss of balance that pregnant women experience is exaggerated in mothers expecting twins. Daily discomforts can be minimized by wearing supportive footwear, bending your knees every time you need to reach down to the floor, and taking care to roll over onto one side so you can use your arms to get up from the floor or out of bed. You should use care in getting out of the bathtub. Mothers expecting multiples find it easy to lose their balance, especially on slippery surfaces, in later pregnancy.

Back-lying, while harmless for a few minutes of moderate exercise, is not a recommended position for pregnancy or labor. The major blood vessels are compressed between the uterus and backbone, which can cause dizziness and nausea in some women. Working on the floor on hands and knees offers a welcome change of position. The uterus is off the backbone and out of the pelvis, which relieves backache. Take care not to let the small of your back sag down into a hollow. Sitting like a tailor with ankles crossed is another comfortable position during pregnancy unless your legs are too swollen to bend at the knees.

If varicose veins run in your family, you may want to take some preventive measures. With twins, the blood volume is greatly increased and hormones relax the walls of the blood vessels, so they are more likely to distend. Veins require the pumping action of the surrounding muscles to push on the circulating blood, so exercise, walking, and frequent ankle movements with the feet elevated will help. Avoid any constriction of the blood vessels, such as tight underwear, garters, knee-high socks or stockings, or sitting with knees crossed. If swelling of the legs is a cause of real discomfort, you can raise the foot of your bed on 10-inch blocks to encourage the return of fluid to the heart at night. You can also try support hose if preventive measures fail. The most effective type of hose is made by Jobst and can be custom-made if necessary. It is important to put on support hose before getting out of bed. Although exercise is important for the "venous pump," rest is also necessary in cases of swelling so the kidneys have a chance to excrete the excess fluid.

Abdominal corsets are occasionally required if the size of the multiple pregnancy is causing severe backache. It is preferable instead to develop good abdominal muscles and to have any orthopedic problem diagnosed. Disk lesions and sacroiliac joint dysfunction (the joints on either side of the rear of the pelvis) respond to mobilization, which an increasing number of physical therapists are being trained to provide. Adjusting joints is usually quick and effective. Beware of practitioners who roster you for an endless series.

The breasts contain no muscle tissue, so if they are allowed to hang by their own weight for prolonged periods of time, stretching of the tissues will result. A bra is recommended for comfort, and

Whenever my back began to ache I would go on all fours on the floor. It was paradise. I spent most of my labor in this position as well.

My therapist recommended a wide belt worn over the sacroiliac joints behind and under the abdomen in front. This gave me a lot of relief.

some women even wear one to bed at night. Nursing twins will increase the milk supply, so your breasts do need extra support. Wait until after the birth to buy nursing bras to ensure the best fit.

Stretch marks vary greatly with the individual and are not always seen in multiple pregnancy. Many mothers of twins, however, complain of intense itching of the abdominal wall. Oil massage has not been shown to prevent stretch marks (I believe that nutrition is the key), but it is a nice treat anyway. Coax your partner into giving you a regular all-over body massage with almond, coconut, or some other natural oil that is absorbed more effectively by the skin than mineral oil. Massage of the vaginal area with cocoa butter can enhance the circulation and increase the suppleness of the tissues to avoid tearing or the need for an incision (episiotomy) during the birth.

My tissues were so stretched that the area at the top of my uterus, just beneath my breastbone, was completely numb for the last weeks.

Relaxation

Massage is a wonderful aid to relaxation, but independent skills need to be developed as well. It is not always necessary to go and lie down on the floor or a bed and work through each part of the body. Simple rest, of course, is extremely necessary in multiple pregnancy, as the body is performing an amazing amount of work. At least twice a day try to find time to lie down or soak in a bath or at least put your feet up for no less than fifteen minutes. Perhaps you can hire a teenager or senior citizen to come in for a little while to mind the other children so you have a chance for some time to yourself. Many excellent audiotapes, vocal and nonvocal, for relaxation can be found in New Age bookstores.

Relaxation has both mental and physical rewards. Muscles that are released allow the blood to circulate more freely, and your body achieves a state of calm that quiets "the chattering monkey of the mind." Incorporate relaxation into daily living, which is easy once you become aware of your own particular patterns of tension. Most people become tense in similar ways. As soon as anxiety develops, the classic body language shows flexion postures. The neck almost disappears as the shoulders are tensed and elevated. The arms and legs are usually bent and crossed, fingers are clenched, and the foot, if not tapping or wrapped around the other leg, points upward.

My husband used to massage my feet every night and I never got leg cramps.

The solution is easy: extend the joints that are flexed. To allow the opposite group of muscles to contract, the tense ones always relax. (This is normal muscle physiology.) For example, making your fingers long relieves tightness in the hands. To relax the jaw, drag it downward actively. The jaw and hands are key areas, as these parts of the body are used so much.

At traffic lights or on the phone, take time to drag down your shoulders, another typically tense area, beginning in early pregnancy with the increased weight of the breasts and continuing through into postpartum with all the mothering activities that require forward bending and lifting. Don't just let go, as that does not demand enough release of the tight shoulder elevators, and shrugging them makes them higher. Pause when you are writing or typing to stretch out the fingers. This way you can monitor your relaxation through the day, trying to perform your tasks efficiently without excess energy diverted by tension. Checking for tense spots enables you to find short cuts while sitting and standing. Mothers who learn hour-to-hour relaxation skills find they cope much better with the postpartum period of disturbed sleep and incessant demands.

Stretch to Relax

The receptors in our joints relay messages directly to our conscious brain. Nerve endings in our muscles coordinate function and relay messages to the spinal cord and the primitive parts of the brain. We are not directly aware of the messages they relay. Close your eyes and focus on your thigh muscle. It is difficult to determine how relaxed or tense it really is. On the other hand, you know immediately if your knee is bent, straight, or halfway between. The joints, then, are more important than muscles in our awareness of relaxation. Movement is an effective way to involve the mind, and yoga, which incorporates many basic stretches, is probably the best example. Yoga also builds strength and balance; its challenges and rewards lie in the confrontation of your own mental and physical limitations. It is real body-mind work. As you stretch into a posture and reach the edge of your pain tolerance, you learn that it is only by continuing to breathe, only by moving slowly toward the pain, only by freeing the body from the resistance of the mind that progress is made. Forcing and determination lead backward, not forward. This letting go is a useful philosophical preparation for childbirth and contrasts with the methods that emphasize distraction and control. The partner exercises in my book *Essential Exercises for the Childbearing Year* (3rd edition) are a good way to involve your partner and to help you learn surrender (not control) for labor.

Relaxation can also be practiced passively, along the lines of transcendental meditation or its modification — the relaxation response, as described by Dr. Herbert Benson in his book on that subject. Here one attempts to do nothing with the body except to sit in a comfortable position. A state of relaxation is developed through mental concentration on a repeated sound or mantra. Other techniques of meditation focus on one's breathing rhythm. Although it sounds easy, it is actually an art to observe rather than to control your breathing. As you learn to let go, you will notice that the breathing becomes slower, more shallow, and you become aware of a pause between the outward and inward breaths. Finding these pauses or moments of non-activity in your breathing cycle leads to deep relaxation. By contrast, concentrating on slow deep breathing may feel like hard work. During labor you want to avoid any degree of unnecessary effort (and I strongly advise you to avoid artificial breathing patterns; see my book *Childbirth with Insight*).

Breathing is an essential component of relaxation and exercise. Exercises in which stretches are maintained (rather than bounced) and movements done slowly enhance your awareness of your breathing. Moving quickly encourages respiratory cheating by breath holding. Breathing is also facilitated by starting with an outward breath, so that the incoming amount of air is spontaneously regulated.

Preparation for Childbirth

Couples who are expecting twins will need to be very well prepared for the birth experience. Confidence and morale are also important as the hospital staff, as well as friends and neighbors, will certainly be warning you about complications. As I have pointed out in previous chapters, many low-birth-weight and prematurity problems with multiples have to do with misdiagnosis and inadequate nutrition. Childbirth education does not guarantee a painless labor, but studies have shown that prepared mothers need less medication and anesthesia than those who do not attend classes. Smaller babies are even more vulnerable to the effects of drugs, so it is important to do without drugs. (A model request letter for natural childbirth, written by an expectant mother of twins and her husband, can be found in Appendix 2.)

The hospital you have chosen may send you details about classes, or your doctor may refer you to classes elsewhere. Look for classes in the community taught by independent educators. Unfortunately, some hospital classes often give no more than instruction in policies and procedures so that you will be a cooperative patient and help things run smoothly for the staff. Occasionally childbirth educators from the community teach in the hospital. These individuals tend to be more consumer-oriented than are the staff from the maternity floor. A nurse from labor and delivery, while she or he may have seen many births, is not always skilled in handling group discussion and helping couples feel comfortable with exercises, massage, and other body work. She or he may be unaware of options and alternatives or believe that there can be no deviation from hospital policy. Those who create the environment in labor and delivery are often the last ones who see the need for any changes.

While most childbirth educators deplore the situation in modern obstetrics, the classes they teach have nevertheless become more and more focused on explanations of clinical procedures. Such information, of course, is necessary and is accorded more emphasis as the prevalence of these procedures increases. As a result, the psychological and experiential aspects of birth tend to be overlooked, as everyone is prepared for what *could* happen. To inform couples of their rights and choices, which in theory they have but in practice often do not, may be considered cruel and misleading. Little will be achieved, however, until the childbearing couples themselves demand the birth environment they desire. Husbands, cameras, and siblings were allowed reluctantly during birth, not because health care providers recommended it to their colleagues but because of consumer pressure. Parents got angry, wrote letters, and changed the practices of physicians and hospitals. Midwives, who have long been a respected tradition in other societies, are reentering maternity services in the United States but deliver fewer than 5 percent of the babies born each year. The role of midwifery is to handle normal births with physician back-up in the case of complications. Abroad, twins would be handled by a midwife in most places, with an obstetrician standing by in case an instrumental or Caesarean delivery is required. Birth attendants in any setting need to feel comfortable delivering twins vaginally in case they are undiagnosed.

Childbirth classes generally encourage a couple to work together as partners. If the father of the baby is unable to attend, you will be encouraged to bring along a sister, roommate, parent, or friend. Whomever you wish to attend the birth should also attend the classes with you. It is important to check with both the doctor and the hospital so that any extra person besides your partner will be allowed to be present at the birth. Many couples have been disappointed by the "only one coach" rule. Find out in good time so you can pressure the

I never got to more than two classes. By the time the hospital would take me in a series, the doctor had changed my due date.

hospital to change its policy or find a room elsewhere. Many hospitals now allow children as well as extra adults to be present at the birth.

Important factors in choosing a class include the experience of the teacher, the size of the group, and the amount of discussion that is encouraged. Often much of the series is taken up with films, hospital tours, and lectures, leaving little time for group sharing and physical activities such as exercise and relaxation. Do not expect the instructor to have special knowledge about multiple birth.

It is a good idea for any couple expecting multiples to attend some classes geared to those planning a Caesarean delivery. The national average for Caesarean is about one birth in four, and if you should have a Caesarean, you'll be glad that you were fully prepared. Considering the reluctance of physicians to attempt what might turn out to be a difficult vaginal delivery, couples must face the unpleasant probability of Caesarean delivery. Caesareans are major surgery and make the postpartum recovery much harder, especially for mothers having to care for two or more babies. Shop around for an obstetrician who is comfortable delivering multiples naturally and read Nancy Cohen's *Silent Knife: Cesarean Prevention and Vaginal Birth After Cesarean*.

The best education starts in early pregnancy and continues after the birth. It is easy for the expectant couple to become confused by the plethora of methods and books advertising various techniques and approaches. Many couples, on the other hand, are not even aware that there are choices in the way to prepare for and give birth. The average adult knows so little about pregnancy and labor that even the most basic course is usually interesting and informative. How, then, is one to evaluate the choices available?

The Lamaze method, which is the most popular and widely available, is geared to control. Specific breathing patterns are taught to help the mother "ride each contraction." Focusing, with eyes open, is an important component of distracting the mind from pain. The Bradley school of thought closely follows the philosophy of the "father of natural childbirth," Grantly Dick-Read. Relaxation, the support of the partner throughout labor, and normal breathing are emphasized. Drugs and medication are explained and discouraged, in contrast with many Lamaze teachers who adapt their teaching to accommodate the medication/anesthesiology practices in local hospitals. Ideally the instructor's commitment is to normal physiology and self-discovery rather than to complex techniques. As Doris Haire, president of the American Foundation of Maternal and Child Health, says, "There's too much hokey-pokey going on in childbirth education today." The simple, universal truths of birth are rarely acknowledged, and almost all birth films present only the roles of the obstetric team. The various methods of preparation are becoming as complicated as the technology that is burgeoning in the maternity units. As a result, most couples want "recipes," charts, checklists, and guidelines to reassure them that they are following the "right" path, as they do not feel free to seek their own style of birth.

The great majority of births have a successful outcome — healthy offspring. Couples are generally pleased with their preparation and, of course, every school of thought claims that its method works. Obviously, students are often self-fulfilling prophecies for their instructors. In our society, not only in childbirth, we have sunk to the point where we trust strangers in a medical institution more than we trust our own bodies. It is to them that we listen rather than to what is happening inside ourselves. The willingness with which the woman in labor, in her vulnerability, turns herself over to those who surround her has encouraged these outsiders to manage the labor and birth. Childbirth is not often painless, but even rarer is a woman who gives birth without fear.

The alternative birth movement has done much to free women of these interventions, however well intentioned, so that they can extend both their minds and their bodies to experience the essence of their own birth. Then they can be conscious of what is happening rather than what they "should" be doing. Birth is a spontaneous event for which it is difficult to rehearse; it is not possible to practice the reflexes that will occur physiologically.

A diligent commitment through pregnancy to nutrition, exercise, rest, relaxation, and education is more significant than the series of classes at the end. One rarely changes lifestyle and convictions in a few sessions. If you have done your best for yourself and your babies for the past nine months, you cannot but approach their birth with courage and confidence to let your body do its best for you.

Treatments to Prolong Pregnancy and Prevent Prematurity

PREMATURITY IS THE SINGLE most important problem with multiple births, occurring ten times more often than with singletons. About half of all twins and three-quarters of triplets are born before the thirty-seventh week. While ever-younger babies are surviving at an increasing financial, emotional, and physical price, there has been little progress in preventing preterm labor or in understanding its causes.

The typical explanations of premature labor — "overstretching" and "overcrowding" — are not borne out by the number of healthy, well-nourished mothers who carry not only twins but triplets to term with good birth weight. As I was writing this chapter, the evening news announced a "breakthrough" in prematurity research. It turned out to be a theory of "silent infection," or infections with no noticeable symptoms (which had been known for years). In one study of mothers with urinary tract infections, some mothers had no symptoms, but when treated with antibiotics their premature labor rate was lowered significantly compared with that of a control group with infections that were not treated. However, I feel that prematurity has multiple causes, and looking for a lone bacterial invader is a simplistic approach. More holistic is the concept of strengthening the "terrain" of the mother physically and mentally. Through my research I continue to find that well-nourished mothers stand the best chance for carrying their babies to term, unless they are suffering from some of the risk factors in the following list.

Throughout the book I have stressed ways to prevent complications, but in this chapter I will give guidelines for recognizing when something is wrong and provide current medical and alternative approaches to treatment.

Excessive uterine activity, cervical effacement (thinning out of the cervix), or dilation (opening of the cervix) prior to thirty-six weeks, especially with a multiple pregnancy, increases the likelihood of preterm birth. The only way to detect any changes in the cervix is by vaginal examination.

Risk Factors for Preterm Labor

Poor nutrition or inadequate hydration

Substance abuse — tobacco, alcohol, street drugs

Emotional stress (no partner, unplanned pregnancy, separation or divorce, recent move, geographic and cultural isolation, chronic illness in family, recent death)

Financial stress, unemployment, inadequate housing

Fear of increased body size by term

Fear of birthing two or more babies

Previous premature labor or delivery

History of premature labor in the maternal line (for example, mother was premature herself, prematurity may be a pattern for several generations)

Chronic cough (risk of premature rupture of membranes)

Obesity or underweight

Placental problems — placental abruption, placenta previa

PIH (pregnancy-induced hypertension/toxemia)

Infection in the genital tract (mycoplasma, ureaplasma, chlamydia); severe kidney and urinary tract infections

Congenital anomalies (gastroschisis), congenital heart disease or defect

Fibroids (benign uterine tumors)

Chromosomal anomalies (for example, Down's syndrome)

Uterine anomalies, cervical incompetence

DES exposure

Diabetes mellitus

Oligohydramnios or polyhydramnios (insufficient or excessive amniotic fluid)

Exposure to ionizing radiation (x-rays), anesthetic gases, lead

Motor vehicle accident or other injury

Physical trauma, abuse

Hard physical labor, tiring travel

Long or rigorous sonograms for higher-order multiples

Two or more second-trimester abortions

Signs of Preterm Labor That You May Not Recognize

---

1. Contractions occurring at regular intervals of 15 minutes or less, about 4 or more per hour. The uterus tightens, becomes hard and peaks — takes a globular shape. Such contractions may bring no discomfort.

2. Menstrual-like cramps, rhythmic or constant, experienced in your lower abdomen.

3. Rhythmic or persistent pressure that may radiate to your thighs.

4. An intuitive feeling that something is wrong.

5. Gas pains, intestinal discomfort, diarrhea.

6. Vaginal discharge — water, mucus, blood.

7. Lower backache, whether it comes and goes or is continuous. It may radiate to your sides or front.

An expectant mother of multiples must be keenly aware of her body and babies in order to detect any threatening changes. The factors listed in the chart may signal that labor is beginning or may just be typical discomforts that women experience in pregnancy. You must know your body and trust your intuition. The number of contractions is rather arbitrary; many mothers of multiples may normally experience up to ten contractions an hour, but not every hour, especially while the cervix is still closed and uneffaced. Twins often settle low down in the pelvis earlier than singletons, and the increased pressure may cause contractions without dilation. Unfortunately, many mothers of twins and almost all mothers of supertwins cannot detect contractions at all. The uterus is stretched so taut that any additional hardening from a contraction may not be felt. Also, they may not be able to distinguish labor contractions from the normal contractions of pregnancy (called Braxton-Hicks contractions) or they may confuse contractions with extra fetal movement. The significant difference between the two types of contractions is that true labor will cause the cervix to thin out and dilate. It is much better to check with your doctor when in doubt (and don't be put off with "You're just carrying twins — of course it's a bit uncomfortable") rather than waiting until it is too late and labor is established.

According to a symposium reported in the November 1988 issue of *Contemporary OB-GYN*, uterine activity increases for several weeks before labor, whether that labor occurs at thirty-four weeks, forty-two weeks, or sometime in between. Baseline activity is higher for women who deliver prematurely, but the difference is not always marked enough to determine which women are at risk.

If you can detect preterm labor in its early phases, before the cervix has undergone significant changes and before the membranes have ruptured, it can sometimes be stopped with rest and increased fluid intake. Just as a marathon runner drinks frequently to prevent muscle cramps, so hydration must be adequate in pregnancy to prevent falling blood volume and the onset of premature contractions. Often, just drinking several glasses of water will take care of the contractions or, in the hospital, you may be put on an intravenous simply for hydration. If there is increased activity of the uterus plus changes in the cervix, tocolytic drugs are usually prescribed to relax the uterus, despite controversy.

Home Monitoring of Contractions

Mothers can observe and record their uterine activity at home with either palpation (feeling with their hands) or a monitor. It is important for each woman to be aware of her normal uterine activity so that she can recognize changes that may signal the onset of labor. If you feel different sensations at any time, lie down on your side and time the contractions. If you have more than four contractions an hour, call your doctor.

Palpation

Lie on your left side, relax your abdominal wall, and use your hands to feel the uterus tighten, become hard, and then relax. Contractions can last from half a minute up to two minutes. Time the intervals from the beginning of one contraction to the beginning of the next.

Monitor

A home monitor (see Resources) can be strapped to the abdomen to record contractions. Recording is usually done every other day for one hour, although some physicians have suggested that it is more meaningful to record contractions for an entire 24-hour period. Janet

My only sign of labor was gas pains. I had been very good with my diet all through pregnancy but I went to a picnic and had a can of soda pop. I thought that was causing the gas. Several hours later my baby was delivered, ten weeks premature.

I had to insist that I be monitored. I told the doctor I wouldn't go home until I was convinced that everything was okay.

I felt a bit funny when my labor began, but I thought it was just from the Chinese meal I had eaten.

Bleyl of the Triplet Connection recommends that mothers expecting higher-order multiples use the home monitor twice a day or until they become aware of contractions without it.

After monitoring the contractions, the woman places the monitor against a telephone receiver and the record is transmitted to a medical center. Several hours of data can be transmitted in a few minutes. The nurse or physician at the medical center interprets the data and decides whether the mother should come in for further checking.

Dr. Michael Katz of the department of obstetrics and gynecology of the University of California at San Francisco has lowered the general preterm rate at his facility by 50 percent with the home monitor.

One study found no difference in preterm labor between those who had their records interpreted by a medical staff and those who used the monitor and were also contacted daily by the hospital staff but did not have their records interpreted. However, the control group, who were not monitored at all, had significantly higher rates of preterm labor. Therefore, it seems that the reduction of preterm labor in the other two groups was associated with the personal support and communication mothers received from the medical staff. The daily communication initiated by the medical center (that is, a doctor or nurse calls the mother rather than the other way around) is very beneficial.

Home monitoring can also educate expectant mothers to detect contractions and thus balance their daily periods of rest and activity.

Fetal Movement

Expectant mothers must become aware of the normal activity patterns of their multiples. As we have seen, medical tests cannot be relied on in every case, and sometimes they may not even be considered. Your ability to pick up decreased movement of one or more babies might be life-saving.

In early and mid-pregnancy, fetal activity is often much more pronounced in a multiple pregnancy than in a singleton pregnancy, but movement gradually declines toward term because of the decreased space available in the uterus for more than one baby. Samueloff found that in multiple pregnancy, mothers experienced an average of 774 movements per day at the peak period of gestation, about twenty-seven weeks. These fetal movements were calculated for a twenty-four-hour period based on the number of movements that mothers counted three times a day for thirty minutes. By the time of delivery, the average number of fetal movements had declined to 224.

If you learn the characteristics of each baby, you will be aware of any sudden decrease in activity. Chapter 6 describes ways to communicate with the babies in the uterus; the more you do this, the more skilled you will become in recognizing each one's individual pattern of movement.

If you are given betamethasone to promote the babies' lung maturity, you will notice a marked decrease in fetal activity, but this lasts only a day or so during the administration of the drug.

Routine Bed Rest to Prevent Premature Labor

The controversy over bed rest continues today. Some studies have found that "rested" babies weighed a little more at birth, presumably because calories were used for fetal growth rather than for maternal activity. However, bed rest does not significantly affect the onset of premature labor. A 1985 study found that bed rest in the hospital, but not at home, increased gestational age and birth weight of twins. In contrast, a 1982 study at the Sloane Hospital for Women in Chicago analyzed thirty-five pregnancies involving triplets, quadruplets, and quintuplets. The study found that bed rest did not increase the gestational age at the time of delivery but it did improve the fetal outcome; 42 percent of the babies were delivered by Caesarean section. (Keep in mind that direct comparison of twins with higher-order multiples is not appropriate.) Yet another British study found that preterm delivery was more common among women admitted (after thirty-two weeks) for bed rest than among controls. That study concluded that "there is at present no scientifically acceptable evidence that this common, disruptive and expensive obstetric policy does more good than harm." Campbell and MacGillivray concluded in their 1988 text *Twins and Twinning* that routine rest in the hospital is unlikely to affect preterm labor, pre-eclampsia, perinatal mortality, or birth weight.

In my opinion, it is better to boost the mother's nutrition so that she has the caloric requirements for both fetal weight gain and her normal activities. Studies not supporting bed rest do, of course, emphasize the need for early detection and specialized follow-up.

One unresolved question is when "preventive" bed rest should be implemented. The most common recommendation is to begin bed rest after the thirtieth week, but at least half of the perinatal mortality in multiples occurs before that time. A 1986 Australian study by O'Shea recommended that bed rest should begin between twenty-one and twenty-eight weeks of gestation because "there is no rational theoretical basis for hospitalization beyond this time." This finding concurred with that of Chervenak's 1984 study in which 81 percent of the perinatal mortality among 385 women occurred prior to twenty-eight weeks. Newton in 1986 stated that bed rest has theoretical advantages and is supported by retrospective studies (such as O'Shea) but not by prospective trials.

I advocate *plenty of rest* for all pregnant women, especially mothers awaiting multiples. Ideally, they should rest in a semirecumbent position or lie down on one side, preferably the left side, to nap two or three times a day. Body size and the number of multiples will determine the necessary reduction in activity.

Definitions of "bed rest" vary greatly, from sitting up in bed for a few days to lying down continuously for weeks without "bathroom privileges." Increased rest for an acute crisis, such as elevated blood pressure or spotting, makes sense. However, prolonged bed rest can have many negative repercussions, such as loss of income, dependence on others, anxiety, guilt, anger, isolation, depression, sexual abstinence, or being labeled "sick." Common discomforts of pregnancy such as heartburn, constipation, swelling of the legs, loss of appetite, thrombosis, backache, and generalized weakness, as well as bone demineralization, can also be increased by inactivity. Studies have shown that these side effects tend to counteract any potential benefits.

In general, bed rest is a conservative approach taken when there is nothing more constructive to recommend. Swedish researchers found that neither hospitalization for bed rest nor a leave of absence from work improved outcome in twin pregnancies. Many orthopedic surgeons recommend bed rest, some of it prolonged, for patients with back pain, especially for pregnant women (such patients should seek physical therapy).

Despite three decades of controversy, some doctors insist on routine bed rest and may put expectant mothers in the hospital if they are having contractions. I suggest that you seek a second opinion if this is recommended to you.

If you feel you have no alternative but to accept medically ordered bed rest, I advocate an individualized exercise program, as im-

Bed rest for six months is hard on the body; I feel I've atrophied. Even eighteen months after the birth, I still haven't recovered my strength.

mobility is not natural for the body. My original training was in physical therapy, and I have treated many expectant mothers admitted to the hospital for prenatal complications. Since I founded the Obstetrics and Gynecology Section of the American Physical Therapy Association in 1977, we have gained more than one thousand members across the country. Large medical centers have physical therapy departments, but smaller maternity units do not, so you may need to arrange an outside consultation. If an individualized exercise program is not possible, you can do the exercises described here.

Exercises for Expectant Mothers on Bed Rest

The only exercises on the "Essential Prenatal Exercise Chart" in Chapter 10 that may increase pressure on your uterus and cervix are numbers 7 and 8 — the curl-ups. When you do these exercises, listen to your body. If contractions increase, ease off. Modify these exercises and instead do frequent head raises on *outward* breath, supporting your abdominal muscles if necessary with your hands as described on page 158. Pelvic tilting on hands and knees (illustrated in the chart) is another alternative that will also give you a welcome change of position.

The typical pregnant woman will be using her arms and legs in normal activities. However, for women on bed rest, the limbs will get progressively weaker from lack of use. Calcium loss from bones is another hazard from prolonged lack of weight bearing. Take the longest route to the bathroom and consider lifting weights for your extremities.

Ideally, exercises against the graded manual resistance of a physical therapist are best. Otherwise you can make weights out of strong, doubled plastic bags of sand or rice. For your legs, fill two bags, tie the ends together and put them on your ankle so that the bags hang down on each side. Wearing a weight like this, you can sit over the side of the bed and straighten one knee or lie down in bed and raise one leg while holding it straight.

Start off with just enough weight to feel mild effort after a couple of repetitions. You should not be tempted to hold your breath. Since rice or sand weights are very easy to adjust, you can always add more as you progress.

You must exhale with each movement. Exhaling will prevent increases in pressure on your abdomen and fluctuations in circulation that occur with straining. I cannot emphasize enough the importance

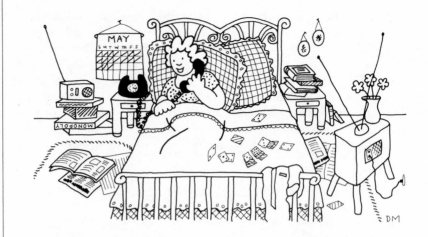

"No, I don't even *have* carpets but you could come for tea." *Illustration by Dora McClurkin, from "Bedrest in Pregnancy" by Susan Greene Hoffman, published by pennypress, Inc.*

of proper breathing. Without it, you may do more harm than good.

Also do frequent free movements with your limbs. Slide your heel up and down the bed to bend and straighten your knee and hip. Stretch your arms over your head. Circle your shoulders, twist your trunk with your arms outstretched, try to clasp your hands behind your back. These exercises will improve your back, open your chest, and boost your appetite. Don't forget to do frequent pelvic floor contractions too.

Suggest to your doctor that you take frequent tub baths or, better still, swim gently in a pool to maintain mobility. A 1990 article by Katz et al. in *Obstetrics and Gynecology* found immersion more effective than bed rest in treating edema of pregnancy.

Making the Best of Bed Rest

If bed rest is unavoidable, you can take a few steps to lighten the sentence. Contacting other mothers of multiples who underwent bed rest for a good outcome will boost your confidence. Home visits by such bed rest graduates, as well as by childbirth educators and ob-gyn physical therapists, are valuable. Try to arrange for a regular massage for circulation and relaxation. A foam wedge to support your belly when you rest on your side is very comfortable (see Spurlin in Resources).

As well as catching up on reading, sewing, knitting, or other hobbies, take this time to educate yourself about twins. In the Resources, I list organizations that specialize in educational materials for pregnancy, birth, and postpartum. Join some of these groups and send for their literature and newsletters.

Some women are extra diligent with bed rest and don't even think to ask their doctor about going out for a quiet dinner with their partner, which in most cases would be a welcome boost to their morale.

Bed rest provides plenty of time for sharing with older siblings and communicating with your unborn babies through touch, visualization, and meditation. In this stressful situation you want to communicate your feelings to them, even of frustration, impatience, anger, or fear. Talk to your babies and explain what is happening.

Daily singing is recommended because it is a joyful activity that will enhance your breathing. It also exposes your babies to a wide range of pitch, which is good for their later learning skills. This will help to compensate for the lack of prenatal movement that your babies will experience.

Castor Oil Packs
Castor oil packs can be used successfully for a number of conditions, such as uterine bleeding, sore throats, bruises, and injuries, although it is not known how or why they work. Gladys McGarey, M.D., cites the case of a baby she delivered with a fine scar instead of a harelip and cleft palate. The condition was apparently healed in the uterus when the castor oil pack was applied for bleeding.

A compress for the abdominal wall is made of wool flannel saturated (but not dripping) with cold-pressed castor oil. This is applied to your belly, and the pack is covered with plastic wrap since castor oil is very sticky and hard to remove from sheets and clothes. Heat from a hot water bottle helps the oil keep warm longer and be absorbed better.

Further details on castor oil packs and the cold-pressed oil and flannel can be obtained from the ARE Medical Clinic in Phoenix, Arizona, or from Women-to-Women in Yarmouth, Maine.

Psychological Issues in Premature Labor, Toxemia, and Other Prenatal Complications

Premature labor can result from an undetected infection or an underlying emotional problem. The following comments are certainly not intended to arouse feelings of guilt but to explore more fully the possibilities for greater awareness. Women tend to feel guilty anyway, and new insights often help move them on to self-forgiveness.

The most important and perhaps most difficult challenge in health care is to understand *why* a person has a particular problem or complication. As mind and body are one, our dysfunction and disease also have a symbolic role — they are trying to tell us something. Besides providing relief from symptoms, holistic health care asks why the person has the symptoms he or she does at this point in time at this location in the body. This approach leads us to understand the phenomenon — not simply to get rid of it.

Ann Evans presented new information about premature labor at the 1989 Congress of the Pre and Perinatal Psychology Association of North America. She found that if a woman had experienced sexual abuse by a caretaker prior to the age of eighteen, she was twice as likely to deliver before thirty-four weeks of gestation and two and a half times more likely to have a newborn with a medical problem. This occurred regardless of the number of previous babies, education, race, alcohol or cigarette abuse, or history of other physical abuse in childhood. Considering that sexual abuse is estimated to occur to one in four girls, this topic should be on every prenatal questionnaire.

David Cheek, a retired obstetrician and skillful hypnotherapist, considers that "premature labor is a preventable disease — if you can talk to the mother." Before he learned to ask his expectant mothers about fear, he had a 7 percent prematurity rate in his practice and often the babies had low birth weight and did not survive. After he learned to help mothers in premature labor to bring unresolved issues to their conscious minds, his prematurity rate dropped to 1.6 percent.

Cheek believes that doctors often arouse anxiety in pregnant women by comments that may seem harmless, such as "well, your cervix is soft" or "you're not very tall." This or some other problem in a woman's life haunts her and causes her to build up a stress response. She dreams at a level that precludes recall, but she tunes in to the normal contractions of her uterus, which she suddenly experiences as painful. This in turn leads to worry about the risks of preterm labor . . . more tension . . . more painful contractions . . . more risk.

Studies on premature labor dismiss such psychological influences. The brain, however, is an important organ to consider, as new research by Candace Pert at the National Institutes of Health has shown that its effects are everywhere in the body. Studies on multiples do not distinguish between pregnancies that were naturally conceived and those that resulted from fertility treatments. Cheek feels that this is an important distinction because he has observed a lack of biological readiness in infertile women under hypnosis.

Cheek and pediatrician Marshall Klaus and social worker Phyllis Klaus all have experience with telephone hypnosis for women in premature labor. When a woman calls with preterm contractions, she is almost in a trance with fear. Over the phone, she is asked to go back to the time when she is comfortable and nothing is going on and then to move forward to whatever it is that tunes her in to her uterus and leads to preterm labor contractions.

Lewis Mehl, M.D., and Gayle Peterson, a social worker, have also been successful in treating premature labor with hypnosis. Cheek, Phyllis Klaus, and Peterson have agreed to have their phone numbers listed in the Resources and to provide phone counseling and hypnosis.

In training graduate physical therapists in ob-gyn (including the care of high-risk pregnancies admitted to the hospital), I emphasize that as they help the mother to stretch and move, they can encourage her to share her emotional concerns. Hospitals are often understaffed and personnel are overworked, so emotional support may be scarce. Many obstetricians believe prematurity is simply caused by an over-distended or crowded uterus and will request a psychological consultation only if the woman is in severe emotional distress. Even then, it is more likely that they would just order sedatives. But physical therapists can visit with mothers regularly and listen actively. Some physical therapists have told me in great excitement how this simple act of humanity has helped some women identify and resolve issues, reducing their symptoms.

As I mentioned in Chapter 3, I have also noticed among countless stories of premature labor and fetal loss that the onset often occurs within hours or days of the mother's discovery that she is carrying multiples. The level of ambivalence and anxiety commonly experienced with single pregnancies can be markedly increased in the case of multiples. It seems that the shock overwhelms the mother and her body acts to let go of the situation. This has significant implications for the manner in which such news is conveyed to the mother and the kind of support she should be given while absorbing its impact. Ideally she should be contacted that same day by a counselor who is a mother of multiples. Even women who have been taking fertility drugs or undergoing in vitro fertilization and other procedures for infertility may feel ambivalent toward their "sudden abundance."

The more pregnancy and birth are controlled by technology, the less women trust their bodies and intuition. Some women go into premature labor because they may unconsciously believe that it is easier to deliver smaller babies or they are fearful of carrying such a load to term. Other women have such financial and emotional stress that they feel they are falling apart, and the babies are falling out, symbolically. Twin Services in Berkeley, California, published a report with the apt title "Twinshock," which discusses the often staggering physical, nutritional, emotional, and economic demands on the parents. Teenage women having their first pregnancy and carrying monozygotic twins (although this is rarely known before birth) are at greatest risk for preterm labor.

Avoid judging and projecting when helping an expectant mother explore her feelings toward the pregnancy. Even reassurance can be a put-down. Feelings are different from behavior, but they are just as real and need to be recognized and affirmed. Much more counseling, education, and support are required for expectant parents of multiples and should continue throughout the first few years after birth.

Tocolytic Drugs

Tocolytic medications attempt to suppress uterine contractions when premature labor is threatening. They have been used for more than two decades and no long-term problems have been reported yet. Some studies show that tocolytic drugs effectively stop preterm labor, allowing the pregnancy to continue for several more weeks, while other studies show that they do not. Campbell and MacGillivray as well as the 16th supplement to *Williams Obstetrics*, the classic obstetric text, conclude that these drugs have no preventive benefit, although they may work as a treatment for premature labor and give the fetal lungs time to mature, especially when the pregnancy is less than thirty-two weeks. An October 1989 technical bulletin by the American College of Obstetricians and Gynecologists stated that although delivery may be delayed for relatively short periods, no reduction in perinatal mortality or in severe respiratory distress syndrome has been demonstrated. Tocolytics may be useful to prevent delivery during transport to a hospital but will have little effect if the cervix is 3 centimeters dilated or 50 percent effaced (see Chapter 12 for a discussion of dilation and effacement).

Ritodrine (Yutopar) was approved by the Food and Drug Administration by the end of 1988 and has been reported as safe, although it may increase the mother's risk of pulmonary congestion. Terbutaline (Breathine) has not been approved by the FDA but it is widely prescribed and some studies have shown it to be more effective than Ritodrine. Possible side effects include increased heart rate for mother and baby, palpitations, tremors, anxiety, and low blood pressure. Both drugs can be given intravenously or by mouth, and terbutaline can also be given by injection under the skin — subcutaneous terbutaline pump therapy. Sometimes the drugs work, or appear to work, for a day or so, and this gains enough time to transport the mother to a high-risk medical center. A steroid, betamethasone, administered at the same time (if under thirty-four weeks), helps the babies' lungs mature and prevents respiratory distress after birth (see Chapter 13). This drug, however, can mask infection in the mother.

I didn't like terbutaline because it made my heart race and I was more keyed up.

I will discuss the effects and side effects of tocolytic drugs in detail because they are used so much in multiple pregnancies in the United States. They are generally prescribed with the attitude that it is better to do something than nothing. While it is preferable to prevent labor before it is established, premature babies will receive more medication in the nursery than they would during pregnancy. Readers are encouraged to follow an optimal diet of nutrients and fluids and have plenty of rest to prevent preterm labor and thus avoid the need for tocolytics.

Michael Odent recommends that women take fish oil capsules, based on his observation that Danish women in the Faero Islands who consume much fish often go beyond their due date. Some fatty acids appear to inhibit the synthesis of prostaglandins and thus may help in stopping preterm labor contractions. Such a simple remedy is certainly worth trying.

Administration of Tocolytics

Intravenous treatment requires hospitalization, often long term, and has significant side effects (discussed later in this section). Usually the drugs are given by IV or injection to stop the contractions; when the contractions have been controlled for at least twelve hours, the mother will be given pills to take every two to four hours, even at night, if her pulse is less than 140 beats per minute. This oral medication may be continued until the thirty-sixth or thirty-seventh week.

The terbutaline pump allows medication to be infused under the skin very slowly and continuously in very small doses to quiet the uterus. Additional larger doses can be programmed for automatic delivery during periods when the mother experiences strong uterine contractions — often in the late afternoon or early evening. The total dose over a twenty-four-hour period is less than 4 mg compared with

---

Contraindications to Tocolytic Drugs for Preterm Labor

ABSOLUTE

Severe pregnancy-induced hypertension
Severe abruption of the placenta
Severe bleeding from any cause
Infection of the amniotic fluid
Fetal death or anomaly incompatible with life
Severe intrauterine growth retardation

RELATIVE

Mild chronic hypertension
Mild abruption of the placenta
Stable placenta previa
Maternal cardiac disease
Hyperthyroidism
Uncontrolled diabetes mellitus
Fetal distress
Fetal anomaly
Mild intrauterine growth retardation
Cervix dilated more than 5 cm

---

up to 30 mg with oral medication. Side effects are reduced and the treatment can be more effective over a longer period of time: about eight weeks on the pump versus a couple of weeks orally.

Management of the pump is easy to learn, but a few days' hospitalization is necessary to determine the appropriate doses to allow the mother to feel comfortable. Together with home monitoring (described earlier in this chapter), women can be followed outside the hospital and there is no need to awaken at night because of the automatic continuous infusion.

Tocolytic drugs have side effects that may be tolerated better if you are forewarned. Your pulse may increase up to 30 beats per minute above normal. The medication also stimulates the nervous system, so you may feel jittery and develop tremors. Dr. Sorger often recommends a glass of wine to stop preterm labor, or wine in combination with terbutaline to reduce contractions and shaking.

Possible fluid buildup in your lungs will be monitored by checking your weight daily as well as your fluid intake and urine output.

Nausea, vomiting, and constipation result from the muscles of the gastrointestinal system becoming less active. Blood vessels expand as a result of this medication, causing you to feel very warm, and headaches can develop. There may be an increase in your glucose level and a decrease in your potassium level as measured by blood tests. All these side effects are more pronounced with the initial treatment but diminish when the medication changes to pills. All medications cross the placenta, and the babies' heartbeats or blood sugar values may be affected to some degree.

Magnesium sulfate is also used to sedate expectant mothers with high blood pressure and threatened convulsions (pre-eclampsia). This medication may cause you to feel warm, nauseated, or sleepy. The babies, if born soon after you take the medication, may have decreased muscle tone.

Indomethacin (Indocin) inhibits prostaglandins, hormone-like substances that, among other things, can trigger the onset of labor. This medication, given orally, has a side effect of initiating the closure of the ductus arteriosus, which allows blood circulation in the unborn baby. However, this effect appears to be reversible when the drug is discontinued.

Cervical Stitchery (Cerclage)

One controversial method of preventing premature labor in twin pregnancies is to close the cervix surgically. A thread, descriptively called a purse-string suture, is inserted around the cervix to hold it tightly closed. This procedure is known as a Shirodkar, MacDonald operation, or cervical cerclage. It is believed to prevent the lower uterine segment from being distended by the extra weight and stretching of a twin pregnancy. But research continues to show that it has no effect in preventing premature labor. Furthermore, the overdistention that supposedly occurs with a twin pregnancy does not recur with subsequent pregnancies. A true "incompetent cervix" (which is associated with fetal loss because it opens during pregnancy) is not caused by multiple pregnancy. This condition results most often from conization of the cervix and in women whose mothers were given the drug DES (diethylstilbestrol) in their pregnancies to prevent miscarriage. Other causes may be prior obstetric or abortion trauma, curettage of the uterus, or treatment to dilate the cervical canal if it is too narrow (stenosis). (Laser treatment is used today for cervical stenosis.)

The cervical stitch, which is usually done in the hospital under spinal anesthesia, carries a risk of infection as well. One study reported that in women who had a *history* of cervical incompetence and subsequently conceived twins, 66 percent of the 43 cases were successfully carried to term following a surgical suture.

The doubled amount of hormones produced by the mother during twin pregnancy softens the tissues, and it is normal for the cervix to be dilated before labor — up to 5 centimeters for mothers who have previously given birth.

Because physicians rarely do an internal examination in late pregnancy, some are not aware of these normal changes. When they find that the cervix is already well dilated, some doctors fear that it is "incompetent" and panic unnecessarily. If the woman is also experiencing strong and frequent Braxton-Hicks contractions, which mothers expecting twins often do in late pregnancy, it may be incorrectly assumed that she is in labor. Examination of the cervix will clarify this. Otherwise, a misunderstanding may be the basis for a Caesarean, particularly if one twin is breech.

In Europe, unlike the United States, it is customary to check the cervix throughout the pregnancy for length of the canal and dilation of the internal opening. A study in 1982 showed that cervical assessment was able to predict 60 to 80 percent of the labors that happened within fourteen days.

O'Grady states, *"Neither routine cerclage nor prophylactic administration of tocolytics in fixed doses appears effective in reducing preterm delivery or neonatal death in twins. In the absence of cervical incompetence or preterm labor, don't use these measures."*

Surveys of Mothers of Twins

Seventy percent of the respondents to a 1987 *Twins* magazine survey spent no time in the hospital during their multiple pregnancies. Of the 30 percent who were hospitalized, 40 percent stayed for one week, the rest for less time. Sixty percent carried their babies thirty-five weeks or longer (some medical authorities consider thirty-five weeks as term for multiples). Thirty-five percent delivered between twenty-seven and thirty weeks, and less than 1 percent gave birth between twenty-four and twenty-six weeks.

12 Labor and Birth of Twins and Supertwins

ALTHOUGH THE POTENTIAL for complications in multiple birth must be acknowledged, the mother's experience of labor was usually no worse, and was often easier, than with a singleton, until the Caesarean epidemic. The extra hormones in twin pregnancy often cause a preparatory dilation of the cervix prior to the onset of labor. It is an obstetric maxim that second deliveries are usually shorter and easier than first, and twins are more commonly a subsequent pregnancy.

Signs of Labor

Contractions of the uterus that increase in both strength and frequency herald the onset of labor. These sensations have been likened to menstrual cramps, gas discomfort, or pain in the lower back or groin.

Sometimes the membranes of one sac rupture as the first sign and, in most cases, contractions follow within a few hours. In a multiple pregnancy, if the first twin is footling breech and prolapse of that cord is a (rare) possibility, you may be asked to go straight to the hospital. If the contractions do not follow ruptured membranes within a half day or so, contractions may be artificially stimulated with pitocin, as most physicians prefer to deliver the baby within twenty-four hours after rupture of the membranes. This precaution is to keep normal bacteria in the birth canal from proceeding up into the sterile uterine environment where they may cause infection. For that reason it is also important to avoid vaginal exams. Dr. Leo Sorger recommends clinical observation of the labor or rectal exams instead. Vaginal exams should be considered only if a sterile speculum is used.

Loss of mucus, often blood-stained, from the cervix, may occur. If it is the only symptom of labor and you have not been advised otherwise, wait until contractions begin (within two to three days) or the membranes spontaneously rupture before contacting your physician.

Deviations from the Due Date

Premature Labor

As discussed in Chapter 11, prematurity is the single most important problem with multiple pregnancy. Every expectant mother should be aware that the signs of premature labor are the same as for term labor. However, they may be confused with other bodily sensations, especially if they occur well before the due date. Mothers often don't recognize these signs, which may be painless, and by the time they finally get to the hospital it is too late to stop the labor. (See page 176 in Chapter 11 for a list of the signs of premature labor that you may not recognize.)

Premature labor is much better prevented than treated, although prevention does not occur from any medical therapy or "magic pills." Healthy nutrition, sensible exercise, rest, relaxation, peace of mind, and emotional support will help to prevent this undesirable experience. The medical treatment for premature labor is hospital admission and tocolytic drugs to diminish uterine activity. (See Chapter 11 for a complete discussion of premature labor and its treatment.)

Postmaturity

The expectation that twins will be premature or at least "early" is so entrenched that little consideration is given to the possibility that they will be overdue. However, a 1990 review of the National Organization of Mothers of Twins Clubs database of 4,445 sets of twins found that 13 percent were born after the ninth month. Even the medical literature has few guidelines on this point. The World Health Organization considers more than forty weeks postmature for twins. Most obstetricians, while they may augment a labor with a pitocin IV, which stimulates contractions, are reluctant to induce labor. Induced labor often lasts longer because the cervix may be unripe and thus more contractions are needed to thin it out and dilate it. Induced contractions are often experienced as stronger and more painful, although the monitor may not show increased intensity. Sometimes induction is not successful and may need to be tried again. You can also try nipple stimulation, making love to orgasm (both of which cause uterine contractions), or taking an ounce of castor oil to get labor started (repeat in one hour if you achieve no response).

The Course of Labor

Labor is divided into three main stages, which always follow in the same sequence, although the nature and length of each stage vary greatly. The first and longest stage has two parts: latent and active. In the latent/early phase, the uterine contractions efface (thin out) the cervix and initiate its dilation. (Effacement is measured in percentages and dilation in centimeters.) With a multiple birth there is usually only one first stage: opening the cervix needs to be accomplished just once if the subsequent babies are born promptly. If there is a delay of hours, contractions will need to open the cervix again if it has closed at all. Women carrying twins are generally a few centimeters dilated before labor begins, so the latent phase of the first stage can be short. Contractions become progressively stronger and last longer after the cervix is effaced and about 5 centimeters dilated. This is the active phase of the first stage. The cervix is fully dilated at 10 centimeters (also termed 5 fingers). The babies at this point are still inside the uterus.

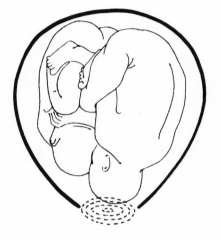

The cervix needs to dilate only once for both babies.

Each baby will have its own second stage, which is the journey down the birth canal through the mother's bony pelvis and vagina, ending with delivery. The third stage of labor follows with the arrival of the afterbirths, one or more placentas and membranes, which should be carefully examined to determine the type of twinning (see Chapter 2) and sent to the lab for microscopic analysis of the membranes.

First Stage of Labor: Effacement and Dilation

In early labor, when contractions may come as infrequently as every half hour or so, you should carry on with your normal activities, which will keep you upright and mobile. If this is your first pregnancy, it may take a while for labor to be established. This will give you time for carbohydrate loading, just like the marathoners. Eat as much complex carbohydrates as you can, such as whole grain pasta, pancakes, and potatoes. This will give you energy for the hours ahead in the hospital, where you will most likely get nothing more than ice chips or water. Talk with your doctor about eating during labor and try to find a doctor who will permit you to eat to appetite and drink to thirst.

Nourishment in labor is a real problem. Many labors become dysfunctional because the "engine has run out of fuel." Most pregnant women cannot go without nourishment for even a couple of hours and to do so for a day or more, under the stress and physical effort of labor, is very difficult. When you are in active labor you probably won't feel like eating, and at that point things move fast anyway. It is during slow, wearing labors that the mothers would benefit from added nutrition.

The reason that laboring women are often denied food and beverages is in the rare event that general anesthesia may be required. Food and drink in the stomach may cause regurgitation into the lungs (the same reason for fasting before surgery). However, regional anesthesia (an epidural or a spinal) is used today for most Caesareans. General anesthesia is more of a risk and and is used only in cases of extreme emergency (where there is no time for a regional anesthesia to take effect) or if the mother has back problems such as a spinal fusion or refuses regional anesthesia, preferring to be asleep. Even if you did need general anesthesia and had eaten, the tube inserted in your throat before surgery theoretically would take care of the potential problem or your stomach contents could be sucked out in case of vomiting after surgery. The midwives at North Central Bronx Hospital in New York have encouraged (often high-risk) mothers to eat and drink freely in labor for over a decade and they have not seen one case of aspiration of vomit.

Staying at home as long as possible in the first stage of labor means greater comfort and autonomy. While some hospitals and birthing suites now have Jacuzzis, double beds, and rocking chairs, most couples prefer the comfort of their own home. You are in active labor and should go to the hospital when you can't talk anymore during a contraction.

Hospital admission is more comfortable these days now that "prepping" (shaving of pubic hair and administering of enemas) has been discontinued. Medical records are usually sent ahead of time, so admission is only a matter of the staff taking a history of the labor and doing a physical exam: checking the blood pressure, urine, dilation of cervix, and presentation of the babies.

The baby lying in the left half of the uterus is usually lower and presents first. When the head (or buttocks) sink down into the pelvis, like an egg in an eggcup, the presenting part is said to be engaged. This, like dilation, may occur before the onset of labor because of the extra weight, pressure, and softening, together with an often smaller head.

Most mothers of twins and supertwins are huge at term and have great difficulty getting comfortable or even walking around without effort. Many pillows and frequent changes of position will help during labor. Lying on your back is undesirable for more than a few minutes at the end of any pregnancy because the uterus compresses the major blood vessels against the backbone, which can lower your blood pressure, make you feel nauseous and faint, and reduce blood flow to the babies. The American College of Obstetricians and Gynecologists has recommended against vigorous exercise on the back after the fourth month of pregnancy but has not advised its members to avoid placing their patients in this position during the most vigorous exercise of all — labor!

Most hospitals now have obstetric beds than can be adapted to a variety of positions. Often these are in a birthing room, however, and mothers of multiples, being considered high risk, may have to go to the delivery room. (Dr. Sorger moves the birthing bed into the delivery room if he is forced to go there.) Some hospitals prepare for potential complications with an intravenous, cross-matched blood, an anesthesiologist, and perhaps a pediatrician or two standing by. Try to find a birth center or hospital as soon as possible that is more supportive of natural birth, with care providers who will view you as "special need" rather than "high risk." This is not an easy task and may require travel to other areas — but it's worth it. Michel Odent, a renowned obstetrician from France, points out that the anxiety of a potentially complicated birth makes it even more necessary that mothers of multiples are supported in a low-key environment. It is not just the equipment in the hospital that is significant, but the attitude of the staff as well. The wallpaper and potted plants may be fancy, but are you allowed to deliver in any position that you choose? The mother should feel free to stand, walk in the halls, sit, go on all fours, or squat. The benefits of being upright for labor and birth have been well documented for so many years that it's a disgrace that so many women spend hours and hours flat on their backs — and they still do in hospitals all over the world.

Gravity improves the drive force of the uterus and increases the effectiveness of the contractions. Shorter labors with less pain are reported by women who are upright or walk around freely. Also, in these circumstances, there are fewer fetal heart abnormalities, less

One of my twins had her head engaged well before the birth. It is a family joke that she only had room to grow hair, because although they are identical, she had a headful of hair and her sister had almost none.

demand for pain medication, and less need to stimulate contractions with drugs. Many physicians will not allow a woman to get out of bed once the membranes have ruptured for fear of prolapse of the cord. However, when the head or presenting part is engaged, there is no room for the cord to slip down.

Medical Interventions

The intravenous (IV) unfortunately has become routine these days. This is "justified" on the grounds that it prevents dehydration because laboring women are not usually allowed to drink. A whole series of "in case" arguments are also offered that include the possibility of hemorrhage and the need for anesthesia, blood, stimulatory drugs, or pain medication. Some women are not bothered by an IV. Others feel that it implies that their body will malfunction without technical help. In such cases, this may be the first step in a whole series of interventions. Some couples maintain their self-confidence better if they refuse an IV rather than submit to it except in the case of complications.

The electronic fetal monitor (continuous ultrasound) is also ubiquitous today. Two or more external monitors mean that the mother is strapped to machines left and right. Also, the babies are exposed to ultrasound for varying amounts of time. The scalp electrode that is used for internal monitoring (electrocardiogram, ECG) can be attached only to the head of the presenting baby. An external monitor may be applied in addition to pick up the second heartbeat. Internal monitoring, while more accurate, carries a greater risk, including infection, accidents, and hemorrhage, as the electrode is inserted into the baby's scalp. In advanced labor fetal scalp blood sampling may be helpful to verify the monitor readings and to establish the status of the oxygen supply.

The IV and the monitor make it difficult, but not impossible, for the woman to move around. The belts can be taken off for a while and the IV bottle can be taken on a rolling pole or detached and carried by your partner or a nurse. A heparin lock (a small plastic tube) may be used instead of the intravenous line to keep a vein open. Radio telemetry now allows the fetal hearts to be recorded anywhere within the range of the nurses' station.

Sometimes the physician will rupture your membranes if they have not already ruptured on their own to speed up labor. Artificial rupture of the membranes, however, puts a time cap on early labor because of the possibility of infection. Cord prolapse, head compression, and bony misalignment are associated with artificial rupture of the membranes.

In addition to faults with the monitoring apparatus and false positive readings, which are fairly uncommon, there can be variations in how monitor results are interpreted. Electronic fetal monitoring is blamed as one of the reasons for the very high Caesarean rate.

Some couples, and most doctors, feel happier with constant surveillance by machinery. However, the information that the machines provide must be weighed against the intervention they entail. One has only to think of the women who still deliver healthy undiagnosed twins! Multiples were born successfully before monitors were invented with traditional noninvasive ways of listening to the fetal hearts, such as with a fetoscope. Rare accidents such as cord prolapse and abruption of the placenta can always be diagnosed by standard techniques of care.

Presentation

The presentation of the babies is assessed by palpation, listening to the heartbeats, and ultrasound. The babies may have been in the same positions for several weeks. Twins arrive one after the other, and the complications of presentation are handled the same way for each twin as if only one baby were involved. As discussed in Chapter 7, nearly 50 percent of twins will both come headfirst (*vertex* presentation), like most singletons. This is the easiest way for the baby and the attendant.

In approximately 40 percent of the other cases, one twin will be *breech*. The second twin, however, can change position after the birth of the first, spontaneously or with manipulation from the obstetrician. Internal version, a procedure in which the doctor manually turns the baby inside the uterus, can also be done if the twin is lying *transverse* (across the mother's pelvis) to bring that baby into a breech or vertex position.

The risks are the same as for any breech baby. The head is the last part to be delivered, the arms need to be brought down, and the shoulders may need assistance through the pelvis. Buttocks may come out first or one or both feet, knees, or legs. Breech deliveries require more skill and dexterity of the obstetrician, although if the mother assumes a squatting position breech babies can be born spontaneously, especially after the delivery of the first multiple. The late Dr. Nial Ettinghausen, a chiropractor and "drugless practitioner" in California, delivered many sets of twins and preferred the second twin to be breech, as he could hold on to the legs better than the head. Unfortunately, the extra difficulty in breech deliveries and the skill required are reasons enough for many obstetricians to opt for a Caesarean. However, because many twins are either early or small for their dates, breech delivery may be easier than in the case of singleton births. Some physicians will not allow the mother to deliver vaginally if the first twin is breech but will if the second twin is breech. Yet other doctors perform a combined vaginal-abdominal delivery. That is, the first twin is delivered vaginally if it is in vertex presentation, but the breech twin is delivered by Caesarean.

Ask your doctor what percentage of his twin and breech deliveries he does vaginally. It is hard to find a doctor today with these skills, as residents are taught surgery instead. However, the medical literature is starting to feature articles reassuring obstetricians that delivery "from below" should be reconsidered for twins, including breech presentations.

Comfort Measures

Mothers expecting multiples often experience more discomfort and pressure in labor than do mothers of singletons. Back and upper thigh massage may help comfort and relax you. Counterpressure against the lower back and pelvis may relieve the pain of contractions, which are usually felt in this area. Hot or cold packs can be tried. Many hospitals have showers and Jacuzzis, and hot water is very soothing. Some hospitals don't allow a bath or shower after rupture of the membranes, but others do. (*Make sure you have help getting out of a slippery tub or taking a shower as you may get dizzy or feel faint.*)

Labor support involves aiding the mother to sustain her courage, to surrender to the intense energy and power of the labor contractions, and to avoid interventions that interfere with normal physiology. In addition to unnecessary medical interference, avoid the (well-intentioned) intervention of breath control. Artificial breathing patterns have been the hallmark of childbirth preparation since the 1950s, despite the fact that mothers become exhausted and anxious when forced to breathe like small dogs during labor. The idea that this helps them feel "in control" denies the true nature of birth, which means no control — trust and surrender are needed. Your body knows how to breathe right now and it will in labor too! Your breathing will be different, with moans, sighs, and other expressive sounds. Artificial breathing techniques disturb this normal physiology. You want to avoid overbreathing because hyperventilation leads to dizziness, nausea, and faintness. If overbreathing is prolonged, the extra oxygen in the body constricts the blood vessels and impairs the release of oxygen from the hemoglobin to the tissues. As a result there is less blood carrying less oxygen, which may affect circulation to the babies. This can be a particular problem if your circulation is already reduced by regional anesthesia or by lying on your back. My philosophy about spontaneous breathing and "sounding" during labor is discussed in detail in my book *Childbirth with Insight* and is demonstrated in a video, *Channel for a New Life,* made of my last birth.

Medication and Anesthesia

The mother anticipating a multiple birth should avoid medication and anesthesia whenever possible. Unless she has been well nourished, her babies may be small or premature and they will have less resistance to the dosages of medication and anesthesia, which will be calculated for the mother's body size. All drugs pass through the sieve-like placentas. Narcotics such as Demerol and sedatives such as Seconal depress fetal respiration. Epidurals (regional anesthesia) lower the mother's blood pressure and slow down labor. A thorough consideration of this subject can be found in *Drugs in Labor and Birth* by Doris Haire, who points out that the package insert for the anesthetic marcaine (used for epidurals) contains five pages of adverse effects.

My labor was progressing well until the doctor ordered Valium because he thought my blood pressure was getting a bit high. After that everything seemed to come to a halt.

If complications occur that require anesthesia, an epidural or spinal (regional anesthesia) is preferable to general anesthesia. An epidural can be administered in the first stage of labor and continued through the birth and recovery phase. This differs from a spinal, which is a single shot done right at the end of labor to facilitate a delivery with instruments or for a Caesarean. Both types of anesthesia — particularly the spinal, which temporarily paralyzes the muscles — abolish the natural bearing-down reflex and thus interfere with the mother's ability to push out the babies. For regional anesthesia you will be asked to curl up on your side to open the spaces between the lower vertebrae of your spine. The area is cleansed with a cold antiseptic fluid and then the anesthetic is administered. You feel a prick and soon your legs tingle and go numb. For an epidural, an indwelling catheter remains so that the anesthetic solution can be added as required from time to time. This tiny tube is strapped down along your back so it cannot be accidentally pulled out by your movements.

Epidural anesthesia is effective for deliveries requiring instrumental assistance. However, the use of epidurals themselves is associated with an increased need for instruments because normal physiology has been disturbed and contractions slow down and become less effective. This leads to further intervention — the need for oxytocin to stimulate the contractions. Acceleration of labor with oxytocin has been linked in one study to postpartum hemorrhage and jaundice in the newborn. The work of the mother's heart is also greatly increased with epidural anesthesia. Other research showed that the use of anesthesia causes delay in the delivery of the second twin and exposes this baby to the effects of the anesthesia for a longer time.

Second Stage of Labor: Descent and Delivery

The second stage of labor officially begins when the cervix is fully dilated. I would like to see its onset redefined as when the presenting baby descends onto the pelvic floor, stimulating the urge to push (in the absence of anesthesia). The only physical assistance that you can provide during this stage of labor is to push along with the expulsive contractions. You should save your effort for the time when the urge is irresistible. You will feel the reflex to push when the first presenting part is low enough on the pelvic floor to stimulate the stretch receptors in the muscles. These receptors relay the message to the brain, which leads to the release of natural oxytocin to stimulate the contractions that lead to the birth. Until this time, while the head or presenting part remains high, maternal effort leads only to fatigue and defeat. There is often a physiological lull at the beginning of the second stage, and if it is not observed by attendants they may force the mother to push before she is ready. Uterine inactivity (inertia) can also be brought on by maternal anxiety.

During the second stage nurses and doctors tend to cheer, instruct, and exhort (which may be necessary for the unprepared woman). Some couples may appreciate this squad of often noisy supporters if their commitment is to control rather than to let go. It is difficult to see how such outer-directed activity can be appropriate when the mother (unless medicated or anesthetized) is experiencing her own inner direction. Of course, she requires peace and quiet to be conscious of her body and to respond spontaneously. Why should she push if the uterus is not pushing? Certainly the purple face and popping eyes reassure the staff that the mother is indeed trying to work hard. Unfortunately, straining with the breath held, as many childbirth preparation courses still instruct, interferes with normal physiology. Forced expulsive effort (known as the Valsalva maneuver) causes severe fluctuations in respiration and circulation. The blood pressure is greatly increased at the onset of strain but within a few seconds starts to fall because blood pools in vessels of the pelvis and legs and cannot return to the heart against such high pressures in the chest. With reduced venous return, the heart has less blood to pump out to the lungs, uterus, and babies. The body, however, has its own inherent wisdom, helped by a lowered respiratory center threshold in pregnancy, and the mother lets out a characteristic grunt. This may annoy the staff, if they are ordering her to hold her breath and shouting at her to relax — as if anyone could relax while holding in so much tension. But the mother's body relaxes on *outward* breath, and only when the pressure is released from above, as air is exhaled, can the pelvic floor relax below and open.

Moaning and groaning — sounds of work with overtones of sexuality — are usually discouraged during childbirth because "air is escaping" and the "force is waning." However, this is the natural way that women respond if they are not holding their breath. Misguided educators and maternity staff dictate that the ideal period to interrupt respiration and push forcefully is considered to be twenty seconds, which allows for a couple of snatched breaths in an average sixty-second contraction. Listening carefully to women in labor attempting to do this reveals that they rarely sustain the strain for more than a few seconds. Uruguayan obstetrician Roberto Caldeyro-Barcia, past president of the International College of Obstetricians and Gynecologists, has shown that women spontaneously push for less than five seconds and often push several times during one contraction. Intervals of normal breathing between pushes maintain normal physiology.

It is a prevalent, but erroneous, belief that you cannot "push" unless a pocket of air is trapped inside to "force down the diaphragm." On the contrary, the abdominal muscles contract on outward breath — most effectively when forcing air out against some resistance. Examples of this include singing, blowing a trumpet, and inflating a balloon. During birth this is achieved by *partially* closing the glottis — which leads to the characteristic guttural sounds uttered by laboring women. If the glottis is shut tightly to hold the breath, a closed-pressure system is formed and the abdominal wall distends and moves outward. The high pressure is transmitted throughout the entire body. This Valsalva maneuver tenses the pelvic floor, strains the abdominals, and reduces blood flow to the babies. In physiologi-

The nurse kept hissing at me to hold my breath. I told her (between contractions) that I had good reasons for wanting to avoid that. Then she said, "Well, at least you don't have to make so much noise." And I replied, "It is my delivery and I'll make as much noise as I like."

I remember the nurses telling me that wasn't the way to push, but my doctor said to go ahead and do what felt right.

Explanation of Abbreviations

G = gravida (number of pregnancies)
T = term (number of infants born at term)
P = preterm (number of premature infants)
A = abortion (miscarriage)
L = living (number of living children)
EDC = expected date of confinement (due date)
Station = descent of baby's head in relation to the pelvis
FHR = fetal heart rate
T = temperature
P = pulse
R = respiration
Prep = shaving of pubic hair
IV = intravenous
VE = vaginal examination
Fundus = top of uterus
1 U = 1 finger above umbilicus (navel)
FF @ U = fundus firm at level of umbilicus
ROA = right occiput anterior (back of baby's head faces mother's right side)
PROM = premature rupture of the membranes
ARM = artificial rupture of the membranes
Oxytoc. = oxytocin (a drug to stimulate contractions)
FHT = fetal heart tones
UC = uterine contractions
A.C. = aftercoming
Nuchal cord = cord around baby's neck
Mec. staining = baby passing meconium from bowel (a sign of potential distress)
AgNO$_3$ 1% = silver nitrate (to prevent eye infection if gonorrhea is present)

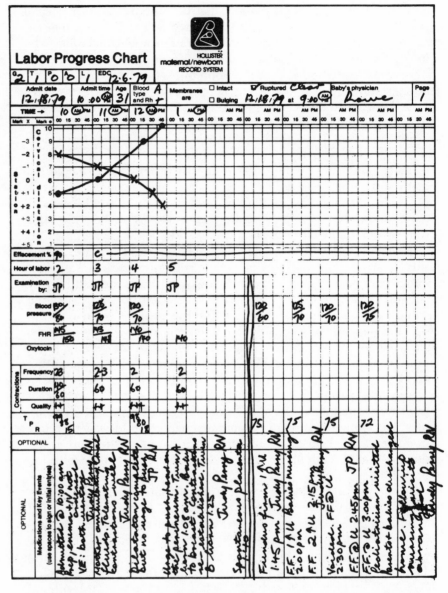

Labor progress chart: a case history. The birth of twins can be easy and uncomplicated.

This record is copyrighted by Miller Communications, Inc., and may not be reproduced without permission of Hollister, Inc., the exclusive licensee under said copyright.

Labor and Delivery Summary *BABY "A"*

HOLLISTER
maternal/newborn
RECORD SYSTEM

Labor Summary

G	T	P	A	L	Type and Rh.
2	1	0	0	1	A

Presentation | **Position**
☑ Vertex   `R O A`
☐ Face or brow
☐ Breech _____
☐ Transverse lie   ☐ Compound
☐ Unknown

Complications   ☐ None
☐ No prenatal care
☐ Preterm labor (≤37 wks.)
☐ Postterm (≥42 wks.)
☐ Febrile (≥100.4°) when admitted
☐ PROM (≥12 hrs. preadmit)
☐ Meconium
☐ Foul smelling fluid
☐ Hydramnios
☐ Abruption
☐ Placenta previa
☐ Bleeding-site undetermined
☐ Toxemia (mild) (severe)
☑ Seizure activity
☐ Precipitous labor (<3 hrs.)
☐ Prolonged labor (≥20 hrs.)
☐ Prolonged latent phase
☐ Prolonged active phase
☐ Prolonged 2nd stage (>2.5 hrs.)
☐ Secondary arrest of dilatation
☐ Cephalopelvic disproportion
☐ Cord prolapse
☐ Decreased FHT variability
☐ Extended fetal bradycardia
☐ Extended fetal tachycardia
☐ Multiple late decelerations
☐ Multiple variable decelerations
☐ Acidosis (pH <7.2)
☐ Anesthetic complications
☐ *Twin pregnancy*
☐ _____

Induction   ☑ None
☐ ARM ☐ Oxytoc.☐ _____
Augmentation   ☑ None
☐ ARM ☐ Oxytoc. ☐ _____

Monitor   FHT   UC   ☑ None
External   ☐   ☐
Internal   ☐   ☐
Medications   Total dosage
_____
_____
_____

Time of last narcotic   :   A P

Delivery Data

Method of Delivery
Cephalic
☑ Spontaneous   Type
☐ Low forceps }
☐ Mid forceps } _____
☐ Rotation _____ to _____
☐ Vacuum extraction
Breech
☐ Spontaneous
☐ Partial extraction *(assisted)*
☐ Total extraction
☐ Forceps to A.C. head
Cesarean *(details in operative notes)*
☐ Low cervical: transverse
☐ Low cervical: vertical
☐ Classical
☐ Cesarean hysterectomy
Placenta
☑ Spontaneous | **Blood loss**
☐ Expressed | ☑ <500 ml.
☐ Manual | ☐ >500 ml.
☐ Adherent | Specify amount,
☐ Curettage | detail in Remarks
Configuration (*300* ml.)
☑ Normal
☐ Abn. _____
Weighed (No) (Yes) _____ gms.
Cord
☐ Nuchal cord x _____
☐ True knot
☑ ③ Umbilical vessels
Cord blood to (lab) (refrig.) (discard)
Episiotomy   Suture
☑ None
☐ Median _____
☐ Mediolateral
☐ Other _____
Laceration
☑ None
☐ ① ② ③ ④ Degree perineal
☐ Vaginal
☐ Cervical
☐ Uterine rupture
☐ Other _____
Surgical Procedures   ☑ None
☐ Tubal ligation
☐ Other

Delivery Data (cont.)

Delivery Anesthesia   ☑ None
☐ ① Local   ☐ ④ Epidural
☐ ② Pudendal   ☐ ⑤ Spinal
☐ ③ Paracervical ☐ ⑥ General

No | Agent/Drug | | Dose
No | Agent/Drug | | Dose

Delivery Room Meds.   ☑ None
Agent/Drug | | Dose | | Route
Time : | A P | Sig
Agent/Drug | | Dose | | Route
Time : | A P | Sig
Agent/Drug | | Dose | | Route
Time : | A P | Sig

Chronology   Date
EDC   *12/7/79*   Time
ADMIT HOSPITAL *12/18/79* *10:00* ④
MEMBRANES RUPTURED *12/18* *9:00* ④
ONSET OF LABOR *12/18* *9:30* ④
COMPLETE CERVICAL DIL. *12/18* *12:30* ④
DELIVERY OF INFANT *12/18* *1:08* ④
DELIVERY OF PLACENTA *12/18* *1:40* ④

Infant Data

Apgar Scores

	Heart rate	Respiration	Muscle tone	Reflex irritability	Skin color	Total
1 min	2	2	2	1		9
5 min	2	2	2	1		9

☑ Spontaneous respiration
Resuscitation
☐ Oxygen
☐ Bag and mask
☐ Intubation
☐ Ext. cardiac massage
☐ Other _____
_____ mins. to sustained respiration

Infant Data (cont.)

Medications
☑ None
☐ Scalp care
☐ Volume expander
☐ Sodium bicarbonate
☐ Drug antagonists
☐ Umbilical catheter
☐ Other _____

Initial Newborn Exam
☑ No observed abnormalities
☐ Gross congenital anomalies
☐ Mec. staining ☐ Trauma
☐ Petechiae ☐ Other
Describe _____

Basic Data
ID bracelet no. *2613*
Hospital record no. _____
☑ Male   **Birth order**
☐ Female   *1* of ① ② ③ ④
Weight *8 lb 3 oz*
Length *22 in*
☐ Vitamin K
☐ AgNO₃ 1% or _____
Sig: _____
Output
☑ Urine *1:15 pm*
☐ Meconium
☐ Gastric _____ (ml.)
☐ Living at transfer to:

Deceased   Date
☐ Antepartum   mo / day / yr
☐ Intrapartum   Time
☐ Neonatal   :   A P
(in deliv. room)

Remarks: *First twin delivered*   *Judy Perry RN*
Nurse

Assisting   Attending   Date completed / /

cal pushing the breath is exhaled during exertion, the abdominal muscles move in toward the spine, and the reduction in volume causes the rise in pressure. It is like squeezing a toothpaste tube instead of blowing up a balloon. As she bears down on outward breath, the mother focuses her attention on the key muscles — the abdominals, which contract, and the pelvic floor, which relaxes as she opens up.

Gradually doctors and hospital personnel are beginning to understand that it is reasonable that women have the choices for responding in the second stage that they have long enjoyed in the first stage of labor. "Gentle pushing" and "controlled exhalation" are even being promoted as new methods, when in fact they are simply what women have done naturally for centuries. Dr. Caldeyro-Barcia is one of the few researchers to look at the effects of forced and prolonged bearing-down efforts on the fetus. His studies have led him to conclude that this well-meant instruction interferes with fetal oxygenation and can increase the need for episiotomy by not allowing time for the pelvic floor to distend. This important research was presented for the first time in 1978 at the International Childbirth Education Association's tenth biennial convention. It is reprinted, along with my articles on the detailed body mechanics involved in these respiratory considerations, in the conference proceedings, *Kaleidoscope of Childbearing: Preparation, Birth, and Nurturing*, edited by Simkin and Reinke.

No one can teach a woman how to push any more than one can teach her how to have an orgasm. Of course anyone can be told what to do, but only she herself can let go. Analogies taught to childbearing women all emphasize "doing" and "control," usually based on cultural ideas about elimination. For example, "Push into your bottom as if you were having a bowel movement" is a common directive in labor. Sexual analogies are far more appropriate and confirm the sexuality of childbirth, which is generally overlooked. The aspects of releasing, letting go, and giving can only happen — by definition they cannot be forced. Those who seek the passion of childbirth must develop a sense of intelligent awareness — the link between body and mind. The first commitment is to learn total trust in your body. Birth, like orgasm, relaxation, and sleep, results from *not* trying.

The custom of creating a sterile field around the genital and lower abdominal area with antiseptic and surgical drapes further removes the mother from her body and the act of giving birth. Prepared women enjoy placing a hand on each head as it emerges through the vagina and feeling the newborn's skin on theirs. The exterior may be

With my first delivery I did what I was told and strained for two and a half hours. The blood vessels in my eyes and cheeks were shot — I looked a mess the next day. With the twins, I just went with the urge when it came. It felt so good compared with the pain I had the last time.

made sterile, but the vaginal pathway certainly is not sterile; thus the rationale for this dehumanizing policy is not clear. Dr. Sorger has not used a sterile field in fifteen years, and there has been no increase in infection among his patients.

Episiotomy, an incision to enlarge the vaginal outlet, should not be needed in most births, but may be done for fetal distress or a difficult presentation. Many obstetricians like to do one "just in case" (to prevent a tear), although episiotomy is a major cause of blood loss at birth, can extend into a tear, and must be sutured. A first- and often a second-degree tear does not need stitches, but larger tears do, just like episiotomies. For most women a tear heals more comfortably.

The parents of twins may be so happy and excited to welcome the first baby that they momentarily forget that the other is still inside. Sometimes it is difficult for the mother to bond with the first twin when the second twin is still in the process of birth, but others may enjoy this interval. Putting the first twin immediately to the mother's breast naturally stimulates contractions. It may not be immediately apparent if the first twin has its own placenta and membranes. These may follow the first birth, or one large placental mass or, less often, two separate placentas may be delivered after the second twin. After the first twin arrives, the doctor will do a vaginal exam and press around the abdomen to determine if the position of the second twin has changed. The mother may be aware of the increased fetal movement with the extra room temporarily available in the uterus. Between the delivery of the first and second twins, the cervix may close down a little if the second twin is not delivered right away. However, in most cases contractions will dilate it again when the uterus is ready for the next expulsive phase, if the physician feels comfortable waiting.

Experimental work with rabbits showed that when 50 percent of the uterine contents were reduced, it took about ten minutes for the muscle fibers to adapt so the uterus could return to normal activity. The special structure of uterine muscle allows the fibers to maintain tension and contractility, although the length of the fibers may vary. Classic obstetric practice, which advises neither undue delay nor haste, recommends that the second twin be delivered within ten to twenty minutes, unless there is bleeding or fetal distress. Although Northwestern University research has shown that an interval of up to five hours is safe, Dr. Sorger prefers to deliver the second twin as soon as possible before the cervix closes or complications develop. In some cases this means rupturing the second sac and, if necessary, turning and extracting the second twin.

After Jason was born, I could feel Aaron inside wiggling around. The doctor was in a hurry to get him out but the baby didn't want to come. First an arm came down, and then a leg. The doctor finally pushed the limbs back and pulled him out by both legs.

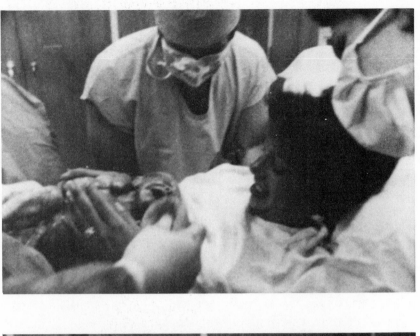

Giving birth to twins is a wonderful accomplishment. *Top:* Greeting the first arrival. *Bottom:* The doctor checks the position of the baby still inside. *Facing page:* The second twin is welcomed into the world.

From the film Having Twins; *courtesy of Polymorph Films, Boston.*

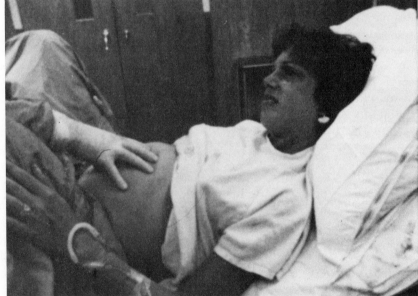

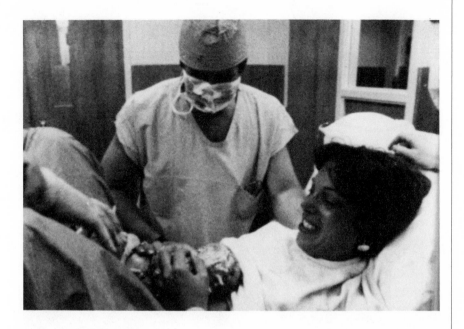

Third Stage of Labor: Delivery of Placenta(s) and Membranes

Each cord is cut after it has ceased pulsing and has been identified so that each twin can later be matched with the appropriate placenta. Samples of cord blood are sent for laboratory analysis. Usually the placentas are separate or fused and are delivered following the birth of both twins. About 60 percent of identical twins have just one placenta. Arrival of the common placenta before the second twin is born is dangerous for this twin. If the placenta is not delivered spontaneously, it can be removed manually before the cervix closes.

Some physicians like to see the placenta delivered within minutes, but in home births and in other countries, up to an hour is acceptable, and tugging on the cord to hasten removal of the placentas is frowned upon. Dr. Sorger waits if there is no bleeding but removes the placenta if bleeding starts.

A uterine stimulant, by IV or injection, is frequently administered during the third stage of labor to augment the contractions of the uterus. The uterine musculature is arranged in different layers, creating a figure-eight effect, so that contractions naturally clamp off any bleeding vessels, preventing hemorrhage from the site where the placenta was attached. Postpartum hemorrhage is more common

I remember that the doctor showed us both this one huge placenta. He pointed out the membranes and where they had been attached.

Our twins were born at home. We buried the placenta in the garden and planted two chrysanthemums above in memory.

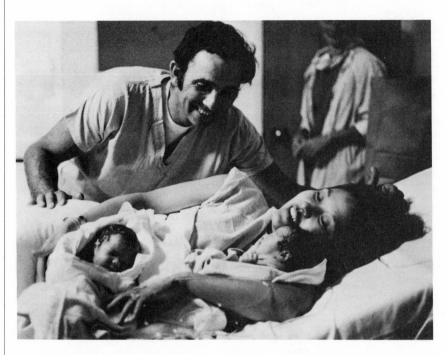

Natural childbirth brings joy to these new parents of twins.

My babies were brought to me alternately for nursing in the hospital, but I think it is essential that both twins be brought in together. This way you don't prolong the fantasy that you gave birth to just one baby, which can delay the bonding with both.

after multiple birth, especially if there is interference in the twin labor or haste with the second baby or the placenta. Excellent nutrition builds an extremely strong uterus that usually can cope with any extra bleeding from the large placental site. Episiotomies or tears are sutured after the placentas are delivered.

Vaginal bleeding may be heavier and last longer after multiple birth owing to the larger area of uterus covered by the placenta.

Breast-feeding, which ideally commences as soon as possible after birth, naturally stimulates the uterus to contract. Newborns at term have the ability to suck very soon, which stimulates an early milk supply and helps prevent engorgement of the breasts. Even if the babies just lick the nipples, this action will raise hormone levels, which helps lactation and aids in maternal attachment to the infants.

Care of the Babies

After each birth mucus is usually aspirated from each infant's nose and mouth with a bulb syringe. A catheter may be used if deep suctioning is necessary. If an episiotomy was done, there is less compression of the baby's chest to help expel the mucus. Oxygen will be administered to the baby if he or she has any breathing difficulties. Heelprints, samples of cord blood, and wristband identification (A or B to indicate the order of birth) are done immediately after birth.

In many states silver nitrate drops or antibiotic ointment must be put in all newborns' eyes. This prevents eye complications that may arise if the mother has gonorrhea. The eye inflammation and blurred vision caused by these drops may interfere with the babies' experience of bonding. Avoid or delay this procedure.

Although parents would prefer to have the babies warm and secure in their arms, hospitals still usually place them in isolettes and take them to the central nursery until their body temperature returns to normal. The cold air conditioning in the delivery rooms is a contributing factor to body temperature problems, but the babies can warm up quickly in your energy field. Thanks to increasing awareness of the importance of parental bonding with newborns, hospitals

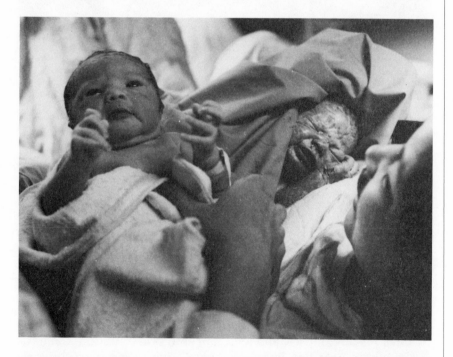

Healthy twins can be cuddled right after birth. The baby on the left has already been washed. The baby on the right is still coated with the protective vernix.
Copyright © Suzanne Arms.

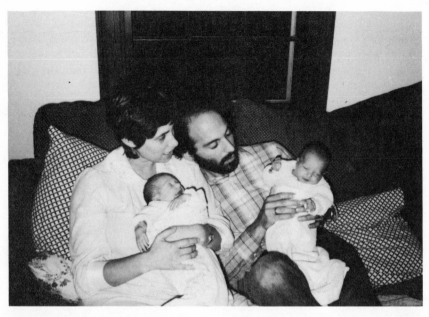

This family left the hospital just a few hours after the birth of their twins and now relaxes at home.

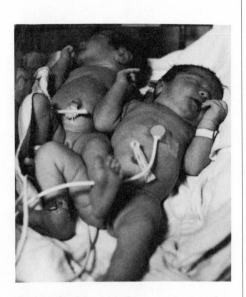

Twinvaluable twinfants — just a few minutes old.
Copyright © Suzanne Arms.

are becoming much more flexible. In fact, some of them actually have adopted a policy, which they may promote as if it were a medicine; for example, "We have instituted twenty minutes' bonding time for all postpartum mothers." Bonding with multiples has special considerations, and the following chapter is devoted to this topic.

Newborn infants are superficially assessed at one and five minutes after birth according to the Apgar scale. Scores of 0, 1, or 2 are given for each category at each time interval.

A perfect score of 10 is rarely given, as it takes a little while for the baby's circulation to adapt, even if the baby is a mature infant born spontaneously. Measurements are made of each infant's weight, length, and circumference of the head. A pediatrician will do a thorough evaluation of each baby's maturity and health. Assessment is made of posture, muscle and joint function, skin condition (some babies are born with fine hairs — lanugo — which disappear in postpartum life), creases in the palms and soles of the feet, development of the genitals, and areola around the nipple and ear cartilage.

Parents are often unprepared for the appearance of the newborn. He or she typically has a disproportionately large head, molded irregularly. The body may be a little blue and covered with creamy white vernix.* Forceps, if used, may leave marks. The large alert eyes are very impressive.

The parents of twins or other multiples become instant celebrities in the hospital. Staff and visitors are fascinated, and the mother receives flowers, gifts, and lots of help. The task of handling two babies seems formidable to the first-time mother, who may wonder if she can learn enough skills in the brief postpartum stay. The first-time mother usually handles just one twin at a time while the staff help with the other. Unless some assistance is arranged for your return home, you will suddenly have the job of both at once.

* Vernix is the baby's protective coating in the fluid-filled uterus.

Apgar Scale	*Score*		
	0	1	2
Appearance (*skin color*)	Blue, pale	Pink body, extremities blue	Completely pink
Heart Rate (*pulse*)	Absent	Below 100	Over 100
Respiration (*breathing effort*)	Absent	Irregular, slow	Strong cry
Muscle Tone (*activity*)	Limp, flaccid	Some flexion of extremities	Active, vigorous movement
Reflex Irritability (*grimace in response to stimulation of sole of foot*)	No response	Grimace	Cry, cough, or sneeze during suctioning

The nearer the total score is to 10, the better the baby's condition

Postpartum Exercises

You should begin postpartum exercises right after the birth. Mothers of twins have a lot of work to do if they are going to fit into their former clothes. Mothers recovering from surgery can do deep breathing, abdominal tightening, and pelvic tilting with the knees bent. Pelvic floor contractions help to restore these important muscles and aid in healing the tissues if there was an episiotomy or tear.

The same exercise program is followed after the birth as before. Check the recti muscles and follow the instructions in Chapter 10. Progress the pelvic tilting and curl-ups as described. *Make sure that you shorten the abdominal muscles before you try to strengthen them.* "Hacking," a type of deep pressure massage with the outer border of your hand, helps to bring life back to the stretched belly. These techniques are demonstrated in my video *Babyjoy: Exercises and Activities for Parents and Newborns* and my book *Marie Osmond's Exercises for Mothers and Babies* (see Further Reading). Many mothers of multiples are so busy with the infants that they often find no time for rest, relaxation, or exercise. As a result they retard their postpartum recovery and feel very depressed that there is no time for their personal needs. It is much easier to start rehabilitation at the beginning. Good physical condition will prevent discomfort and injury as you lift and care for the babies. It may be a long, long time before you get to sleep through the night, so rest periods and the ability to let your body relax for a short while need to be cultivated.

Because of the novelty of twins, you can expect more attention and cooperation from the staff, especially with breast-feeding. If this is not forthcoming, contact La Leche League. Some mothers have a problem making sure their babies are brought to them for night feedings, as it is often easier for the nursery staff to give an infant a bottle and let the mother sleep. You will need as much practice as possible during your hospital stay, learning to put one or both babies to the breast together. Breast-feeding is especially encouraged after multiple birth to help the uterus return to its former size. You may feel postpartum contractions in the early days, and they are often stronger while you are breast-feeding. They can be particularly uncomfortable in a second or subsequent pregnancy. The feeding of multiples is discussed in Chapter 15.

After my quads were born, I could just pick up my abdomen, like a mountain of dough. It would just go, "blub, blub, blub" when I let go. I did frequent abdominal contractions, within a binder for support, and it was amazing. The muscles were back to almost normal within a few weeks!

All the new mothers of twins in our club are in awful shape. Postpartum exercise evenings are really popular because these women really need them.

Before my twins were born, I never realized how important my abdominal muscles were. I couldn't even stand up when I got off the delivery table. I was bent over at a forty-five degree angle and my inside organs all went "slosh."

My abdominal muscles after the birth were unbelievable. I felt I could put my hand in and touch my backbone.

No matter how tired you are, try to do your postpartum exercises every day. They are really important to help you feel well and able to cope.

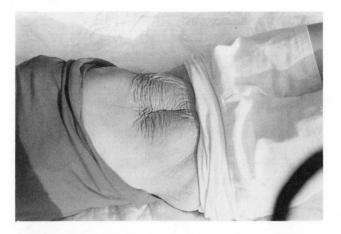

"Twinskin" will improve with abdominal shortening.

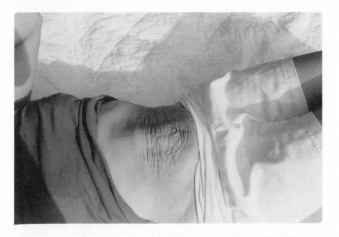

Breath holding strains and bulges the abdominal wall, showing the separation between the recti muscles.

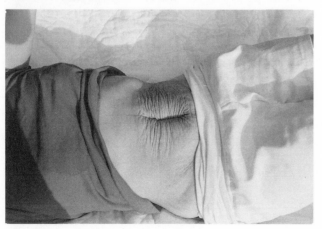

Shorten the muscles on outward breath; pull your belly button to your backbone.

Natural Childbirth for Twins and Supertwins

Just as more and more singletons and twins are being delivered by Caesarean, triplets and quadruplets are almost invariably brought into the world by major surgery.

It is extremely important that women know that natural birth for multiples is possible. The more women abdicate responsibility for their births to the medical profession and the more it is wrested from them by interventions, the worse the malpractice situation will be as their anger surfaces later. Insurance companies unfortunately are increasingly dictating medical practice, to the detriment of the doctor-patient relationship. But taking responsibility means taking informed risks, and expectant mothers need to hear about good outcomes as well as bad ones.

Interestingly, in a survey of the records of the Chicago Maternity Center from 1901 to 1933 presented at a 1988 Northwestern University conference, the perinatal mortality rate was about the same as today. All of those multiples were born at home, delivered by midwives, nurses, and medical students to a population consisting mainly of immigrants living under adverse socioeconomic conditions.

It is not my intent to encourage home birth for twins and supertwins. I never advocate the place of birth for anyone under any circumstances: women have to deliver where they feel safe. I simply wish to keep a balanced perspective that includes the historical fact that before the recent advent of hospital obstetrics, all multiples were born at home (albeit with some mishaps). Furthermore, all the high-tech intervention and enormous expense that surround the delivery of supertwins today have not significantly improved outcome. In Chapter 19 I describe natural births for supertwins in Japan.

The following anecdotes may inspire couples to shop around for a physician who will consider vaginal delivery, vertical or squatting positions, and nourishment during labor. The mothers whose cases I cite here all enjoyed excellent nutrition and good prenatal care, gained adequate weight, and went close to or even beyond their due date. Good nutrition, support, and the couple's belief in the mother's innate ability to birth normally are essential, too — after all, the mother wants to birth the babies, not have the doctor "deliver" them.

Spontaneous Delivery of Triplets in the Hospital

Dr. Leo Sorger assisted in the spontaneous delivery of triplets at thirty-five and a half weeks. The hospital insisted that the birth take

When you are besieged on all sides with advice on how to cope with twins, it is easy to forget that what every baby needs, most of all, is a healthy mother. Extra rest and good nutrition are absolutely essential.

Don't be discouraged by people who say, "You poor thing" or "I'm glad it's you and not me." Later, your ego will be boosted when they exclaim, "I don't know how you manage so well!"

My twins' birth was uneventful and happy. Both were delivered by our midwife while our OB sat in a corner of the room and did nothing. We all went home three hours later and cuddled up to sleep in our own bed.

I asked the hospital to put in a heparin lock instead of an IV so I could move around freely.

place in the delivery room, but the staff managed to wheel the flexible birthing bed from the labor room so that the mother could remain in an upright position. She chose to be on her knees, embracing her husband, who in turn helped support her. With gravity assisting, each baby (all were headfirst) dropped out very easily. They all weighed between 5 and 6 pounds, and the time interval between the arrival of each triplet was about 20 minutes. The mother received no intravenous or anesthesia, and the doctor did not perform an episiotomy.

Professor Robert Derom, a Belgian obstetrician and long-time expert on multiple birth, delivers almost all of his triplets and quadruplets vaginally. He described to me in the fall of 1988 how he had recently delivered a set of quadruplets vaginally — and all of them were breech! As a singleton breech is an indication for a Caesarean for the overwhelming majority of obstetricians in the United States, it is important for American mothers to know how obstetric practices differ in other countries. Dr. Louis Keith, who wrote the Foreword to this book, vaginally delivered two sets of triplets, at about thirty-five to thirty-six weeks, at the Cook County Hospital in Chicago during the first years of his residency. All infants did well.

It took a lot of planning and talking to get my wishes approved by the hospital. I simply wanted the birth to be as near to a home delivery, which I had originally planned before the twins were diagnosed, as it could be.

When I arrived at the hospital, the contractions were still light, and I had no urge to push even though I was completely dilated. Suddenly there was one strong contraction and a baby was there — in the labor bed, as planned. The second baby had been transverse but the doctor turned the baby to feet first and I pushed him out. I had twenty-four-hour rooming-in, which is something the hospital doesn't usually allow. This occurred only because I had a nurse friend stay with me during the night. Planning ahead of time paid off. I left the hospital twenty-eight hours after the births, and of course my two bundles went with me.

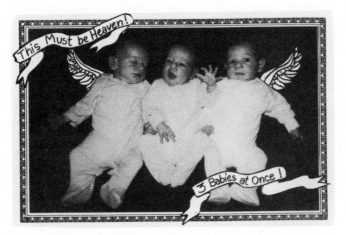

Triplets Born at Home after a Previous Caesarean

The three bouncing babies shown in the birth announcement were all born at home. Women and their partners who seek home births are generally highly informed and assume much responsibility for planning the event.

I was extremely upset that I had had a Caesarean and it was my desire to have a nonintervention, natural birth. I felt the only way to get this was by having a home birth and was taken by the beauty and simplicity of it all. I knew I could never have that in a hospital.

After our three babies were born I was contacted by a woman who had triplets about the same time. She had gone through the hospital and at thirteen weeks her doctor had told her she would have to have a Caesarean. He never discussed diet or its importance with her. So they went that route and she had her babies early, I think around thirty weeks, with twenty or so people in the delivery room and a bill for $50,000.

This story began when the pregnant mother simply sought a natural birth after her first child was delivered by Caesarean. While the general policy held by the doctors in her small town was to allow a trial of labor for a subsequent birth, rather than automatically schedule a repeat Caesarean, Mary would have had to find a doctor who actually practiced natural childbirth in such situations, and her pregnancy and labor would have had to fit his or her standards of "normal." She could have hoped for a vaginal birth, but that's all she felt she would have had — "hope with a very uncertain outcome."

So Mary sought midwives who would assist her at home. When it become apparent that "twins" were on the way, she felt it would be impossible to achieve the vaginal birth she wanted if she "plugged in to the medical establishment." Thus, she decided against an ultrasound, feeling that it would be only the beginning of a lot of medical interference. As the midwives would never have considered a home birth for triplets, Mary is glad that she did not have the ultrasound!

Carrying twins under the care of any of her local doctors would have meant a Caesarean at thirty-eight weeks "to avoid uterine rupture from the uterus growing too large." Mary's midwife says, "I agreed to help Mary and her husband do their prenatal care and see what things felt like when she got closer to term. I didn't feel right sending her off for a lot of obstetric technology she didn't want and a C section she didn't need, so we started looking for ways to make it feel safe at home. They didn't want an ultrasound and I didn't take the possibility of more than two babies very seriously, although the father asked if I thought there could be more than two after reading *Having Twins*."

Mary's husband was working in the home and was available to help at the end of pregnancy. During the last few weeks, Mary rested in bed most of the time and was lucky to have a good woman friend staying with her. She helped feed Mary and gave her and her husband invaluable emotional support. Eating every couple of hours, Mary never had a long stretch without food. She took in about 200 grams of protein a day and gained nearly 70 pounds.

Two midwives took turns visiting Mary every other day to check her urine and blood pressure, which remained normal. One week after the due date, labor began. The first two babies were born, headfirst and uneventfully, nine minutes apart. At this point the family doctor, who had been taking fetal heart tones and checking her belly, said that she felt a head. The midwife reached in and felt a foot way up high, but the baby was facing Mary's front so the midwife turned her around to face the back. This breech baby was delivered ten min-

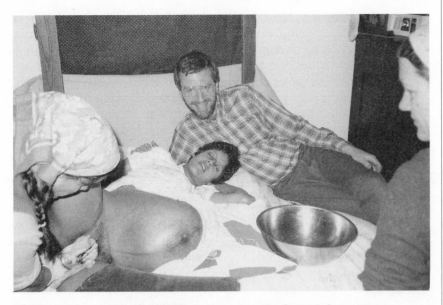

The midwife protects the mother's tissues as the first triplet emerges.

Every night my husband would make me a plate of sliced turkey with raw apples, carrots, or green peppers. He would wrap it in plastic and put it by the bed. When I got up to go to the bathroom — at least three times a night — I would eat a little out of the plate. No one can really understand how tough a job it is to eat like that when I was so full of babies. I was convinced that the only way to have a healthy home birth with twins was to have a term birth.

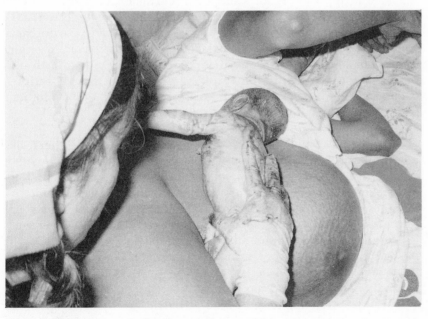

The midwife lifts the first triplet up to her mother.

A relaxed, loving atmosphere was just what I needed to have such a positive and wonderful birth.

utes after the second. Next, with three umbilical cords dangling from her vagina, Mary pushed out the one single placenta and the two that were joined. No episiotomy was necessary, and there was only a slight tear after delivering the breech baby. The first-born was a boy of 6½ pounds. The second-born was a girl who weighed 6 pounds, 14 ounces, and the third, the largest, was a girl weighing 7 pounds. The total weight of the three babies was over 20 pounds! All three babies nursed within the first hour and were entirely breast-fed for five months.

Mary had a little trouble urinating at first, as the stretch reflex of her bladder was diminished from months of great pressure. This cleared up within a few hours after birth. For a week or so, her balance was shaky when walking because her skin and muscles were so loose that "her belly swung back and forth when she moved." Today she is still concerned about her abdominal wall. But she has three wonderful, healthy children, born without any medical intervention and for a total financial outlay of only $1,000 (although the midwives did not ask for that much).

As midwifery services were not covered in her state by health insurance, the family practice doctor billed the insurance company. However because there were no complications or special equipment, the insurance paid only for a single birth. This is deplorable, when a hospital birth of a singleton cannot even be had for as little as $1,000. Ironically, the insurance probably would have paid any astronomical sum had it been incurred in the hospital. This kind of insurance reimbursement is yet another way that competence in giving birth normally is not rewarded. In the "triple high-risk" pregnancy — triplet, vaginal birth after previous Caesarean, home birth — the mother's competence and self-reliance were penalized.

Some mothers of twins have had their babies at home. Others, like noted childbirth educator and author Gail Brewer, who had two other home births, felt safer in the hospital with twins. One woman in Kansas delivered dizygotic twins at home, not without complications. Although it was her second pregnancy, the first baby took four hours to push out. The second twin's cord prolapsed, so the mother went in the knee-chest position and was given oxygen while the midwife pushed the cord back up. During the discussion about hospital transfer, when the mother was left alone, her instinct to birth the baby naturally reemerged and ten minutes later she delivered a very alert and relaxed, completely pink little girl. The first twin weighed 5½ pounds and the second 6 pounds, and they were born at forty weeks, one day after the due date. The five-foot-tall mother had eaten well in pregnancy and had gained about fifty pounds. She taught aerobics until six weeks before the birth and nursed the twins for three years.

Jeannine Parvati Baker, author of several books, including *Conscious Conception and Prenatal Yoga*, delivered her twins at home. It was her second pregnancy, and she had experienced some bleeding in early labor and went to the hospital. After the bleeding stopped, she checked herself out, went home, and delivered the babies within a few hours with the obstetrician (who had followed her home from the hospital). The second baby was breech and she describes the experience: "I had the least pain of all my births with my breech baby. It even felt to me as if this was the right way to birth rather than vertex!"

Sheila Kitzinger, noted British childbirth educator and author, elected to have her twin daughters at home. There has always been a tradition of home birth in England, endorsed by the medical profession, which dwindled as birth moved into the hospitals. Birth at home is currently being revived again there, as in Holland.

Nancy Sutherland, founder of Parents Centres in New Zealand, delivered two sets of twins. The first experience in the hospital led her to insist on a home delivery for the second set. After much searching, she found a midwife and a physician to provide back-up care if required. She delivered a breech baby and a vertex baby without complications. (One of those twins is Diony Young, a renowned childbirth activist and author in New York State). Nancy made sure she found attendants who were old enough to have had a lot of experience and also to have worked with the native Maori women so that they would have an appreciation and respect for natural birth.

Dr. Nial Ettinghausen delivered more than twenty sets of twins at home without mishap. Family practitioners, such as Dr. Greg White in Chicago, have attended home births for decades. His book *Emergency Childbirth*, written for fire fighters and police, is an excellent guide in case twins arrive at home — planned or unplanned.

One Nevada mother delivered one of her twins — "by God and me" — in the car. The doctor had time just to roll up his sleeves to catch the other twin when the mother arrived at the hospital. In Arizona, a nine-year-old boy telephoned an emergency number when his mother went into rapid labor at home. While he followed the instructions of a dispatcher, both babies were born uneventfully.

Twins are routinely delivered at home at The Farm, an alternative-lifestyle community in Tennessee. Its midwifery program has gained national and international attention for its amazing statistics

I knew I wanted to have my babies at home. We had three midwives coming to the birth, plus a friend who was a nurse, and we live five minutes from the hospital. I decided that if something so tragic or awful happened that we couldn't make it to the hospital, then we would be better off at home anyway.

of excellent outcome and low intervention. Ina May Gaskin, chief midwife and author of *Spiritual Midwifery* and *Babies, Breastfeeding, and Bonding,* explains that the usual 7- or 8-pound weights in births at The Farm are due to the quality of prenatal care and nutrition. By the end of 1988, twelve sets of twins had been born at The Farm and only two had required transfer to the hospital. None have been born by Caesarean.

The Maternity Center and its branches in El Paso, Texas, provided midwifery services for expectant mothers of twins at home or at the homelike center from its establishment in 1976 until it closed for financial reasons in 1987. The midwives had delivered more than one hundred sets of twins, with a very low rate of transfer to hospital. Many of the pregnant women were poor and high risk, so the staff at the center stressed nutrition, especially additional protein and iron.

I believe all women should be supported in their birth choices. It is much better to plan intelligently with committed caregivers than to do as one mother of twins did and trick the doctor into coming to a motel room for a "single" delivery.

It would be an interesting experiment if government authorities and researchers would take a population of expectant mothers of twins and provide them with the best possible prenatal circumstances. In this fantasy, the women and their families would live all together in pleasant surroundings for sharing and moral support. They would be provided with the freshest, natural food of a wide variety, a pool for swimming, and classes in gentle exercise, relaxation, meditation, and education for birth. Midwives would take care of the women in consultation with obstetricians, so that these expectant mothers would have the support of another woman, experienced in birth, through the entire labor and delivery. I feel sure that the problems of multiples would occur less frequently in this utopia!

13 Caesarean Section and Alternatives

BEFORE WE LOOK at the use and overuse of Caesarean delivery, I would like to explore some nonsurgical alternatives such as instrumental delivery (forceps or vacuum extraction), external version (turning the baby), and VBAC (vaginal birth after Caesarean).

Instrumental Delivery

In cases of headfirst babies who do not descend properly, Dr. Leo Sorger uses forceps or vacuum extraction in the squatting position. With forceps the doctor places metal "tongs" on the baby's head to pull the baby through the birth canal. Vacuum extraction involves a suction cup.

The squatting position avoids problems with the mother's circulation that can occur if she lies on her back with her legs in stirrups. It also has the benefits of gravity and improved drive angle of the uterus, requiring less force from the doctor.

External Version

Dr. Sorger has also successfully turned several breech twins to a headfirst position. With this technique, the mother lies in a tilted position, head down, so the babies come out of the pelvis into the abdomen. With gentle manual pressure, the doctor coaxes the baby who is breech or transverse to change position. Sometimes the midwife or woman's partner helps with another pair of hands. This procedure is usually done in the doctor's office, but if the office attempt fails the mother may choose to try again in the hospital with an injection of terbutaline to relax the uterus.

Combined Vaginal-Abdominal Delivery

Caesarean section for the second twin after the first twin has been delivered vaginally can be done as a last resort if difficulties arise. For example, the second twin may remain too high in the abdomen to be delivered vaginally or the cervix may begin to close following the first birth. If the presence of the second twin is not diagnosed prior to delivery and a drug has been given to the mother after the birth of the first twin to make the uterus contract before delivery of the placenta, fetal distress can develop in the second twin that may necessitate an emergency Caesarean. Of the mothers who responded to a 1987 *Twins* magazine survey, 4 percent had combined vaginal-Caesarean deliveries. Dr. Sorger has never needed to do a combined vaginal-abdominal delivery in any of his own multiple deliveries, but he did two such deliveries when he was called as a consultant for second twins who were in trouble. He believes that skill and confidence in breech birth and prompt delivery of the second twin avoids this unnecessary surgery.

Vaginal Birth After Caesarean (VBAC)

Many obstetricians are reluctant to consider a vaginal birth after a previous Caesarean, despite the recommendation of the American College of Obstetricians and Gynecologists. The fear is that the scar will rupture, particularly in a multiple pregnancy where more stretching of the uterus is anticipated. The transverse lower uterine incision used today, however, is stronger than the vertical or classical uterine incision done in the past. (The incision that is visible on the abdominal wall is not necessarily in the same position as it is in the uterus.) Nonetheless, some apprehensive doctors have scheduled earlier repeat Caesareans for twins than for singletons, and this unnecessary intervention before term has contributed to a higher death rate for twins.

As long ago as 1962 Dr. Alan Guttmacher described four VBACs and stated that the indications for a subsequent vaginal delivery were the same for twins as for a singleton: the absence of any conditions in the current pregnancy that constituted criteria for a Caesarean. Many obstetricians believe that the scar will withstand labor in a multiple pregnancy and thus support VBACs for mothers of twins.

A 1988 report by Flamm et al. in the *American Journal of Obstetrics and Gynecology* showed the safety of VBACs. Not one case of rupture occurred in more than 5,000 VBACs, including 89 women whose scar was of unknown origin. No case has been reported of a mother dying from rupture of a lower uterine incision. If the scar were to rupture, which is extremely rare, immediate surgery would be done to deliver the baby. What actually happens is that there is a slight opening of the scar (dehiscence), but even then the risk is only 2 percent in singleton pregnancies and 4 percent in twin pregnancies.

Some obstetricians pay lip service to the idea of "allowing" women to go into labor ("trial of labor") after a previous Caesarean but are often quick to find some reason to do another surgical delivery. The phrase "trial of labor" suggests a lack of confidence in the natural mechanisms of the birth process. Not enough doctors encourage their patients with the high success rate of VBACs, agreeing too readily to the anxious, poorly informed woman's desire for another Caesarean. Although the VBAC rate of at least 80 percent is possible, currently it is only 10 percent.

Women who want to give birth vaginally after a Caesarean should have the chance to do so with a supportive obstetrician. Not only is this important for the mother's mental and physical health, but babies need to experience labor contractions. *Different Doorway* by Jane English explores this theory in detail and explains the effect of nonlabor Caesarean birth on the developing personality of the infant.

Caesarean Section

Many obstetricians are turning to Caesarean section to avoid delivering difficult presentations vaginally and supposedly to make delivery less traumatic for very high- and low-birth-weight babies. Thus, they are becoming less experienced with breech and twin births and are more likely to continue to do Caesareans in these cases. (Several researchers, however, have found this not to be the case with low-birth-weight twins.) Premature babies do not do better after a Caesarean; on the contrary, the challenges of a vaginal birth may enhance their lung maturation and chances of survival.

The loss of one quintuplet after a Caesarean delivery at a European hospital in 1977 cautioned obstetricians in that unit against the Caesarean policy. It turned out that the highest-birth-weight baby was the only one who did not survive. The physicians concluded that nature had arranged for a certain baby to engage in the pelvis and be born first — if delivered vaginally. However, with surgical delivery this doomed baby was delivered last.

An x-ray showed that one of the triplets had a hyperextended head rather than flexed. I had a Caesarean delivery even though each baby was in a vertex position.

Numerous articles have appeared in recent medical literature to persuade obstetricians to reconsider vaginal delivery for twins. However, Caesarean section remains widespread for multiple births. The rate of Caesarean delivery in the United States has been climbing steadily and by the end of 1988 was 28 percent of all births. The National Center for Health Statistics predicted that if the present rate of escalation continues, 40 percent of deliveries will be Caesarean by the year 2000 and for women thirty-five and older, the rate will be almost 50 percent. In eleven states courts have ordered Caesareans in individual cases, overriding the mothers' wishes. Fifty-two percent of the mothers of multiples in the *Twins* magazine survey had Caesareans; only 44 percent gave birth vaginally. (The other 4 percent had combined vaginal-Caesarean delivery.) The actual Caesarean rate for twins will not be known until mid-1990 because the method of delivery was not listed on birth certificates until 1989. Samples by the National Center for Health Statistics are not helpful because twin births are too few. For many obstetricians, Caesarean section for twins is routine, and for supertwins the rate approaches 90–100 percent.

Michel Odent, an obstetrician known worldwide for his natural childbirth practices, delivered 72 sets of twins among 15,000 births while he was chief of the state hospital in Pithiviers, France. He did only six Caesareans (two of them for the second twin only), making a rate of 8.5 percent (lower than the rate of most U.S. obstetricians for singletons). His secretary had twin girls born naturally in his hospital, and she was a wonderful resource for the other mothers of twins.

The expectant mother of twins has an extremely high risk of Caesarean birth in the United States because half the time one twin is breech. The most common reason for a Caesarean section today is history of a previous Caesarean, which, as has been pointed out, is usually not a valid reason. Other reasons include abnormal labor (a loose term that encompasses "failure to progress" or "obstetrician distress," especially if the doctor expects an "overstretched" uterus to "fail to progress") or prematurity. Many obstetricians consider multiple pregnancy per se an indication for Caesarean birth! Pelvic disproportion, another cause for Caesarean in singleton births, rarely occurs with twins because the babies are often smaller than singletons. However, maternal disease, such as herpes, diabetes, and pregnancy-induced hypertension may require Caesarean birth.

Surgical delivery should be done only for special problems such as fetal distress, prolapsed cord, placenta previa (in which the placenta blocks the cervical opening), transverse lie presentation of the

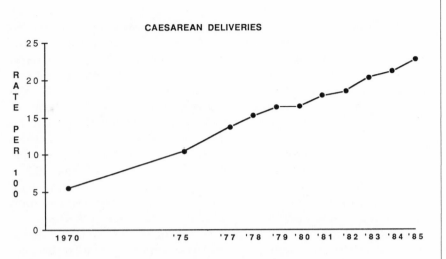

CAESAREAN DELIVERIES

RATE PER 100

25
20
15
10
5
0

1970   '75   '77 '78 '79 '80 '81 '82 '83 '84 '85

The Caesarean rate has been escalating alarmingly in the past two decades.
Source: National Center for Health Statistics.

first multiple,* and placental abruption (premature detachment of the placenta).

Delivery of twins by Caesarean is not without risk to the babies. Respiratory distress may be increased without the squeezing of the chest and lungs and other stimulation that occurs during vaginal delivery. Either baby can suffer trauma during a Caesarean, especially if a breech baby is wedged in the pelvis. Parents are often unprepared for the amount of physical manipulation doctors may have to do — it is not simply a matter of making a cut and lifting out the babies. Texas obstetrician Ronald Cole offers an "ultimate Caesarean birth experience." Believing that babies are highly aware, he describes what is happening while calm music plays and the lights are dimmed. It is important for the doctor or the father (but he may be too overwhelmed at a Caesarean) to talk to the babies and explain what is happening. If you know you will be having a Caesarean, begin right away to prepare your babies for this type of birth experience. New York psychiatrist Rima Laibow was amazed one day when her young son suddenly asked her why, when he was born, the people looking down at him had "half-faces" (wearing masks)!

A 1988 study in San Francisco found no difference between Caesarean and vaginal delivery with regard to perinatal mortality, need for resuscitation, duration of newborn stay in the hospital, or trauma. A 1987 report in Israel did not regard breech presentation of the second twin as an indication for Caesarean section; nor is this recommended by skillful obstetricians.

I did not want a Caesarean unless the babies were in danger. A sonogram revealed that they were both head down; my doctor still wanted to do a C section, but I finally got my way.

* An experienced obstetrician can turn a transverse lie second twin by internal version.

Dr. Marilyn Riese of the Louisville Twin Study reported in 1988 that Caesareans did not offer any advantages or disadvantages for infants that she followed up. The only difference observed between Caesarean and non-Caesarean twins was that the preterm Caesarean infant was more active during sleep, and this activity was related to temperament at eight, eighteen, and twenty-four months of age.

Cetrulo's 1986 study claims that Caesareans have decreased the perinatal mortality rate of twins with other than headfirst presentations to that of singletons and have eliminated the differential in mortality between first-born and second-born twins. Other, larger studies have shown no improvement in perinatal outcome with increasing use of Caesarean section. I am convinced that the length of gestation is more relevant to perinatal mortality than the mode of delivery.

A 1981 study found that the fetal outcome for triplets and quadruplets was similar whether they were delivered vaginally or by Caesarean at any point during the pregnancy. The risk of maternal death during Caesarean section is from 3 to 11 times higher than with vaginal delivery. A study in the *Journal of the American Medical Association* reported 1 to 2 maternal deaths per 1,000 operations. Morbidity (nonfatal complications) are 8 to 10 times higher than after vaginal birth.

Recovery from major surgery is an added burden to the mother. Although no muscles are cut and the incision may be very low in the abdomen, just above the pubic hair (bikini cut), the trauma makes it harder to get your very stretched abdominal muscles back to their original length and strength.

Interview your doctor carefully about his or her feelings about these issues and his or her usual practices. Hoping for the best is not enough; unnecessary Caesareans have to be actively prevented. You will remember your birth experience forever; so will your babies. You want them to enter the world spontaneously, without unnecessary drugs or surgery. Be prepared to change physicians or hospitals and to write letters to hospitals, the Board of Health, politicians, and others to achieve the birth setting you desire.

Caesarean Section Procedures

Caesarean delivery is usually performed under regional anesthesia — a spinal or epidural* (described in Chapter 12) — so that the mother

* If the mother has had an epidural prior to the Caesarean. If she has not, the quicker spinal will be done. Spinal anesthesia, in contrast to epidural, will often paralyze some respiratory muscles, which leads to feelings of restriction or suffocation. Despite these sensations, breathing is invariably adequate.

How to Avoid a Caesarean

1. Choose a physician who is completely committed to natural childbirth and who is comfortable and successful with vaginal breech delivery and versions (turning the babies before or during delivery). Beware of "wait and see" attitudes; ask for statistics. Your doctor should inspire you with confidence and have trust in the birth process, and his or her Caesarean rate should be under 10 percent.

2. Make sure that you have excellent nutrition throughout your pregnancy to have the best chance of carrying your twins or triplets to term.

3. Have optimal labor support by a midwife or other experienced birth professional, in addition to your partner, even if you have to find and pay the midwife yourself.

4. Stay upright and mobile during your labor as much as possible. Determine beforehand whether your doctor and hospital support active birth squatting and other positions to deliver both vertex and breech babies.

5. Choose a hospital where you have the freedom to eat, drink, and walk around as you wish during labor.

6. Be as informed as you can about birth and medical interventions. Choose private childbirth classes that are oriented toward you, the consumer, rather than those offered by the hospital that may emphasize interventions.

7. Write a birth plan like the example in Appendix 2.

8. Explore, with assistance if possible, any unresolved issues that you have about birth, fear of labor, previous abortions, unplanned conception, imprints from your own experiences of being born, or problems with your partner. (See Resources.)

9. Communicate with your babies throughout the pregnancy and labor. Let them know that you trust the birth process and their ability to be born in their own style.

10. Believe in your own power, strength, and knowledge to birth your babies naturally.

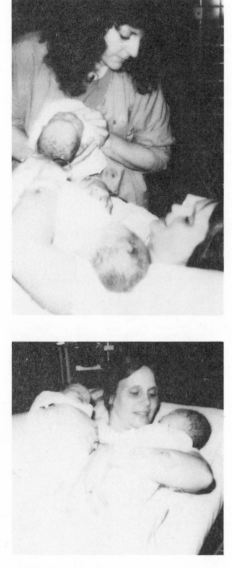

Regional anesthesia means that the mother can be awake and aware to greet her newborns.

is awake and can share the event with her partner. Thanks to the tireless efforts of consumers and childbirth education groups like C/ Sec, Inc., and the Cesarean Prevention Movement, partners are now allowed to be present, which enhances parental attachment to the babies. In the event of complications, the mother needs the support and presence of her partner. It is not always possible to find supportive doctors and hospitals, but do shop around.

The pubic hair is shaved for a Caesarean, and most incisions today are a "bikini cut," which is covered when the hair grows back.

An intravenous is always given prior to surgery, and a blood pressure cuff is wrapped around one upper arm, as blood pressure tends to fall when regional anesthesia is used. Oxygen is administered and a catheter will be inserted into the bladder.

General anesthesia is used only if there is a great need for speed or some problem with the mother's backbone, such as a spinal fusion, that prevents administration of the regional anesthesia. Prior to the anesthetic gas, sodium pentothal or a similar drug is administered through the IV to put you to sleep. Then a tube is placed in your throat (which is why your throat may be a little sore the next day) for the anesthetic gas. To diminish the effects of the anesthesia on the babies, the anesthesia is given as late as possible.

The actual birth takes only minutes. Although you will not feel pain, you will be aware of pressure and tugging sensations, especially if the babies are firmly wedged in your pelvis and take some effort on the part of the obstetrician to get them out. If the lower twin lies transverse, a vertical (classical) incision may be made in the uterus. After the delivery, completing the uterine and abdominal closures can take up to an hour. Sutures or staples may be used and removed up to eight days later, although dissolvable stitches are more comfortable. Pitocin is added to the IV after the surgery to make the uterus contract, preventing hemorrhage.

If you had regional anesthesia and the babies are in good condition, you should be able to fondle and nurse them before the anesthesia has worn off; otherwise you might be distracted by pain. Ask for TENS — transcutaneous electrical nerve stimulation — usually administered by a physical therapist. This is a small battery-operated unit with electrodes that are placed on each side of your incision. Electrical currents are delivered to the skin and travel faster to your brain than the slower sensations of pain; the effect is rather like scratching an itch. The increased comfort from TENS means less or no need for narcotics, which pass into the breast milk.

Some hospitals routinely place Caesarean babies in the nursery

Essential Exercises Following Caesarean Birth

Commence as soon as you recover from the anesthetic. Do each exercise twice to start, progressing at your own pace through the phases. Relax and breathe deeply between each exercise. The sequence can be repeated in reverse order.

Phase I

1. Breathing Exercises: upper chest, mid-chest, diaphragmatic with abdominal-wall-tightening.

2. Huffing. These two are very important if general anesthesia was used and will help prevent gas pain.

3. Foot Exercises: bend, stretch, rotate.

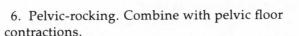

4. Leg-Bracing: tense and relax legs. Continue these for as long as you are confined to bed.

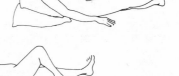

Phase II

5. Bending and straightening alternate knee.

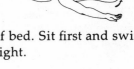

6. Pelvic-rocking. Combine with pelvic floor contractions.

Before standing: Bend knees; use arms to turn toward edge of bed. Sit first and swing feet a few times. Brace abdominal muscles as you stand upright.
Posture check.

Add Phase III

7. Bridge and twist.

8. Reach to the knees.

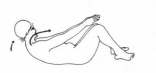

Add Phase IV

Check for separation of the recti muscles. Check stopping and starting the urine flow.

9. Straight curl-up.

10. Leg-Sliding.

11. Diagonal curl-up.

12. Relaxation on front when comfort permits.

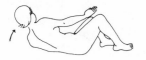

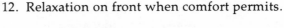

Phase V

Progressive abdominal exercises.

My abdominal skin was extremely sensitive. I nearly screamed from the pain as I moved in the bed. I know other mothers of multiples who had the same weird experience.

After the birth of my twins, it was obvious that my abdominal wall was too weak to support my spine. I felt dizzy and nauseated if I tried to stand or walk even a few steps without a binder. My doctor said no exercises for six weeks, so all I could do was wear a girdle. I know I would have gotten around much better if I had exercised.

I was very dissatisfied with the hospital treatment I received after my Caesarean. They refused to give me any pain medication, so I never got to sleep. Once the twins arrive, the staff don't seem to care about Mother anymore. I could have used a lot more support and help trying to care for both babies after the surgery.

for observation. Ask to have your babies with you if there is no medical problem.

Nursing after a Caesarean is not only possible but highly desirable. It may be a little slower to get started after general anesthesia. Sucking stimulates the uterus to contract so that it recovers faster, and nursing a Caesarean or premature baby always raises the mother's self-esteem. She feels that even though the birth did not turn out as planned, at least she can fulfill an important biological function and satisfy mutual emotional needs. Rooming-in is one positive way to use the extra time you will need to remain in the hospital. You will enjoy extra contact with the babies as breastfeeding becomes established. Hospitals now permit sibling visitation, which is even more necessary after the separation caused by surgery. An electric bed is a necessity, not a luxury, especially with twins. Caesarean mothers also appreciate sharing a room with a woman who has had a Caesarean rather than a vaginal birth.

For more information about Caesareans, see Suggested Reading or contact C/Sec, Inc., or Cesarean Prevention Movement, whose addresses are in Resources. Detailed information on clearing the chest after surgery with general anesthesia or if you had a cold may be found in the chapter on Caesarean birth in my book *Essential Exercises for the Childbearing Year*. Deep breathing, ''huffing'' (a deep, rapid, forced outward breath instead of a cough), and abdominal contractions are important to prevent the formation of gas. In the absence of normal intestinal movement (which temporarily ceases after the surgery), gas accumulates in your abdomen. This can be extremely painful, especially around the third day. Deep breathing and abdominal wall tightening exercises, which help substitute for the lack of peristalsis, should begin in the recovery room.

Rehabilitation after Caesarean birth, especially for mothers of multiples, with their more distended abdominal muscles, is essential. It must be started immediately, although unfortunately mothers are often advised to wait six weeks before beginning an exercise program. In the hospital, demand to see a physical therapist who can evaluate and supervise your program. Those first few days are very important, so don't waste them. Although you may feel ill, depressed, and in pain, pulling your body back together is the first step before you can start caring for your new multiples and other children. (See Chapter 12 and the chart of exercises on page 229.)

14 | Bonding with Multiples

THE PROCESS OF PARENT-INFANT attachment has received much attention in recent years thanks to the pioneering work of pediatricians Marshall Klaus and John Kennell and obstetrician Frederick Leboyer. Most hospitals now recognize the importance of bonding and encourage contact between parents and offspring immediately after birth. Some maternity care professionals, however, are still quick to separate mothers and infants. Remember, they are *your* babies.

The term ''bonding'' implies a seal or a process of attachment, apt associations for understanding the significance of this postpartum stage. However, bonding does not always take place automatically, and mothers anxiously awaiting the experience may feel guilt or disappointment if it is not attained according to their expectations.

Ideally, babies should experience a smooth transition from life inside the uterus to life outside, with as few changes as possible. Therefore, skin-to-skin contact is important while an infant is carried, bathed, rocked, and nursed. But we live in an imperfect world where ideals, while they should be strived for, cannot always be achieved. So if you had a Caesarean or your babies have some problem that necessitates that they be taken from you for hours or even days after birth, do not worry. Human beings are adaptable and you will be able to bond with them, especially if you have developed a good foundation of prenatal bonding.

Prenatal Bonding

Everyone would agree that all newborns have distinct personalities, yet most find it hard to believe that those personalities form during the nine months of pregnancy. Books such as *The Secret Life of the Unborn Child* by psychiatrist Thomas Verny, *Babies Remember Birth* by psychologist David Chamberlain, *Life Before Life* by psychologist Helen Wambach, and my forthcoming *Inside Experiences* tell us that babies are aware of a great deal within the uterus. They sense whether they are wanted, whether they are the gender their parents desire, whether mother is planning to leave father, or if she is still grieving a prior miscarriage.

As we saw in Chapter 6, bonding begins in the prenatal phase (which mothers always knew and researchers are just discovering!). Mothers who lose one baby through miscarriage or stillbirth can describe how much they had already bonded with that baby. If two or more babies were present, two or more bonds existed. Mothers of twins generally have a clear perception of each baby, its individual position, level of activity, and sometimes the gender.

Surrogate mothers, who are trying *not* to bond, nevertheless do so at an unconscious level. One mother who conceived twins and relinquished them to her sister-in-law for adoption described to me how she hardly slept the last few weeks of the pregnancy because "there was so little time left to be with them and I didn't want to miss any of it." One surrogate mother felt relieved to discover that she was carrying twins because she knew that when they went to their new home, they would have each other.

In the past, twins were commonly separated by adoption and the mothers who relinquished them were treated with little sensitivity by social service personnel and adoption agencies. Frequently, they were not consulted about separation since adoptions were generally closed and anonymous. Today adoption agencies are more cognizant of the twin bonds and have discontinued such separations.

Because mothers carry their offspring within their bodies, bonds are experienced on an intuitive and hormonal level as well as a conscious one. The mother identifies with the child while it is in her body and the desired result is an expanded sense of self. The challenge is for a mother of twins to expand her identification to include two babies. Parents can bond with twins prenatally through physical touching and games, singing, meditation, prayer, visualization — whatever means they choose that unites them emotionally and spiritually with their babies. Initially, it may be a challenge to realize that there are in fact two babies. Parents can take turns making contact with one of the babies or work together as a pair bonding with a pair. This process will change and evolve as they distinguish differences between the unborn babies. The challenge is not to view the babies collectively — as two halves of a whole — or, the other extreme, to see them as diametrically opposite. Often mothers of triplets regard them as a pair plus one and after birth one triplet frequently is the odd one out, for both good and bad reasons.

Ideal bonding starts with conscious conception, which is ex-

When everyone learned I was having twins as a surrogate, they were much more interested and supportive. I guess twins just made the whole arrangement seem way out. People would say, "Now there will be one for the other family and one for you," but that never entered my mind. I wanted the twins to be together.

I knew from the ultrasound that the upper baby was a girl. The gender of the other baby was not identified. Throughout the pregnancy I used to stroke the top of my belly, talking and humming to Sarah. After the birth I immediately felt a strong bond with Sarah but Susan seemed always whining and demanding, especially needing to be touched a great deal.

plained in a book of that name by Jeannine Parvati Baker and explored in a forthcoming book of mine, *Channel for a New Life*. However, for the already pregnant readers of this book, I will now consider the factors that play a role in early attachment and suggest ways in which the bonds can be initiated and strengthened.

Diagnosis/Disclosure

Parents' ease in adjusting to the news of an extra baby or babies depends greatly on the timing of their discovery and the manner in which it is conveyed. The public is aware of the great impact of the news because the most common question that mothers are asked is "When did you find out you were having twins (or triplets)?"

As we saw earlier, most mothers of twins do suspect that they are carrying multiples. However, the confirmation of this intuition can still present some problems. As I warned in Chapter 11, sometimes the unconscious bonds with the babies are so fragile that a woman goes into premature labor shortly after learning the diagnosis. The news should be disclosed with the utmost sensitivity, in an open-ended session, with ongoing support including immediate contact with parents of multiples. Joking over the ultrasound machine is an undesirable form of disclosure.

Ideally, the multiple pregnancy should be diagnosed at least by the second trimester so that parents have several months to prepare adequately for the babies and the health care providers can make necessary arrangements for special care. Obviously, the more information and support that can be gathered, the better. Good planning for the postpartum period is essential.

If ultrasound and amniocentesis are performed, the couple should benefit from as much information as possible. Why should the lab technician know that you are carrying monozygotic boys and not inform you and your partner? There will be enough surprises around the birth! With knowledge of the babies' genders, you can name them and get to know them on a more personal basis, thus enhancing the prenatal bond.

Nutrition

Eating well and carrying your babies to term are very important for optimal bonding. Good nutrition before and after the birth can also prevent fatigue, one of the factors that further impairs bonding. Pre-

It was a big shock to me when I saw on the ultrasound that I was carrying twins. Worse, though, was the news that one baby was very small and had a major congenital defect. I felt very ambivalent. It was hard to enjoy the celebrity status of expecting twins when I secretly hoped that the malformed twin would not live. I actually searched around for a physician who would not perform heroic rescue measures. When this baby did survive, I had a terrible time trying to bond with him.

maturity interrupts the prenatal bonding phase. Then, since low-birth-weight babies are usually kept in an isolette, they are separated from the mother after birth as well. The appearance of premature babies can make bonding difficult.

Counseling and Support Before and After the Birth

Obviously the best role models are other mothers of twins or triplets, and expectant parents should contact twin families and attend Mothers of Twins Club meetings before the birth. Empathetic counselors can also make a significant contribution. (Twin Services in California offers free telephone counseling, 10 A.M.–4 P.M. Pacific standard time, on its Twinline; see Resources.) With adequate preparation and ongoing support, mothers of twins can be open to receiving and loving two babies.

Postpartum Bonding

Bonding, as we have seen, occurs on a continuum from conception to birth. The moment of birth happens to be one of the key points along the road where peak emotions facilitate deep attachment. Shock and negative experiences in pregnancy and birth should be avoided. The more directly the mother can experience each event of the pregnancy and birth, the more power she has to follow her natural instincts. If things happen too fast or without the mother's full understanding, she may withdraw and become less conscious of events and feelings, leading to "missing pieces" in her recollection of these important events.

Any such unfulfilled transitions during the childbearing year inhibit the mother's freedom to explore the subtleties of any birth experience, especially a multiple birth experience. Because twin and other multiple births are often considered high risk, anxieties, emotional shocks, and physical traumas that change the parents' hopes and plans are not uncommon. For example, late diagnosis or a sudden Caesarean section do not allow adequate time for psychological processing of the change of plans. After the birth the parents may find a lack of support and understanding of the impact and adjustment involved with a multiple birth. It is crucial to avoid any unnecessary intervention in the birth process, as one interference can lead to many others.

Bonding After Normal Delivery

A pediatrician and a nurse for each baby as well as for the mother will be in the delivery room. You may want to handle just one baby at a time at first, but you need to hold both to affirm the reality of birthing two babies.

Babies in good condition will be placed skin-to-skin on the mother and may begin nursing at this time. Drops or ointment in the babies' eyes should be avoided if you are sure you don't have gonor-rhea, or at least they should be delayed as long as possible — hospi-tals will usually wait twenty-four hours — until parents have had a long, intimate time together to get acquainted with their newborns with good eye contact.

It was a "magical experience" to be nursing one baby while laboring with the second.

Bonding After a Caesarean

With regional anesthesia mothers can be awake and aware when their twins are delivered by Caesarean. Unfortunately, many Caesarean babies are placed in the intensive care nursery for 24 hours of routine observation, delaying the bonding process. It has been found that Caesarean mothers who were routinely separated from their infants in the past were more likely to abuse them later. But it is unclear whether this is due to the separation or the Caesarean.

Even though time is short when an emergency Caesarean is being set up, it is important to explain what is happening to the ba-bies, to reassure them that they will be delivered safely, if not in the way they instinctively anticipated their birth. It would be helpful if maternity care providers could provide emotional support for the par-ents, helping them to express disappointment and self-forgiveness. In my experience, mothers who have gone through a Caesarean with this kind of support do not experience the typical feelings of guilt, resentment, and other unfinished psychological business that linger for months or years afterward. These mothers can get right on with affirming and enjoying their babies' existence. Unfortunately, many maternity care providers are drawn to the profession to heal their own unconscious birth anxiety. They are not available to support you with yours at a time of crisis because they are unconsciously repress-ing their own primal pain — usually with "efficient activity."

Breast-feeding after a Caesarean helps mothers restore their self-esteem and hormonally assists mother-infant attachment. It is na-ture's way of continuing the process of bonding begun prenatally.

We simply refused the eye drops and just were overwhelmed by the magnificence of our babies' eyes. They looked so calm and wise!

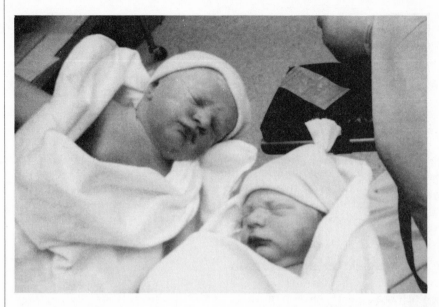

With identical babies, it is easier to bond with the unit at first.

I found it difficult to bond with the unexpected twin, as all through my pregnancy I had related to just one baby.

It took me many months to feel that I had really become attached to each baby. I'm sure it would have been easier if I had held them both right after birth. The hospital staff want to be helpful and take over much of their care, but it is better if they help you with each baby so the bonding process gets off to a good start.

The hospital nursery interferes in this continuum with its bright fluorescent lights, the crying of other babies, the separation of twins from mother and co-twin, and often the swaddling of infants to prevent movement. Keep your babies with you if they are healthy.

Rooming-in with both babies facilitates attachment and breast-feeding. If the infants are bottle-feeding, it is particularly important to establish close eye and body contact (skin-to-skin as much as possible). Ongoing physical contact can be achieved by sharing the family bed and the family bath, by massaging the babies, and by wearing baby carriers (one in front and one in back, or a baby per partner).

So much equipment today is designed to separate mothers from their babies. Playpens, swings, and jolly jumpers are useful at busy times, especially for mothers of multiples, but babies prefer and need body contact. Spend some time alone with each baby, bathing, nursing, playing, and repeating his or her name, as well as with the babies together.

Postpartum Support

New parents, in the absence of complications, do not need medical care, but they do need rest, good food, and lots of help. A first-class

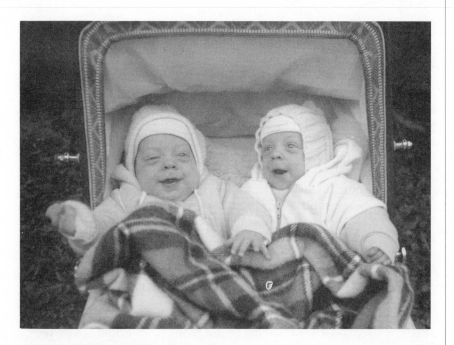

Next, parents search for differences.

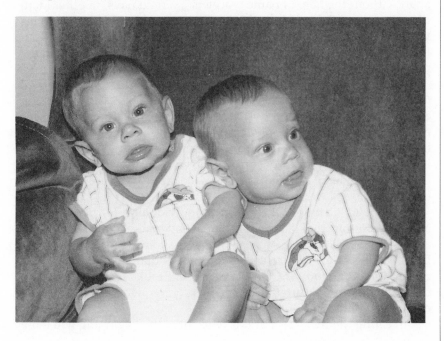

hotel is much cheaper than a hospital. The bathroom is close, the sheets are changed daily, and the food will be much better. You will have privacy without curious visitors. I strongly recommend that you ask family members who want to give a gift to consider a hotel stay! (Postpartum with the babies, two years later without them.) Some health insurance companies pay for "mother care" at home if you leave the hospital early. Ideally, expectant parents of twins will have extra labor support from a midwife, and that support should be continued for the first days or weeks at home.

New parents need help with household chores so they are free to rest and enjoy the babies, but ongoing emotional support is equally important. Some mothers of twins have a friend or relative stay for the first week after birth to fulfill both needs. Mothering the mother is the best way to promote attachment and to establish breast-feeding. It would be a wonderful experience for an expectant mother of twins to spend a week or two helping a new mother of multiples. There is so much more that we can do as women to help each other without hiring experts.

You need help, more help, and even more help!

It takes time for mothers to bond with more than one baby, and at first it may be easier to attach to the twins or the triplets as a unit. It may be impossible for the parents themselves to tell the babies apart without the help of name bracelets, painted nails, or other identifying marks. (Don't admit this in front of the babies — the twins will hear it all their lives if they look identical!) When feelings of attachment and parental self-confidence are strong and secure, then the parents can begin to differentiate individual personalities.

Pediatrician Marshall Klaus and Karen Gromada, a mother of twins and the editor of *DoubleTalk,* emphasize the necessity of making comparisons and finding physical and personality differences to see the babies as separate people. Gromada points out that dressing babies alike may actually help the attachment process and lead to earlier individualization. The advice to avoid comparing the babies and dressing them alike can make mothers feel guilty because it is almost impossible to follow.

Monozygotic twins take longer to individualize for two reasons. Not only do they look alike, but they behave more similarly than dizygotic twins. Moreover, they may reverse roles from time to time. In a 1987 interview with *Twins* magazine, pediatrician T. Berry Brazelton quoted a study in which researchers took 70 minutes to perceive the behavioral differences between twins, whereas their mothers needed only 15 minutes.

Treating the twins as a unit is efficient at the beginning while the mother sorts out the differences between them. While it is important to handle, play with, and photograph the babies alone as well as together, too much emphasis on individuality can put great pressure on parents as they try to meet the demands of their twins with different schedules and different levels of development.

Complications

A negative birth experience can be detrimental to bonding in the same way that a good birth experience promotes maternal self-esteem and confidence. Sometimes the birth may proceed smoothly for the first baby but complications develop with the second that require assistance with instruments or even a Caesarean delivery. The second twin may also need to be rushed to intensive care or to another hospital while the first may not.

Hospitalization of One or More Multiples

It is difficult for parents to bond with an infant in intensive care, as they understandably wish to protect themselves from a potential loss. They typically refer to the baby as "it." But even if the baby does die, the healthiest process is for the parents to love and affirm the baby's existence, however brief, so that they can let him or her go peacefully and can move on with their lives. Parents may receive less than adequate support in the case of death or disability of one or more babies. If the grieving process is delayed, then so too will be the attachment to the living baby or babies. For this reason the grief must be acknowledged and supported. (Chapter 17 discusses the experience of loss in detail.)

Labels such as "premature" and "brain-damaged" or incorrect identification of zygosity can have an impact long after the birth and can interfere with parental attachment and with the children's self-esteem. Pediatrician Elizabeth Bryan, author of *Twins in the Family*, stresses that "uncertainty is agonizing and is made worse if the parents feel that something is being hidden. For instance, when the doctor is plainly worried but continues to say that all is well."

Photographs of the baby or babies are essential if they are confined in the intensive care nursery, and one picture of both babies together is ideal. When possible, the mother and father should stay in the hospital to provide care and contact. Babies can tell their own

My triplets came home from the hospital one at a time, and I felt this staggered timing was a great help in allowing me to know and bond to each baby in turn.

I think twins bond so strongly with each other that they don't need mother-father bonding as much — or they use mother-father bonding to a different purpose.

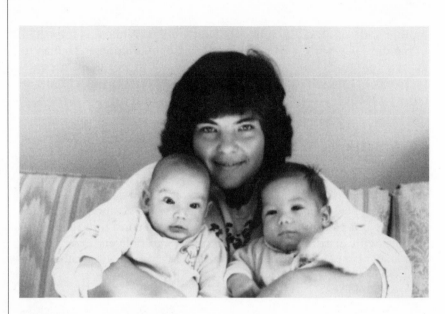

Bonding is easier when twins look different.

mothers by smell (through chemicals called pheromones), as shown in the film *The Amazing Newborn*, and the parent-infant bond is an important constant when the babies are exposed to multiple caretakers. Parents can visualize their love and energy going out to their babies when they are physically separated and keep the emotional and spiritual ties strong.

If a mother has a tendency to attach more to the first-born (some mothers experience the second baby as an ''extra''), she certainly tends to bond more strongly with the baby who comes home first. If the babies must be separated to come home, not only will the relationship between the mother and the second-born likely suffer, but it may carry over and impair the twin bond as well. Some mothers, however, like the gradual adjustment that separate homecomings provides.

Mothers almost always experience unresolved feelings about pregnancy, the birth experience, and the transition to mothering twins. Mothers of multiples often feel socially and psychologically isolated as well as physically burdened. Priorities must be set so that the mother can realize her human limitations and avoid the guilt and anxiety that she is ''not doing enough.'' A mother needs to be reassured that it is better to confront and work through any negative feelings than to suppress them. A baby always senses the truth of the situation whether before or after birth. Expressing and sharing this truth heals the relationship.

Differences in appearance may not be observable in monozygotic twins, and while they respond similarly to their environment, there will always be differences in personality and temperament. A better position in the uterus may give one twin an advantage for nutrition, movement, or touch from the mother. The effect of the environment after birth is not necessarily the same, especially if the mother, for example, favors the first-born, the one with lighter birth weight, or the one who came home first.

A 1988 Italian video study of a mother with her two monozygotic first-born girls showed quite a variance of gazing and smiling patterns for each member of the pair; one twin was ten times more reciprocal.

There is sometimes a conflict about how to treat twins differently yet fairly and if not with the same kind of attention, at least with the same amount. But meeting the needs of each twin will constantly vary.

Parents often feel that because their love is divided between two babies, each one is getting only half of what he or she would as a

I had a hard time believing the twins were mine for keeps. I felt I was just babysitting them for someone else.

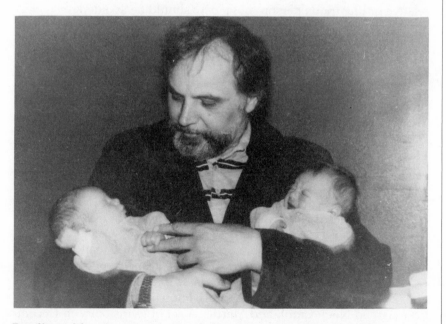

Bonding with twins means extra challenges . . . and extra rewards.

singleton. But parents do learn to fully love more than one child, even when the children arrive all at once. Twin parents can be reassured by compensating factors such as the special bond between the multiples themselves and the lifelong extra attention from outsiders. Also, parents of twins receive double love in return, and the father is typically (and essentially!) much more involved than with a singleton where the maternal-infant bond tends to be more exclusive.

Naming

Infant names are usually finalized before you leave the hospital. Each state has its own requirement for completion of the birth certificate and if you wish to change the names later a fee is involved.

If you knew about the twins in advance, you will probably have picked out a number of names. Most couples have a few alternatives for a single birth, but with the arrival of unexpected multiples they may change their minds and choose names that are "twinlike." It's a good idea to have at least two male and two female names before the birth, and three may come in handy in case a triplet was hidden on your ultrasound. Favoritism in one name, such as that of a special relative or illustrious person, obviously should be avoided.

We chose Ezekiel and Zachariah for our twin sons' names. We call them Zeke and Zach for short.

Every individual's identity is connected in some way with his or her name, so the choice of names needs careful consideration. Although twins are part of a pair, and they share that social unit, their names should be clearly their own. "Tweedledee and Tweedledum" names, which emphasize twinship over individuality, do not help the process of differentiation, and parents as well as children often regret them later. Avoid rhyming names like Rigby and Digby, Marlene and Darlene, Elaine and Germaine, Helen and Ellen, Dale and Gale, Wendy and Wanda, Ronald and Donald. Also avoid names that may not rhyme but are clearly couplets: George and Georgia, Robert and Roberta, Francis and Francine. Occasionally parents favor fancy names of famous couples such as Samson and Delilah, Mary and Joseph, and, for triplets, Franklin, Delano, and Roosevelt, or Faith, Hope, and Charity, or just Tom, Dick, and Harry. Frequently multiples share names with the same first letter: Jenny and Joanne; Richard and Roland; Timmy, Tommy, and Tammy. All such combinations can cause confusion. I know of a set of quadruplets called Annette, Suzette, Bernadette, and Yvette. Triplets born on Christmas Day have been named Noel, Carol, and Merrie. A set of twins born on December 7, 1941, were called Pearl and Harbor. Birth order is sometimes indicated in the names, as in Anthony and Barrie or Oliver and Timothy. More obvious are the triplet names Primo, Secondo, and Terzo (first, second, and third in Italian).

Repeat the infant's name as often as possible to confirm his or her identity and enhance bonding. Another reason for repeating the name at every opportunity is that multiples themselves are often slower than singletons to refer to themselves by name.

Bonding and Gender

In most cases, parental bonding is easiest with a boy-girl pair and hardest with babies who look alike. However, some women have strong gender preferences, especially if they already have other children, and these expectations may or may not be fulfilled in their twins. Ideally, disappointment about the sex of the babies can be worked out prenatally, now that technology can often verify gender. However, as I have said before, own and explore your feelings. Don't deny them. They will gradually change.

I didn't feel as close to the boy twin as the girl, but I made a special effort to try to see his positive attributes.

Do not try to hide facts that the baby or babies may have picked up in the uterus. It is far better that a mother say, "You know, I didn't want two more girls, but now that I know you as the special people you are, I wouldn't change you for anyone else in the world," than that she deny her initial feelings of disappointment. It is harder to love a baby of the less preferred sex or one with a defect, and it won't get any easier until the real feelings are addressed and the attachment can begin to unfold and flourish. Gender disappointment is very common. I have led groups for expectant and new parents to address this issue and have been amazed at the enrollment!

Changing Attachment

Twins often have very different personalities, and there is nothing wrong in feeling differently toward them. Feelings are feelings; it is how we express them in our behavior that counts. Parents typically favor one twin over the other at different times, so the favored twin or multiple changes frequently anyway. Understanding this process makes it easier for parents to spontaneously express their feelings. Twins, like all siblings, must learn to take turns, and this concept can be introduced from the very beginning. Often mothers of twins have said that their babies seem to understand the situation!

In response to that often-asked question about favoritism, I have to admit, yes, I do have a favorite. My favorite twin is the one who gives me a piece of grilled cheese sandwich from his mouth, the one who picks up and comforts his brother, the one who watches the bird on the windowsill.

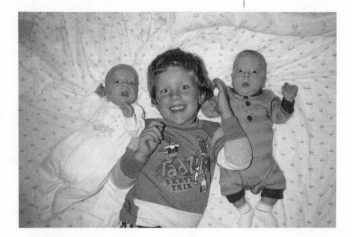 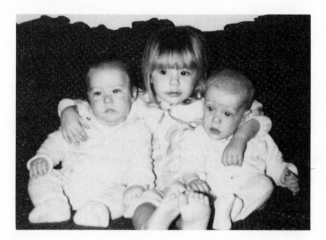

Older siblings enjoy the twin bond too.

A mother may favor one twin because she feels guilty for having favored the other in the uterus, just as a parent may give more attention to a fussy baby while benignly neglecting the other. It is far better for a mother to say, "I couldn't hold you after the birth because you needed special care away from me, and I need to hold you right now to make up for that," than to continue to feel distanced from one of her babies. Of course, she wants to protect herself against those negative feelings of frustrations and disappointment, but if she is still carrying that kind of emotional baggage, she needs to let it go.

Bonding with multiples is a challenge with fantastic rewards. Only families with multiples have the opportunity to experience both the bond between babies and the bond between the multiple unit and other siblings too. Although each family will have its own difficulties and compensations, they can take pride in the fact that they belong to a special group where God surely chooses the members!

15 Caring for Two When You Get Home

MOST MOTHERS LEAVE the hospital on the third or fourth postpartum day, although earlier discharge is becoming popular. Mothers of twins often like to prolong the period during which others are bringing them meals, assisting with baby care, and providing regular rest — especially if there are other children at home. (Consider a hotel; see Chapter 14.) If you had the twins at home, your family unit has not been interrupted and neighbors and friends ideally will provide help. Call Careteam or Gentle Care (see Resources) to determine your eligibility for home help.

Experienced mothers have the advantage of confidence and knowing what to expect from newborns. First-time mothers are learning their skills under more difficult circumstances with twins, although they do not have extra siblings to care for as well. Some think that raising twins is easier because when the behavior of one might worry them, if two are doing the same thing, they figure it is normal. This chapter presents an overview of the special aspects of caring for multiples. Further information on child care can be found in the multitude of books for parents today, some of which are listed in Suggested Reading. Specific details on raising multiples can be found in the many Mothers of Twins Clubs publications, *The Care of Twin Children* by Theroux and Tingley, and *The Joy of Raising Twins* by Pamela Novotny.

During pregnancy the body had many months to prepare for the various changes it underwent and ultimately for the birth itself. Afterward, the changes take place in hours and days. Physiological adaptations must merge with the psychological anticlimax that often follows an exciting and long-anticipated event. Hormone levels change as the milk comes in around the third day after birth. All of these changes, including the arrival of two babies, can make the most placid mother feel overwhelmed and depressed. If her partner is unable to lend much support, it is essential that the budget be manipulated where possible to arrange for some household help. The first

"If It's Quiet, I Must Be Sleeping!"

A is for the alarm clock that I don't need anymore.

B is for behavioral psychology. I've thrown the book out the window; the only one being conditioned was me.

C is for colic and cheese curls. They go together; the louder the babies cry, the more cheese curls I eat.

D is for diet — the one I need after all of the cheese curls.

E is for exercise to go with the diet. I've said good-bye to the health club. The most exercise I get now is chewing a bagel.

F is for the 5:00 shadows — the one on Dad's face because there's no time to shave and the twin who thinks that 5 a.m. is the very best time of day.

G is the *The Gong Show* — the only thing that is on TV when I'm up with the five o'clock shadow.

H is for humor. "Keep your sense of humor" was the only piece of sensible advice I received after my twins were born.

I is for insomnia — something that I don't have to worry about any more.

J is for justice — something that my father prayed for when I was busy giving him white hair; I wish he hadn't prayed so hard.

K is for kangaroo — the one that I feel like after I've walked around with a baby in a carrier all day long.

L is for *Love Boat* reruns — the favorite show of the night owl, the twin sister of the 5:00 shadow.

M is for mess — the household variety.

N is for the night owl who believes that midnight is the very best time of day. N is also for nosey neighbors who can't imagine how you can cope so they wake you up to see how you are doing.

O is for the obstetrician — the one who told you that you were absolutely, positively, only having one baby.

P is for the pediatrician — the one whose kids you'll put through college.

Q is for quiet that there is little of; if it's quiet, then I must be sleeping.

R is for romance — something that I used to enjoy when I spent more than two hours a night in bed.

S is for sitters who are highly enthusiastic at the beginning of an evening and shell-shocked at the end of their stay.

T is for taxes — at least this year we'll have extra deductions.

U is for all of the things that I used to do — I used to knit. I used to take long naps. I used to sleep 8 hours a night. I used to exercise.

V is for volunteers — people who ask if they can help without thinking first.

W is for wash and wash and wash and wash — the laundry, the dishes, the squirmy babies, the floor, etc., etc.

X is for extra everything — cribs, toys, diapers, car seats, food, money, and most of all patience.

Y is for yes, and it's what I say to the volunteers before they have time to reconsider.

Z is for zwieback which has been chewed on and smeared and now resembles concrete; and Z is also for Z

Z
Z
Z
Z
Z
the nap that I'm going to take some day!

by Paula Brigham
Kankakee, IL

few weeks are crucial, but some lucky mothers of multiples have help for up to a year. *Fatigue is the biggest contributor to postpartum depression, and the job of feeding two babies around the clock is exhausting, especially if you burden yourself with bottle-feeding.* Triplets and other children are even more work for the mother to handle.

Family Stress

Most expectant parents worry about the extra work of multiples and the effects on older children. Very few anticipate the effects on the marital relationship. These effects may begin prenatally with problems in the pregnancy, bed rest, or concern about premature delivery. After the birth, the father may have an extra job, one twin may still be in the hospital, and there is no time for shared activities except baby care. Few mothers believe that depression will ever happen to them. It tends to come on a few weeks or months after the birth, which is surrounded with so much attention and excitement that any hormonal baby blues in the first few days may hardly be noticed. Bringing home just one baby or an ongoing medical problem with one or both can cause a severe let-down. Mothers who feel too tired or too busy or can't be bothered to go anywhere may be showing early signs of depression.

Nurturing the mother during this early phase of adjustment is very important. Sometimes relatives or friends can come and stay for a few weeks or the father can take off time from work or go on flextime. Housekeeping services, more than child care services, are required. The mother wants the joy of looking after the babies — not handing them over to a professional so that she is left with the chores. Washers, dryers, crock pots, pressure cookers, and microwave ovens are valuable time savers.

Don't worry about the house; babies grow up so fast and they will be gone before you know it. Collect the clutter in plastic crates or laundry baskets and soak the dishes in the sink until you have time to wash them or load the dishwasher. The housework will always be there. One mother of twins received an embroidered sampler with the message "A tidy house is the sign of a misspent life." You can ask your husband when he comes home to a zoo, "Would you rather have a clean house or a loving wife and mother?" The big challenge of parenting is to respond to the child when the child needs you and not to postpone it until you are ready.

Twins are really a strain. You wonder if you'll ever get enough sleep or even have any time for yourself again.

My pediatrician's advice to us when we left the hospital was "Cancel all engagements for the next eighteen months."

I had no experience in child care at all, and there I was at home with my twins — outnumbered. I could have used an extra pair of arms.

You have to set priorities every day. I often used to take the telephone off the hook, especially when the babies were asleep and I took a rest.

We had a live-in graduate student to help with the twins. We did not have to pay out anything, as we took care of her room and board. I don't know how we would have managed without her cooking and babysitting.

People you haven't heard from for years suddenly come to visit you now that you have had twins.

Twins are simple to take care of — if you are prepared to give up sleep.

Sometimes I just have to lock myself in the bathroom or scream at the top of my lungs. It helps to talk to another mother of twins because she's the only one who can really understand.

I found stress management techniques helpful — deep breathing, deep muscle relaxation, imagery, self-hypnosis, and meditation.

People are so inquisitive. They will let a door slam in your face while they ask about your twins.

How Families and Friends Can Help

---

1. Give baby clothes (at least 12-month size unless the babies are premature) or equipment. A rocking chair, a video camera, and a cordless phone are ultimate gifts for a family with multiples. Please, no stuffed animals or receiving blankets!
2. Give a few weeks or months of a diaper service.
3. Bring food, such as a casserole or a whole meal.
4. Organize the neighborhood to cook a meal per day for the first month and give the parents a calendar so they know what to expect each day.
5. Offer to bathe, feed, and babysit the multiples.
6. Offer to grocery shop, and take the babies with you.
7. Help clean the house.
8. Give a gift certificate to the mother for a massage, facial, exercise program, or swimming pool membership.
9. When the babies are older, invite one or more to stay overnight; give the parents a weekend away.
10. Invite other siblings out for treats.

Friends and relatives should not be permitted to visit unless they are prepared to help. Let them prepare snacks or fold laundry. A liberating aspect of breast-feeding is that only the mother can do it; bottle-feeding mothers may find that they are fixing afternoon tea while the visitor enjoys giving the bottles.

Fathering Multiples

One Mothers of Twins Club surveyed fathers of twins and found that although they are more nervous and anxious in the beginning than fathers of singletons, they were compensated by the admiration of others. First-time fathers of twins are particularly happy and proud of their complete family unit in which each adult has a baby. Fathers of twins all report much greater involvement in child care, as well as in play, than fathers of single babies. It is well known that fathers who participate in the birth experience, like mothers, develop very close bonds with the offspring. Some parents exhibit wonderful team-work as they constantly interchange twins. It's very important not to get into a rut with one parent always taking a certain baby. The most welcome assistance from the father comes during night feedings. He can bring the babies to the mother so that she can nurse without hav-ing to get out of bed, or he can give one twin a bottle. The father can also help by changing diapers afterward and returning the babies to bed. If the twins tend to fall asleep while nursing, as most babies do, it may be easier to change them first to avoid waking them up after they're fed.

An expectant mother's perception of how much support she will receive from her partner is central to her ability to cope with multi-ples. Fathers feel much additional pressure — to bring in more money, to help more at home, and to give loving support to the mother despite perhaps no more than a couple of hours sleep at a stretch for months. The exhaustion and constant care of the multiples mean that sex is often pushed aside for longer than it is after singleton birth. This is a phase in which the couple become parents first and foremost and spouses second; but this phase will pass.

The Parents of Multiple Births Association (POMBA) in Canada surveyed 348 fathers of multiples in 1981. More than a third worried about the reduction of family income to one salary when expenses would be doubling. Also, many were dealing with a move to a larger house, and more than half had to buy a larger car. Nine percent felt there was a direct effect on their careers owing to restricted mobility, less time for studies, and, of course, fatigue. More than half were concerned about their wives' health or ability to cope under the heavy workload that accompanies multiples. Twenty percent felt that their marriages had deteriorated after the birth of the multiples, but five percent thought they had improved. Forty percent of fathers did not share in the workload, although 60 percent did help with feeding. Fathers generally become sole providers for the household.

Suggestions for fathers include the following:

Check your financial situation before the birth and arrange for extra expenses, house renovation if required, and perhaps a bank loan to pay for extra help.

Organize household and child care help, especially for older sib-lings. Request help from family and friends. Get friends to

I really missed having time for myself. Even getting a shower and brushing my teeth required planning far ahead. I spent a lot of time crying in those early months, mostly because I was physically exhausted. If I had to do it over again, I would cry out for more help. I would tell others how desperate I was instead of saying I was doing fine.

The small size of our twins made my boyfriend apprehensive about handling them.

I gave up the idea of being a superwoman long ago and enjoy being a single mother of twins.

After a few months of flaunting my single motherhood, I settled into the role more comfortably. By the time the twins were nine months old, I was just another mother. No one knows if I'm single, married, or divorced.

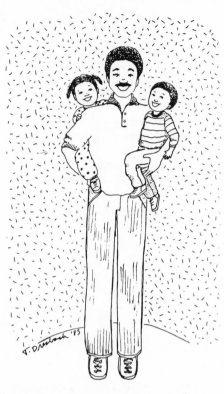

Line drawing by Terry Dresbach. Reproduced with permission from Twin Services, Inc.

I gained two children but lost my wife, and I didn't particularly like this zombie who looked like her but had no time for me or our marriage. It took me about three weeks to realize that if we were to keep our marriage intact, I'd better pitch in and be a partner. Once that brilliant thought was turned into action, I became a zombie too, but at least then we were a matched set again!

My husband took a while to get used to my neglect of him and the decrease in our domestic standards.

pledge work or food (not just verbally — have them fill out cards).

Spend more time with your babies. This will increase your confidence as a father and your ability to see them as individuals and not just as twins. Look after the multiples by yourself so your wife can have a break.

Don't just help with the babies, but share the housework too.

Be prepared for your wife's total absorption in the babies for several months. Get together with other fathers of multiples — join a parents of twins club.

Breast-Feeding

The Advantages of Nature's Bounty

Breast-feeding is the simplest, cheapest, and most convenient way to feed twins, triplets, and quadruplets* if the mother is committed to the idea. It is emotionally and physiologically satisfying for mother and children and provides the ideal food for your babies. All breast-feeding mothers require plenty of support and encouragement, however, in our society. Although the stores of fat laid down in pregnancy provide energy for breast-feeding, lactation is a nutritional challenge. At least 400 extra calories per baby are required in addition to the daily requirements for twin pregnancy (a total daily intake of about 4,000 calories), as well as a similar amount of extra protein (at least 100 gm per day). Mothers are thus forced to take care of themselves, to eat nutritious well-balanced meals, to drink plenty of fluids, and to get adequate rest and relaxation.

Nursing offers a special time to cuddle and bond with babies — only the mother can do it. And breast-feeding is convenient. Breast milk is always available and it is the perfect food (which changes continuously in the first few weeks to adapt to the infant's maturation). It is always at the right temperature. The money saved by not buying formula and all the equipment can be used for a diaper service, clothes dryer, or household help. Some of the many benefits for the babies include less indigestion and colic, fewer allergies, and better development of the palate and facial structure by the vigorous sucking required by the natural nipple.

* Higher-order multiples may need supplementation — but always give the breast first.

Breast-fed babies have softer stools, which, like their vomit, are not offensive as are the harder stools of bottle-fed babies. The American Academy of Pediatrics supports breast-feeding as the most desirable method.

Breast-feeding is no problem physiologically, as the supply of milk keeps up with the demand. However, it takes some practice in the beginning to position two babies who may sometimes want different amounts of milk and who may suck differently at the breast simultaneously. The twins may not coincide in their growth spurts and time spent nursing. Any problems with breast-feeding are usually twin problems rather than nursing difficulties.

A 1986 survey of Mothers of Twins Clubs in the United States found that three-quarters of the mothers breast-fed their twins. But it was as high as 83 percent in the farm states of Iowa, Wisconsin, and Indiana. A 1985 Parents of Multiple Births Association survey in Canada found that half the mothers who breast-fed did so for four or more months and 14 percent breast-fed for more than eleven months. About half the mothers supplemented their own breast milk with either formula or breast milk from others.

Demand feeding is regulated entirely by the infants: you feed them when they want to be fed. This is clearly the best situation from the babies' point of view, but few mothers of multiples manage it because it is such a time-consuming occupation that they can do little else through the day. Two babies often want to be fed simulta-

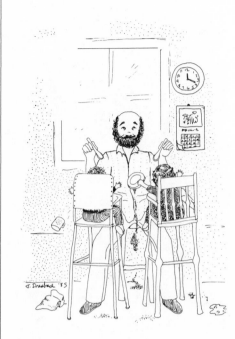

Line drawing by Terry Dresbach. Reprinted with permission from Twin Services, Inc.

I could never have survived without my husband's help — especially at night. I just nursed the babies in bed and he did the fetching, cleaning, and changing.

The first few months are the worst. Then life becomes much easier, and the joy and pleasure of the twins outweigh the workload.

I often tried to be supermom and paid the toll in fatigue. My family paid the price in lack of attention.

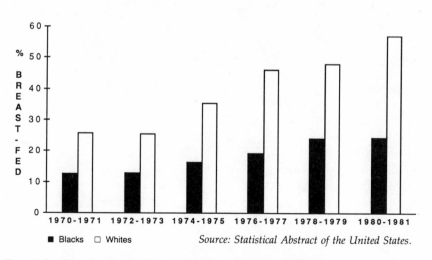

Source: Statistical Abstract of the United States.

■ Blacks □ Whites

Breast-feeding is slowly increasing for whites and blacks.

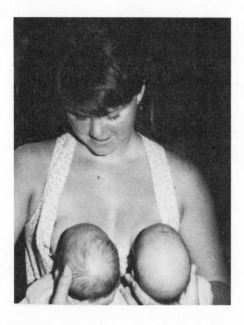

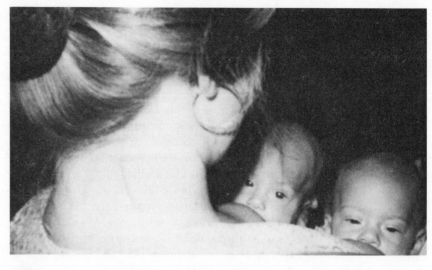

Feeding twins simultaneously saves time.

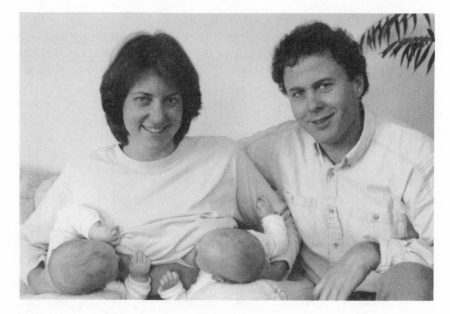

I had a difficult time losing weight after my first pregnancy as I bottle-fed. So I was determined to breast-feed this time.

I regret that I never breast-fed my twins, but my doctor discouraged me.

In the beginning I nursed my babies both at once, although I confess I felt like a cow. As they grew I found they were simply too heavy to feed together.

For the first six weeks, all you are really doing is feeding. I watched a mother who bottle-fed her twins and figured that she got only one extra hour off. Nursing twins means more frequent feeding at shorter intervals, but the convenience outweighs that extra hour.

neously, in which case most mothers feed the one who screams louder first, at the fuller breast, or both together.

Simultaneous feeding takes less time than demand feeding but requires waking one twin when the other awakens ready to nurse. Most mothers prefer simultaneous feeding so that they can get more sleep, but some don't like waking a sleeping baby. See whether it works best to wake up both babies or to feed them as they wake naturally. Mothers of triplets usually find that the most satisfactory solution is to encourage the babies to adopt similar schedules. Triplets are fed "on the circuit," that is, rotated on the breasts, often two at a time. Quads are nursed two by two, no more time-consuming than triplets.

Occasionally the babies' conditions place them on different schedules. For example, a weaker twin may need feeding every three hours while the stronger twin can wait four hours. Mothers may find it helpful to keep charts of each baby's feeding. These can also be used to record bowel movements, baths, temperatures, and so on.

Troubleshooting

It is often easier to nurse multiples than a singleton, as the additional demand increases milk production. (Breast size has nothing to do with the ability to nurse, as sucking builds up the supply.)

Night nursing is very important to establish and build a good milk supply. If the babies are small, they may take less at night but nurse more often. Mothers often get off to a poor start with breast-feeding because hospital staff find it easier to feed the babies themselves overnight than to awaken the mother. This causes the mother's breasts to become engorged and, if the babies are filled with formula and have no interest in sucking on the breast, the mother will then have to express the milk. An engorged breast is difficult for the baby as well as the mother because the nipple cannot protrude adequately.

If the milk supply is plentiful, when the first twin starts sucking, the let-down reflex may cause milk to spurt over the second twin. So it may be easier to nurse one at a time at the beginning. Women who experience an inadequate amount of milk often simply need to increase their fluid intake and improve their nutrition. Brewer's yeast, nonalcoholic beer, and wheat germ can help too. Many babies have gas or colic, are fussy, and spit up if the mother is consuming dairy products or if a milk-based formula is being used. The mother may find that the situation improves if she cuts out all dairy products from

A container of liquid by your bed, especially at night, helps a nursing mother to keep up her fluid intake.

I used to make lunch at breakfast time so that I never missed a meal.

I always kept a bottle of juice on the kitchen table, and every time I walked by I would pour myself a glass.

Going out with twins often was a prolonged expedition. It was a great help to take along small snacks for me, like cheese and fruit, for when I started to feel tired and weak.

Nursing twins is not the same experience as nursing a singleton, but for each baby it is just as important. And when you look down at those four little eyes and see two mouths break into milky smiles it's worth it all!

When I nursed the twins together, they always went on the same breast. If one nursed singly, I would alternate.

I know you are supposed to do all that sterilizing, but as a single mother and a full-time student I would rather spend my time with the twins.

The books say you are not supposed to prop their bottles, but, coping on my own, propping makes a big difference.

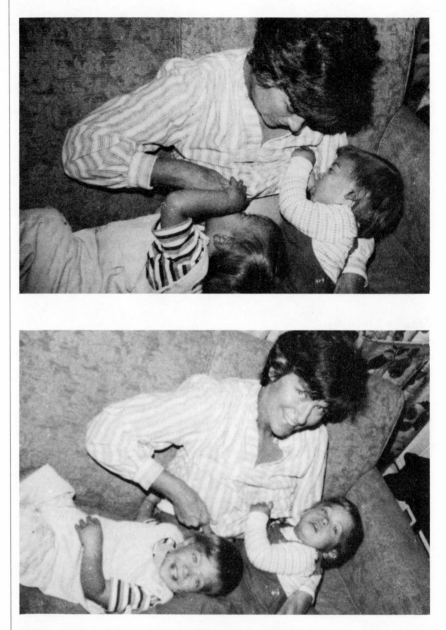

I enjoyed feeding the babies with one on each side of me. This way I could feed one and entertain the other. Lying on a couch or bed also enabled me to elevate my tired and overworked legs.

It's important to alternate the first baby at mealtimes, as the baby fed last usually gets more time and attention.

I found that one of the great bonuses of nursing, especially when they were toddlers, was the way it would calm them both down if there were any conflicts.

Both mother and twins enjoy breast-feeding together.

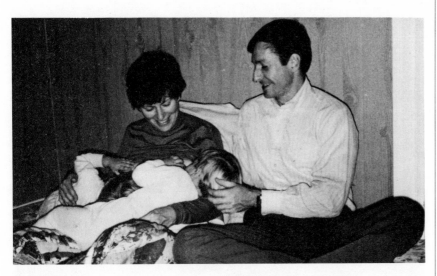

The same twins, two years old here, are nursed before bedtime.

her diet and the babies'; soy formula can be substituted for the babies. Never give cow's milk during the first year — it contains much higher proportions of protein and salt than breast milk and infant formula and can strain infant kidneys. Cow's milk is best for baby calves.

It is a good idea to air your nipples occasionally; sunlight is best. Soggy pads inside a bra lead to skin breakdown and infection. Vitamin E oil or lanolin helps to prevent dry skin and cracking. Further advice on caring for the breasts may be found in *Nursing Your Baby* by Karen Pryor, an excellent book on breast-feeding. Also highly recommended are Sheila Kitzinger's *Breastfeeding Your Baby* and *The Womanly Art of Breastfeeding* by La Leche League. Another good source is *Breastfeeding Twins, Triplets, and Quadruplets: 195 Practical Hints for Success,* published by the Center for the Study of Multiple Birth. See page 297 for information about using a breast pump.

Nursing Logistics

Breast-feeding twins means that you can complete both feedings at one sitting. You can let the hungrier twin nurse first or nurse both at the same time; either way avoids feeding all day long.

If someone helps you at the outset to get the twins into position, you may be more inclined to nurse your twins simultaneously. Some

Breast-feeding, which means a lot of close contact with each twin, is really helpful for learning to bond with each baby as an individual.

At first I kept charts on everything, as you're supposed to. I soon dropped all of that. I just nursed my triplets when they wanted to be fed and I never had any problems. Maybe I overfed one and underfed another — but it worked out just fine.

My doctor said that if God had meant for me to nurse triplets, I would have been given three breasts. I'm really angry that I didn't try because I have met other mothers of triplets who really enjoyed it.

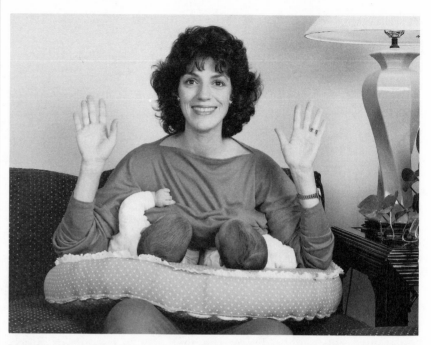

Nursing two babies at once is much easier than giving bottles. The cushion ties at the back and has a zippered removable cover. The mother's hands are free to burp a baby, help dress siblings, or read stories. *Courtesy of Four-Dee Products.*

Doubters would say to me, "I guess you're not breast-feeding" when they saw I had twins. "Why not?" I would reply. "It's the most natural thing in the world — two babies, two breasts."

The needs of the babies should be top priority, not what suits mother's needs, limitations, or lifestyle. Women have breasts so we can nurse our babies and this must be emphasized.

mothers find it easier to wait until the babies develop head control, around the third month. You can try a variety of positions, and pillows really help (see Resources). The "football hold" is popular: the legs of each baby are directed backward under your arms while you cradle a head in each hand. This comfortable position leaves your hands free once the babies can stay attached on their own. The twins' bodies can also be crossed on the your lap and held in your arms. Another option is to position the babies so that their bodies are longitudinal, lying on each side of you on their bellies, or both lying parallel toward one side and the other. Pillows can be placed under the babies to support their heads and trunks or under your elbows. When you want to be discreet or don't have the space, put one baby on the left in the traditional position and the other on the right in the football hold.

Mothers who can master the art of breast-feeding twins while lying down can really enjoy a relaxation session. Breast-feeding in this position is very useful for night feedings in bed.

Most experts recommend switching breasts at each nursing to maintain a good supply in both and to give each baby left and right visual stimulation. I believe that it is important to give your infants as much variety as possible. Look for opportunities to nurse the babies separately for one-on-one bonding.

Some pediatricians, however, recommend always using the same breast for one baby at each feeding. This preserves the correct relationship between supply and demand but may mean that your breasts end up a little different in size. If for any reason the milk supply in one breast is diminished, the baby who sucks more strongly can be placed on the other breast to increase milk production.

It depends on your personality and the advice of your pediatrician whether you nurse the babies intuitively or fill in charts to keep track of the babies' feedings. Half a dozen wet diapers a day and weight gain will indicate that each baby is getting enough to eat. It is not necessary to put the babies on the scale all the time. This can make mothers anxious. Babies soon become very efficient at sucking and can drain the breast in five minutes or so, although they often like to linger at the nipple, sinking deep into an alpha wave level of consciousness, their lips quivering with what Wilhelm Reich called oral orgasm. Mothers often experience orgasm too — or at least pleasurable sensations. Nature designed it that way, to ensure survival of the species. Many women feel alarmed — even guilty — by their response and, not understanding its natural purpose, may opt for bottle-feeding.

You can express your milk and store it in the refrigerator for the babysitter to use or for bottle-feeding extra multiples. Avoid or use great care with bottle holders and propping bottles. If you supplement with breast milk or formula in a bottle, nurse first. In the beginning it is better to spoon-feed the substitute than to confuse the baby between breast and bottle. Adding water, especially sugar water, to milk in a bottle not only is unnecessary and unhealthy for the infant but interferes with the breast milk supply. You may feel a lot of pressure to supplement with formula, or you may be subject to jokes and remarks of disbelief about nursing multiples. Moral support is very important, especially if you are nursing multiples, and counseling and encouragement from La Leche League is recommended if any difficulties arise.

A mother's milk supply is typically down at the end of the day, from fatigue and perhaps inadequate fluid intake. This is the time to have a teenager come in and pick up the mess and start preparing the meal while you put your feet up and have a drink and a snack.

Many articles for mothers of twins rationalize the bottle-feeding of twins to help mothers be guilt free with the decision. More helpful information is needed so that women will have the knowledge they need to have successful breast-feeding experiences.

I'm a walking, talking, breathing example of a woman who successfully nursed twins, worked full time, lost 87 pounds, and lived to tell about it. My eight-month-old identical boys have only recently started to wean from the breast. I can honestly say that breast-feeding was the most relaxing, natural experience I have ever had. I nursed both using the football hold mostly.

My husband was very supportive. We both strongly agree that breast milk was meant for human babies. I fed both babies at the same time since this saved time and neither twin had to wait. Seeing both satisfied simultaneously is a pleasure.

Breast-feeding was a very rewarding experience. Some of my boys' first interactions occurred at these times.

Relactation

Milk has been produced by women who adopted an infant years after they gave birth or even by some women who have never been pregnant. So if your milk was dried up with medication and you changed your mind about breast-feeding, or if your twins were in the intensive care nursery and pumping was difficult — have faith. With enough motivation and support, especially from your partner and doctor, you can do it. You can find other mothers who have accomplished relactation through your local La Leche League or your pediatrician.

Relactation is initiated with a device known as Lact-Aid. It is a plastic bag with a tube for the baby to suck. This bag can be filled with donor breast milk (preferably) or formula. The baby sucks on both your breast and the Lact-Aid tube, stimulating your milk production. As your supply builds up, you can gradually reduce the Lact-Aid fluid until it is not needed, which usually takes a couple of months. The process is faster and easier with twins because they provide double sucking stimulation.

Some advantages are claimed for bottle-feeding twins, such as equal sharing between both parents and more sleep for the mother. However, the father can do his share of parenting by changing diapers or bathing the babies so that the infants can be completely breast-fed. Some parents try to do both, which is much more of a hassle in most cases. Every attempt should be made to support the mother in the ways described here so that enough milk is produced even for supertwins.

Bottle-Feeding

Considerable work is involved in preparing formula, particularly for twins. Sometimes each twin requires a separate formula, in a ready-to-use or concentrated form. Usually a batch is made up for at least a day or two at a time, which is less effort if everything must be sterilized. Some pediatricians consider the heat of an electric dishwasher or microwave oven adequate for sterilization. Certainly many mothers of twins discover short cuts to save the work involved in sterilization.

Most mothers use the terminal method of sterilization, where the filled bottles (about fourteen to sixteen for twins) are put together in a large pot or a couple of sterilizers for about half an hour and then

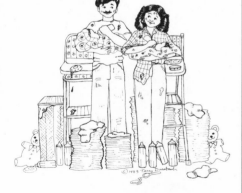

Breast-feeding can save a lot of work.
Line drawing by Terry Dresbach. Reproduced with permission from Twin Services, Inc.

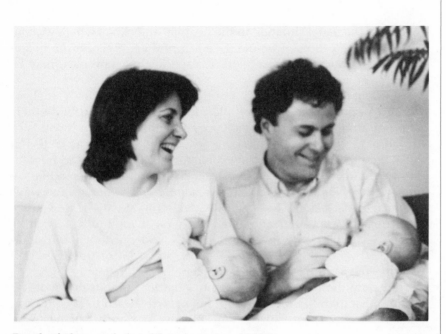

But the father can help with an occasional bottle.

left to cool. Disposable plastic liners for bottles cut down on the soaking and cleaning involved. Special soaks remove the milk residue from bottles to make for easier cleaning. Playtex nursing kits are quick and easy, but they are expensive, as are professional formula services, which supply everything. Remember: it doesn't hurt to ask if there is a discount for multiples.

When the twins are bottle-fed, the father, or perhaps a visitor, usually feeds one. If the mother is alone and feeding the babies together, she can position them on a sofa or her lap or place them in infant seats and sit between them. One baby may be fed by hand, while the mother keeps an eye on the bottle propped for the other.* When the twins can sit alone, the mother can hold a bottle in each hand. If they are not both hungry, one twin may be content to watch from a swing chair.

I strongly advise breast-feeding and in this book I have devoted more space to support it than I have to bottle-feeding. This is the

* Never leave a baby alone in case he or she chokes on the milk.

reverse of the usual situation in the hospital and clinic, where women are encouraged to use formula (free samples are given in the hospital), and support for breast-feeding, especially of multiples, may be scarce or nonexistent.

Of course, breast-feeding is difficult, for example, for a single or working or poor mother of multiples. It is also a challenge for mothers who commute to and from the neonatal intensive care unit with sick newborns and who often have other children at home as well. But these are predominantly social problems that need to be addressed. Showing a mother how to fix formula only adds to her outlay of money, time, and effort. Instead we should ask: What are the ways in which breast-feeding can be facilitated in this situation? Preventive measures for expectant and new mothers of multiples — such as home help, child care, travel assistance, and nutritional subsidies provided by health insurance — could save a lot of intensive care costs as well as providing intangible benefits for the family.

Burping the babies is considered a harder job by some mothers of multiples than the feeding. Parents of twins learn to become ambidextrous. One twin can be lying in your lap on his or her side, having his or her back rubbed, while the other twin is spitting up over one shoulder. Twins who need to be fed and burped simultaneously can create a hectic time!

My twins nursed quite differently. One sucked more vigorously. The other never needed burping.

Dental Care

If you bottle-feed your infants you will need to take certain precautions to minimize later tooth decay. First, a child should *never* be allowed to go to bed with a bottle of juice or milk. This bathes the teeth and results in "nursing bottle mouth" — a typical pattern of cavities the child develops at four or five years of age. Likewise, never give a child a pacifier dipped in sugar or honey, however tempting it may be with more than one child to care for. Tooth decay begins between eight and twenty-four months, long before the average child is first taken to a dentist. It is essential to adhere to a daily cleaning routine, which should be begun when the child gets her or his first tooth. A film of bacteria, known as plaque, covers teeth and should be removed twice a day to ensure healthy gums and teeth. Parents of multiples may feel that this is yet another burden in their busy schedule, but it takes only a couple of minutes to wipe the gums of each child vigorously with two-inch nonsterile gauze squares. This will pay off in later years with great savings in dental bills.

Introducing Solid Food

Don't be tempted to introduce solid foods too early. Consuming solid food does not affect sleeping patterns and makes a lot more mess and work for you. Solids need not be introduced before five or six months or even later. Until the second half of the first year, most of the food particles simply pass undigested through the baby's system.

Twins often have different food tastes and even different food allergies. Wait with this messy step until the babies have some teeth, are clearly interested in food (grabbing at your plate, utensils, and so on), and can bring the food with their tongue to the back of their mouth to swallow. Breast-feeding, of course, may be continued along with solid food up to two years or more.

The babies may differ in their solid food requirements. An iron-fortified cereal is usually advised by the pediatrician to begin with. After the babies accept this, other foods can be added, but only one or two per week. When the twins gain enough balance to sit, usually at about six months, they can be placed in highchairs or portable seats that attach to the table, with seat belts. Keep the chairs away from the walls and place them on sheets of newspaper or a large plastic tablecloth if you want to spare yourself the trouble of washing the floor every day. Sometimes it may be less work to bring the food to the

My babies were breast-fed prior to the meal, but they were still very hungry. Meals became a hassle as both babies demanded food yet were unable to do any self-feeding. I shoveled food into them as fast as I could using one spoon while alternating bites. Sometimes I used two spoons simultaneously! A suction cup toy on each highchair helped to distract them. An improvement was seen at eight months when they could gnaw on finger foods while I alternated spoonfuls.

We use "Sassy seats" for our ten-month-old twins. They are collapsible chairs that clamp onto the table and are held in place by the child's weight. They are cheaper and take up much less space than regular highchairs. Also our girls are very small and the chairs fit them better. They are easy to transport and have proved invaluable in restaurants since many seem to have only one highchair and we have two babies!

In the grocery store, people make comments like "Stocking up for a year?" and "Buying for an army?"

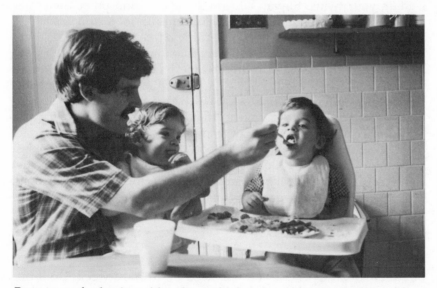

Parents can feed twins with only one highchair and just one spoon.

It didn't take long for the novelty of having quads to wear off as far as shopping is concerned. I am afraid I just push right on now to avoid time-wasting encounters with the public. People never think of quads; they always ask if I have two sets of twins.

To help weaning, introduce the concept of taking turns with everything including nursing. Do other activities than nurse when you sit down, and look for opportunities to nurse them separately.

We received two Carri-Cradle infant seats as gifts when our twin boys were born seven months ago. They are fantastic. I could put one in the seat on the floor and rock it with my foot as I fed the other.

I prepare as much as possible early in the day, because by late afternoon my energy level is very low. The crockpot is a big help, as are two pressure cookers, and both keep the nutrients in the food.

twins' room instead of bringing them to the kitchen. The food doesn't fly as far if you all sit on the floor. Some babies will be happier side by side, or you can sit between them. One dish and one spoon are all that are required — even for quintuplets — until they want to feed themselves. One baby will be swallowing his or her mouthful and getting ready for more while the other baby is being fed. With multiples, it is much easier to avoid forcing food on babies. Twins quickly learn to eat independently, so they don't have to wait their turn and can help themselves instead. Bibs with a container flap at the bottom to catch many falling morsels are recommended. I sewed "raincoats" made of quick-drying parka fabric that covered the baby from neck to ankles, with long sleeves. This saved much laundry of baby clothes. However, the parents could use such a garment too! One mother of twins recommends feeding the twins in the bath so that the mess goes down the drain! (Make sure you kneel or squat to avoid backache.)

Even monozygotic twins can have different tastes and appetites. If one twin is always hungrier and asks for snacks or juice, the mother may automatically supply the other twin as well. Apart from over-feeding, this can lead to a social setback, where one child never asks for anything because she or he doesn't need to. One twin need only request and both receive.

Processed commercial baby food is the most expensive way of feeding your twins. Sugar, salt, preservatives, and other chemicals are often added except in brands sold in health food stores, such as Earth's Best, which are certified organic and free from pesticides, herbicides and fertilizers. Foods can be ordered in bulk from Earth's Best (see Resources). It is easy and much more economical, however, to prepare portions of food cooked for the rest of the family in a baby grinder or blender, or else do what we did for our children — simply chew what we eat and give it to them, partially digested, like the birds do! This is very convenient, especially when dining out.

Do not add sugar and salt to food that you cook for the babies and remove the babies' portion before seasoning for the rest of the family. Vegan mothers should add vitamin B_{12} for the infants. Cooking large quantities saves time, and the extra can be stored in the freezer. Small portions for the babies can be frozen in ice cube trays.

Diapers

Buy prefolded diapers — you will need up to 200 a week. Until the babies have solid bowel movements, just put the diapers through two cycles of the washing machine. Use bleach only in the last cycle, as it can mix with the ammonia in the urine and cause diaper rash. If rash develops, dry the babies' bottoms with a hair dryer (on low setting) or put the babies in the sun for a few minutes and use castor oil. Use Biobottoms and other natural-fabric diaper covers that air better than plastic pants. Cotton sleepwear can be ordered from ads in the back of *Mothering* magazine and from addresses listed in Resources.

Twins Can Be a Hard Happiness

Postpartum depression is undoubtedly greater for mothers of twins or higher-order multiples. The LaTrobe Twin Study found depression to be five times more common in mothers of twins than in mothers of singletons; 76 percent of mothers of twins reported being constantly exhausted, versus 8 percent of mothers of singletons. In addition to David Hay of LaTrobe, Marilyn Riese of the Louisville Twin Study is researching the incidence of postpartum depression in mothers of twins. Pat Malmstrom of Twin Services calls the condition *twinshock*.

Caesarean delivery, with its medication, anesthesia, and separation from the newborns, is a major contributing factor. It is hard for a mother to be ecstatic over her babies when she is in pain trying to recover from major surgery. Most mothers of multiples wonder how they are going to cope with two or more babies at once, a worry that is exacerbated by the need to recover from a Caesarean or to deal with one or more babies in the neonatal intensive care unit.

Breast-feeding, which can elevate a mother's self-esteem in the face of these problems, is not always supported enough by medical staff. Depression can understandably set in while a mother struggles through the early weeks, but the ongoing fatigue and sleep deprivation, which continue for months and sometimes a few years, are also a threat to a mother's mental health, unless she has good support, especially from her partner, and plenty of home help.

Caring for two babies is exhausting, more so for higher-order multiples. The mothers who have two sets of twins born in twenty-four months — and there are some — have it even harder than mothers of quadruplets. Research by the Louisville Twin Study showed that the psychological dynamics between twins is basically the same as between any other siblings less than two years apart in age.

Guilt feelings may arise from giving unequal attention to the two babies, neglecting other family members, and showing preference toward one twin or disappointment in one or both. Every mother does her best even if it may not seem so in hindsight or measure up

Being hugged by four arms makes up for 160 diapers a week!

Sleep charts are a sanity saver. It's reassuring to see that you have a right to feel lousy because there's been only three hours in twenty-four when they've both been asleep. You also start to see sleep and nap patterns more readily.

The hardest thing about twins is comforting both when both are fussy.

When I was able to have more physical contact with the babies, I became more responsive and less depressed. But my depression did not really go away until I was able to nurse them all.

Infafeeders were a godsend for those hectic feeding times when I was alone.

My best advice is to just do the best you can. No one can expect more from you. If your house is a wreck and you have sandwiches for supper, who cares?

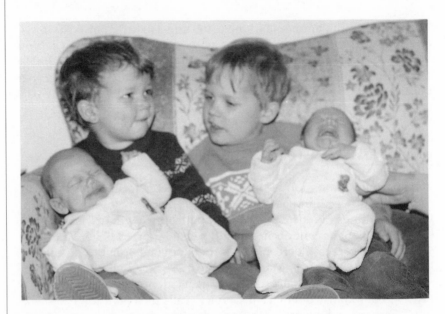

It's hard enough to figure out why one baby is crying, let alone two!

Some days my husband would come home and find me sitting in the playpen, alone, crying, while the babies crawled around the room. I'd explain, "This is the only place where they can't attack me."

It might be "twice as nice" when twins are older, but at first it sure is "double trouble."

to her ideal. When worrying about spending the same amount of time with each baby, Karen Gromada, editor of *DoubleTalk*, advises: "Stop worrying and think — if these children were a year apart, would I be so worried about treating them exactly the same at all times?"

More than three-quarters of mothers report being constantly exhausted after their twins' arrival. Mothers of twins do a lot of crying and screaming from the emotional stress of juggling two babies or more alone, without help. Those who don't often develop jaw problems! Counseling helps mothers who feel too burned out to be rational and acknowledge their own needs.

Parents of twins are at higher risk for drug and alcohol abuse, family violence, and divorce. Child abuse can be physical, verbal, or emotional, or it can simply be neglect. A 1985 study of 48 families with term twins found nine times more abuse than in families without twins; in half the families only the sibling, but neither of the twins, was abused. Parents Anonymous and other hot lines for times of crisis are listed in Resources.

In different countries and states, support may be available through community nursing services, day care, grants and allowances for families with multiples or special twin agencies such as

Twin Services in Berkeley, California. Contacting the local high school or senior citizen center might turn up someone who can help you for a few hours.

All parents feel very tied down in the beginning, but parents of multiples especially so. A chorus of crying babies is much more grating on the nerves than the howls of a singleton. Twins frequently cry together. They may disturb each other or one twin may scream for attention and the second may start up even louder. No wonder their parents are forced to exclaim, "I've just got to get away for a while." Yet so many mothers of multiples feel it is just too much trouble to go out in the early months. They would rather have people come to them, even if the house always looks as if a hurricane just passed through. In retrospect, these same women will emphatically advise others to have a break from their babies as soon and as often as possible. It is worth any manipulation, they advise, to get out even to the hairdresser or to have a candlelight dinner alone.

Parents also need to get out with the babies so that the infants receive their share of fresh air and admiration. An Australian study found that 74 percent of mothers did not go out without the twins and 92 percent never went out alone without their partner. Some mothers of twins avoid going out without another pair of arms because of having to handle two babies who may both cry and want to eat at the same time. You need to be flexible and make the babies your top priority — but it is important for your sanity to get out of the house. It is easy to feel isolated, especially in winter if your babies get constant colds, coughs, and ear infections, and it is a challenge to bundle them up to go outside.

Family and friends are essential to prevent feelings of isolation, and it helps to have them visit when the babies are still small and babysitters may be hard to find. You may need two babysitters or have to pay one person one and a half times as much. To help sitters, write down details of each baby's schedule and particular preferences. Of course, two babysitters are more expensive, but hiring high school students or calling on relatives can reduce the cost. Because it is more difficult and expensive to find care for more than one baby, mothers of multiples usually suffer great social isolation in the beginning, especially if they have recently moved. Live-in help is the best, as it is the ongoing maintenance that helps keep the house and laundry clean and tempers calm. If you have a spare room, consider getting an au pair from abroad (see Resources).

Two or three newborns can fit in a baby carriage or pram and can sleep there, inside or outside. This expensive equipment is soon out-

Parenting multiples is more stressful than parenting singletons. It's awfully hard to keep your cool when there are two voices screaming for something. If you try to discipline them at the same time one is always grinning or giggling at the other. If you have to move both forcibly, it is harder to carry two crying kids than one.

Having twins was extremely stressful for the first three to four months. Between the two of them I got no more than one hour of sleep at a time. I became impatient and violent and I often got confused about where I had left a baby. I came dangerously close to abusing all three of my children.

I wish I were an octopus and could hold both babies and the two-year-old and catch up with housework with the other arms.

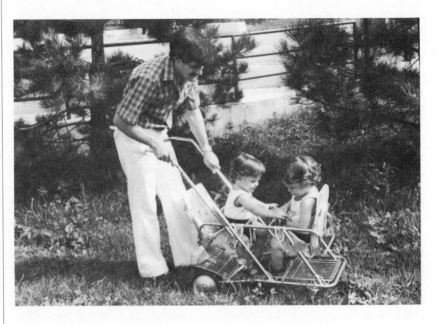

The twin limousine lets twins ride in style.

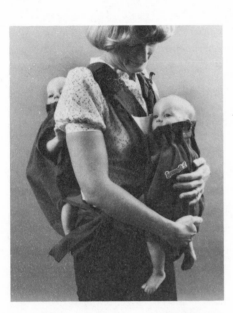

This mother of twins is carrying one in front and one behind. *Courtesy of Snugli, Inc.*

People stare when I go out with our children. When they ask how old the twins are, I say, "Which ones?" They just about faint!

Trimming forty nails on wiggling fingers and toes wipes out the whole morning. Tying shoes, fastening pants and hats and mittens means I need another person to help if I want to take a ride in the car.

I was so tired by the end of the day that the thought of entertaining friends was out of the question. Instead, we would invite people to brunch, which suited us much better. If we did invite guests to dinner, my husband would always get take-out Chinese food.

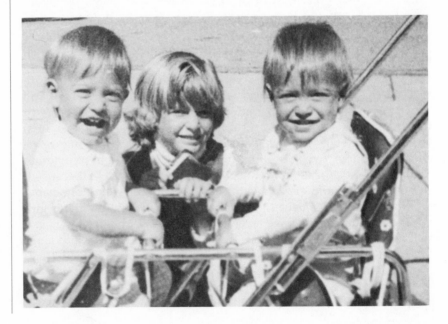

grown, so check secondhand stores or Mothers of Twins Clubs. Twins often use a stroller for a longer time because of the challenge for parents to run after toddlers going in different directions. Limousine strollers allow face-to-face interaction — which has its pros and cons — or the babies can sit in tandem. The leg room becomes limited as the twins grow bigger. Side-by-side strollers are more difficult to handle and are too broad to pass through some doors. Umbrella-type single strollers can be hooked together. These are compact and portable, and they can be used singly when needed. A booster seat can be attached to single strollers when the twins are toddlers.

Babies prefer body contact, so when possible try to carry one or both babies on your body. A variety of soft fabric carriers, backpacks with metal frames, and slings that can be worn in various ways are available. Do move a baby from your front onto your back after the first few weeks. Most of the carriers have head supports, or you can just use a length of cloth or a towel or receiving blanket. Many mothers wonder why they are carrying a baby in front who is six months old! Some carriers (Double Cuddle and Gemini) are designed especially for twins. Carrying anything on the back tends to improve pos-

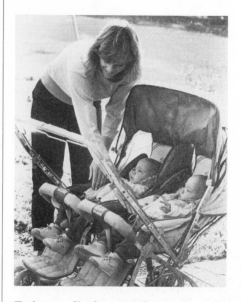

Twins can lie down to sleep . . .

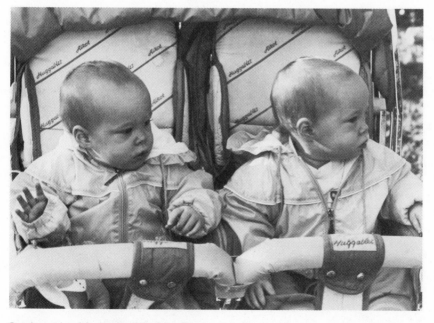

Or sit up in this Huggables stroller.

I resented advice to get away from my babies. Bonding with twins takes much longer than with a singleton, and I needed all the time I could find to adequately mother each infant.

Nobody expects triplets, and people are always asking if I have twins, as the boy is a bit bigger than his sisters. So I say, "Yes, they're twins," and keep on going.

Initially we put all the triplets in one carriage. Now two fit in the carriage and one of us takes the other in a backpack.

ture; try using a backpack sometimes instead of a purse, which will leave your hands free for the twins.

In the grocery store, you can put both babies in one shopping cart, lined first with a thick blanket, and push that cart while you fill another one with groceries. Alternatively, one twin can sit in an infant seat inside the cart while you carry the other one on your back. Small children can sit side by side with both legs in the space intended for one leg. Use blankets at each side to help prop them up. Bring toys to the store and tie them to the cart so you don't have to pick them up off the floor constantly. Some mothers use harnesses for toddlers who like to run off in different directions.

Sometimes mothers of multiples resent outsiders' curiosity and questions. Often people don't know how to react to multiples and make comments that are dumb or sarcastic. Most mothers are pleased to be sociable with interested, polite people and enjoy the opportunity to feel special.

Beginning with the trip home from the hospital, whenever you take the babies in the car they should be secured in infant car seats, which is law in most places. It is essential to train children to accept

Make a foam mattress for a folding playpen and the twins can sleep as well as play when you are visiting.

I found that a large single pram, with a twin at each end, was more convenient than a double pram. Separate back rests are a good idea so that one baby can sit up while the other sleeps.

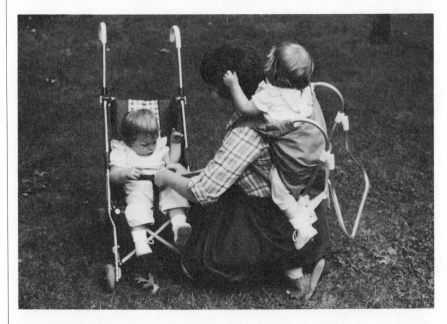

Mothers of twins enjoy getting out: with a twosome . . .

restraints in automobiles, as the number of children unnecessarily maimed or killed in car accidents is tragic. An excellent examination of the various types of car seats is contained in *The Care of Twin Children* by Theroux and Tingley (see Suggested Reading). They also provide helpful information on strollers, carriages, highchairs, and playpens.

Babies always break down barriers of social reserve. Strangers even go out of their way to accommodate parents with twins. One couple was getting out bottles to feed their babies in a restaurant when people nearby offered to feed and amuse the babies so that the parents could enjoy a peaceful meal together.

Sleeping

Some twins disturb each other, but most do not. Parents usually place them in the same crib on the excellent rationale that they have already spent a long time in close proximity. At first parents may put them at opposite ends, only to find later that they are snuggled together, perhaps even sucking each other's thumbs. When twins awaken, they often entertain each other, watching overhead mobiles or playing with each other's toes or fingers.

Some parents like to swaddle the babies when they first come home. Avoid this restrictive practice. Multiples, more than singletons, were cramped enough in the uterus. Other parents use one crib but divide it in half with a padded board. This interferes with the twin bond, which should be honored. Parents who own two bassinets, especially on wheels, can use these to separate crying twins. The age at which an infant first starts to sleep through the night varies widely. With twins the situation is more complex but not always worse than with singletons. Some twins both sleep through as early as eight weeks.

Ideally, parents of twins try to arrange for both babies to nap together and not to have such a long nap in the afternoon that they do not want to go to bed at night. On difficult days, it may help to put the babies in the car, as the motion usually lulls them to sleep. Then the mother or father can just relax or read while parked, until the babies awaken.

One child may want more nursing and cuddling time than the other. While the mother is attending to the more demanding twin, her helper, if she has one, can entertain the other or just let him or her fall asleep in her arms.

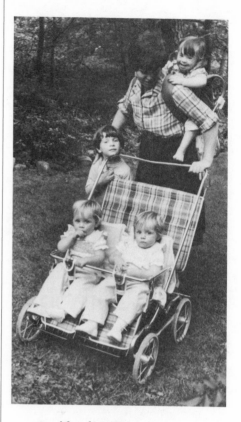

. . . or with a foursome.

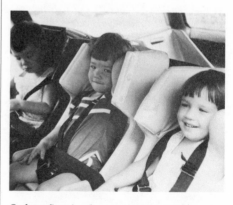

Safety first in the car for the Kiernan triplets.

I think our twins somehow know there are two of them and compensate with good behavior. They have both slept through the night since they were eight weeks old.

Our triplets did not sleep through the night for over a year. It was a mistake, I think, always to nurse them when one baby woke up hungry and disturbed the others.

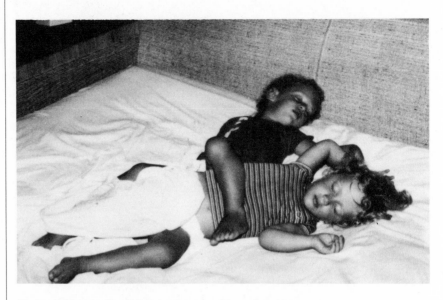

Twins enjoy each other's company when asleep too.

Our society seems to fear dependency in a pathological way. Tiny babies are separated from their mothers, and multiples are further separated from each other. Someone suggested that I put a barricade in the center of the crib for our twins and nearly dropped dead when I said they slept with us.

Alternative sleeping arrangements in the parents' bedroom are discussed in an interesting book called *The Family Bed* by Tine Thevenin. One of the best features of the family bed is the potential for more sleep. Some parents complain, however, that they cannot even have the babies in the same room because they are disturbed by every sniffle. Newborns do take a few weeks to settle into a steady, quiet breathing rhythm and they may make irregular sounds. On the other hand, if your babies are sleeping safely beside you, you don't have to worry that they have smothered or been struck by SIDS (crib death).

From the babies' point of view, sleeping in the parents' bed provides continuity of the warmth and body contact they enjoyed in utero. Jean Liedloff has explored this concept in her fascinating book *The Continuum Concept.* Babies who feel secure in infancy go on to become more trusting and independent children and adults. Twins need the continuum with their mother and each other.

If the babies are sleeping in your bed, you don't have to get out of bed to nurse them. It is convenient to just roll over and nurse them — after a while you won't even have turn on the light — and everyone enjoys more rest. Questions about sex, rolling on the babies, persuading older children to sleep alone, and so on are thoroughly addressed in Thevenin's book.

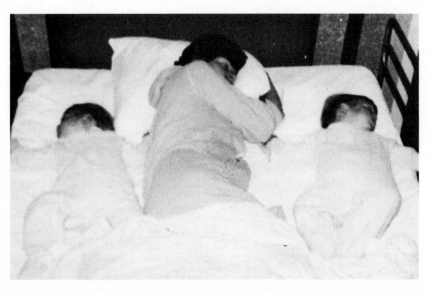

Sharing the bed means more sleep for everyone.

Whether you plan on a family bed or not — it will happen anyway!

Most mothers of twins had better get used to not getting much sleep for a while. If you accept this, it doesn't bother you as much as if you fight it. Attitude is so important! My twins are two and a half and just started sleeping through the night.

Bathing

Baths are fun for babies and parents, especially a family bath together. I have never bathed a baby except in the tub with me and I wouldn't want to deal with the slippery baby, aching back, and extra equipment, and mess. The family bath is a great place for baby exercises. Support just the head as the baby floats on his or her back and watch the baby move with delight. Baths also help to calm restless infants. Many parents do not bother to bathe both twins each day. Some compromise by bathing just one baby a day and others bathe both babies every few days. It is necessary only to wash a baby's diaper area and face regularly and to provide clean clothes, but many people feel that once all the bath equipment is out you might as well bathe both twins at once, particularly in the evening when your partner is there to help.

The kitchen sink or laundry tub may be used for bathing babies until they can sit independently. These save much back strain as they are higher than a bathtub. Later some parents use bath seats attached by suction cups to the regular tub. Get on your hands and knees to spare your back.

Never leave your babies unattended, especially in a bath. Two can get

I used to bathe both babies each day. After all, you need only one tub of water and they seemed to sleep better.

Changing two or more wiggly babies can be wearing. I keep a bowl of small toys near the changing table to occupy little hands and minds while the diapers are being changed.

I arranged for help with morning baths when my triplets were very young. I could then give each baby undivided attention during the bath and dressing.

We both enjoy watching the babies play together. This must be one of the most special treats for parents of twins.

The essentials of caring for twins are simply making sure that they are well fed and well loved. I found things went better if I fitted in with the babies' pattern, instead of trying to force them to fit into my idea of a schedule.

My husband and I take turns to take one of the twins out individually once a week.

When the baby twins learn to sit, put them in individual laundry baskets with a few toys next to each other.

up much more mischief than one baby, especially turning on the hot water. Choose bath toys carefully so that there is nothing that could become a dangerous missile or weapon.

Twinproofing the House

A single child is obviously much easier to keep an eye on than two or more. Multiples may all go in opposite directions — one turns on the taps in the bath, another unravels the toilet paper, and a third gets into the cabinet under the sink. Twins can join forces and create dangerous situations. For example, together they may be able to drag furniture, pull over a highchair, or tug a tablecloth onto the floor. Safety hints for childproofing a house are found in many books. (See Suggested Reading.) Install collapsible gates for doorways and stairwells, safety caps for electrical outlets, and locking devices on all doors, especially cabinets. All poisons and other dangerous substances should be stored at a high level. Beware also of plants, as some leaves and berries can be poisonous if eaten. Babies explore the world around them by putting everything in their mouths to taste.

Although crawling multiples are a big challenge, restrictive de-

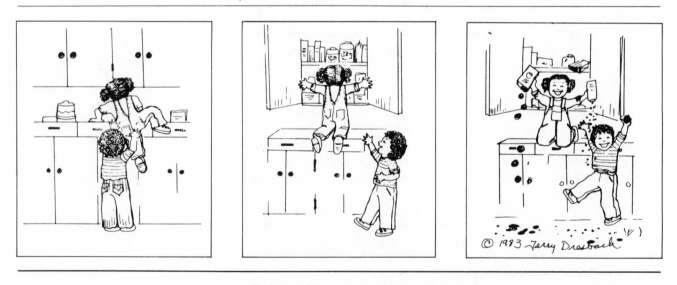

Twingenuity. *Line drawing by Terry Dresbach. Courtesy of Twin Services, Inc.*

vices such as playpens, jump seats, and gates interfere with curiosity and mastery of body skills, so if you use them, do so sparingly. Children learn quickest if they are allowed to complete an activity and then move on to something else. As Joseph Chilton Pearce points out, a child who is constantly stopped from taking out pots and pans, for example, will seek the experience again and again until the "circuit" in his brain is complete. Keep the telephone number of your local poison center handy. Educate your twins about "Mr. Yuk," a comic face on luminous green stickers for marking dangerous substances. Keep some ipecac in the house; it will induce vomiting if a baby has swallowed anything undesirable (but call the poison center at your hospital first — some substances should not be regurgitated). Ipecac may be bought over the counter in any drugstore.

We put up seventy-five feet of welded fencing with a locked door for $90. It's not the most attractive fencing, but it does the trick. It encloses a sandbox, swing set, children's pool, and other weather-resistant toys. We can easily remove the fencing when the triplets are older, but it's great for peace of mind now.

We found that a playpen was very confining for two babies, so we bought a Kiddy Korral, like a portable fence, which gave them a larger, safe area to play in.

Toilet Learning

No child under about eighteen months will have reached sufficient neurological development to learn toilet independence. Before that time, lucky breaks may occur or, more often, it is the parents who become toilet trained. Twins may be slower than singletons in learning sphincter control. Most authorities do not recommend attempting to toilet train twins before two years of age. Parents use two potties or sometimes one potty and one toilet seat. It is worth trying only a few times in the beginning. If the babies don't seem ready, abandon training for another month or so. When they are ready, it won't be difficult. Small plastic jars around the house are handy for boys.

   Children, as they are great imitators, learn more quickly when they can observe adults. When toilet training, use plenty of praise and never punish.

Our twins took longer before they were potty trained than our first child. But the job was much easier with the twins as they learn a lot from each other.

We found it handy to keep a glass jar in the bathroom to score a catch when our twin boys were in the tub.

Sharing

Twins learn to share and take turns earlier and easier than do singletons. Parents often comment that twins also play together better than do other siblings. The ability of twins to amuse themselves is one of their great advantages from the parents' point of view. Of course, there are times when biting and fighting can overwhelm the most patient parent. Time out (use a timer; a few minutes should do the trick) is one of the most recommended forms of discipline. Shouting and spanking show that the adult has lost control and is resorting to

Providing several duplicate toys, especially in the first few years, makes life easier for the parents. If my twins were squabbling over the red racing car, then peace could reign if I produced the white racing car too.

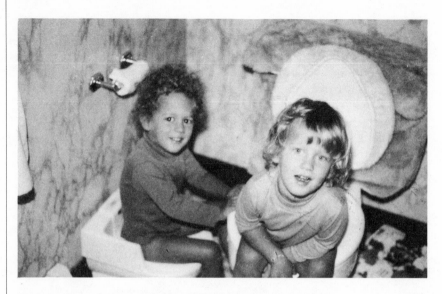

Twins learn to take turns — even at toilet training.

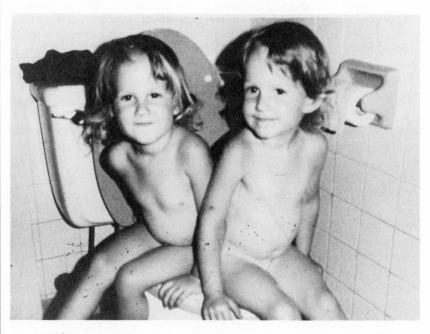

. . . sometimes.

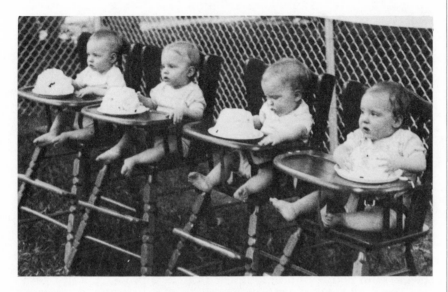

When there are four in a set, a whole cake is better than a quarter.

A mother of twins learns to be alone — when she scolds one daughter and the other buries her little head in the rug and moans. With triplets, two will hold the scolded one or try to spank the parent.

superior (thus unfair) physical power. Each twin should have his or her toys, labeled with his or her name. A set place for each twin to store personal toys is a good idea. Any unlabeled, identical toy in better condition may be claimed by the dominant twin. Many twins, however, are able to tell their identical toys apart, often by smell (soft toys). Of course, arguments can always ensue over two toys as well as one. Multiples need toys that promote cooperative play — jigsaws, Legos, seesaw, balls, games — as well as individual coloring books, pull toys, and building blocks. Hammers and ''weapons'' are not a good idea for multiples, but otherwise let them choose their own toys, pets, and hobbies.

Parents of multiples strongly advise that twins should not be given one gift to share, but something for each child. Twins sometimes complain that Christmas or birthdays are not very exciting for them because they tend to receive identical gifts. If Peter opens a package from Grandpa and finds a baseball glove, John, who is watching, has a pretty good idea what his present will be. Similarly, multiples prefer to give separate gifts rather than give one gift from both or all of them.

For twins' birthdays, some parents choose to celebrate the occasion on different days for each twin, alternating the actual birthday

The mother of twins learns to discard conventional math formulas about multiples. Mothers of twins do not have to be twice as patient, ambitious, or loving as mothers of singletons. Rather, the mother of twins observes, somewhat arrogantly, that her life is a thousand times more interesting and she knows she is a million times luckier.

The days are long, but the years are short.

I try to alternate where the twins sit at the table, which one is fed first or dressed first — wanting to be as fair as I can.

Our twins each have their own cake and invite their own friends and sit at opposite ends of the table.

each year. Some parents go to the trouble of giving back-to-back parties or celebrating one birthday a week later, so that each twin will feel unique and special. Parents usually make a birthday cake for each of the multiples, but one father's solution was one large cake with two halves decorated differently with its own set of candles. Some parents feel that sharing is better encouraged without duplicate cakes. Sometimes multiples have different birthdays if they were born around midnight. A birth on New Year's Eve may put twins' birthdays in different years. A mother of triplets decided to celebrate the birthday on the day when two out of the three were born. Other hints about twin birthdays include sending out separate invitations and taking a photo of each twin with his or her separate cake.

It is a dilemma for the parents of twins to decide whether to punish both or neither when a culprit will not confess or when one twin insists that it was teamwork. Most parents feel that punishing one twin leads to bad feelings on the part of the other as well as themselves. With higher-order multiples it can be a problem of just gathering them all together and trying to work out what happened. Most parents try to let multiples sort out their own disputes. Questioning rather than commanding will often draw out the facts. Punishing

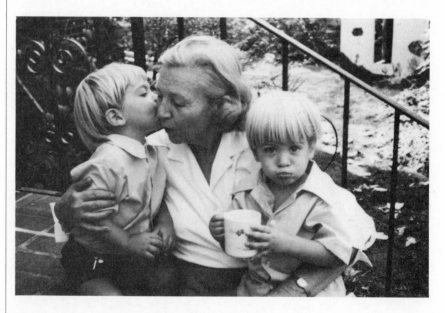

Grandmothers of twins get twice as many hugs.

both is never a good idea, according to twin psychologists Judy Hagedorn and Janet Kizziar, who are twins themselves. They recommend that parents punish the child they see misbehaving and explain, "You were the one I saw hitting your sister. Next time you may hit her first, but if I catch her hitting you, she will be punished." Further discussion of twin issues, with many interesting case histories, can be found in their book *Gemini*. Experts agree that punishment should never involve sending a child to bed, depriving him or her of food, confining the child to a playpen, or separating one twin from the other. Such measures can lead to difficulties with bed, meals, play, and twinship. I personally share the view expressed in *How to Talk so Kids Will Listen and How to Listen so Kids Will Talk*: punishment only breeds resentment and loss of self-esteem. The authors suggest hundreds of more creative alternatives to punishment.

The Older Siblings

Each position in the family has its advantages and disadvantages. The single first-born is the most displaced by the arrival of twins. As this

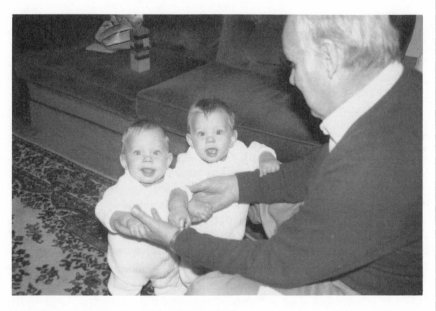

Grandfathers of twins have four hands to hold.

I've learned to seize the moment, stop whatever I am doing, and give my full attention to the child who interrupts. When I do this, these snatches of quality time give me a chance to enjoy that one's uniqueness.

I always felt guilty because I couldn't give two children as much love and attention as one. My pediatrician made me feel a lot better when he said that public attention would make up for it.

Whenever passers-by stop to ask the twins' names and ages, I always introduce their older sister.

We heard our young twins name-calling, and one of them said, "I can't even call you ugly — you look just like me!"

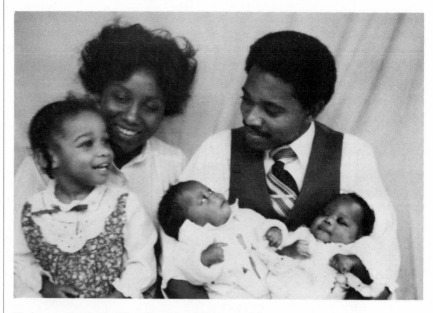

Twins are "two-rific," but the older child is special too.

Every time someone says to my twins, "How cute," I add, "Yes, and aren't Sarah's blond curls pretty?"

child lacks a sibling companion, parents need to provide special attention and privileges for him or her. Thoughtfulness for the feelings of the other children are essential during family outings. People will make a fuss over the multiples but will ignore the other child. This goes on for years. Many parents will meet someone after a long absence who will inquire about how the twins or triplets are doing but neglect to ask after the other children.

The LaTrobe Twin Study found that two-thirds of parents reported problems with older siblings in the first six months after the twins were born. Bed wetting was the most common, but parents reported physical aggression too. Avoid changing the child care, playschool, or sleeping arrangements of the older siblings around the time of the twins' arrival to mitigate feelings of resentment in the older children. Involve siblings in prenatal visits and hospital tours and in activities described in Chapter 14 that facilitate prenatal bonding, such as singing and reading to the babies. Have a babysitter for the twins sometimes so you can be with the older siblings. Explain to your other children when you feel overwhelmed. Include siblings in photos and in labels and name tags you might make for the twins. However, dressing the siblings like the twins, as with dressing the twins the same (see next section), gives the impression that it is important to look like someone else.

Siblings of twins feel that they are an attraction for their friends, but few want to be twins or to have twins. In the study, girls tended to have a close relationship with twin siblings, whereas boys tended to think the parents fussed over the twins too much. Also, siblings age two to five presented significant problems about half as often as siblings age eight to eleven. Some siblings are outwardly hostile, but others become withdrawn or perfectionistic, avoiding attention-seeking behavior and making sure they are not an additional burden. Early diagnosis of multiple pregnancy, if it is accompanied by bed rest or hospitalization, is also disruptive for children at home. Nowadays, twins take up much of the family's time and attention before the birth as well as after, and this can be a source of stress.

Home help is essential so that the parents can spend time with older siblings. If adults appreciated more the reality of being a sibling of twins, they would not ignore the older children as they focus on the multiples. A lone sibling may feel that he or she is the only family member without a partner. Preschool and school teachers are sometimes aware of problems that may escape parental attention at home, so keep communication open between home and school.

Resentment and jealousy are common among siblings in any family. It has been generally observed that monozygotic twins are more cooperative and dizygotic twins tend to be more competitive. Parents of multiples are usually prepared for the worst. Often these conflicts appear not so much between the twins or triplets but between other children in the family and the multiples. Regressive behavior such as biting and bed wetting is not uncommon. Sometimes the older child will want a bottle or demand to be dressed like the twins. (It must indeed be bewildering for the child at home who has been prepared for twins when triplets arrive.) Parents have shared some funny stories about the suggestions these children have: "We could always sell one" or "Couldn't we tie them both together and make one?"

Multiples and other siblings should be encouraged to air their feelings but not be permitted to turn them into physical abuse. Dolls or puppets are sometimes an aid to learning the child's true attitudes through play acting. Encourage family members (parents too) to hit pillows — never each other. Anger is a very real and important emotion; it must be expressed safely.

The first question people usually ask is "When did you find out you were having triplets?" Next they say, "How adorable. May I hold one?"

When people ask, "How do you tell them apart?" I reply, "I look at them!"

I think parents of twins have a difficult time in the beginning when they try to become attached to more than one baby. Dressing the babies alike can help the parents bond with the unit. Later, it becomes easier to discover each twin as an individual.

Mum and Dad have each other, the twins have each other — but I have no one.

My toddler won't come to the store with me if I am taking the twins. Everyone makes such a fuss of them, he might as well be invisible, even though he is standing right beside their stroller.

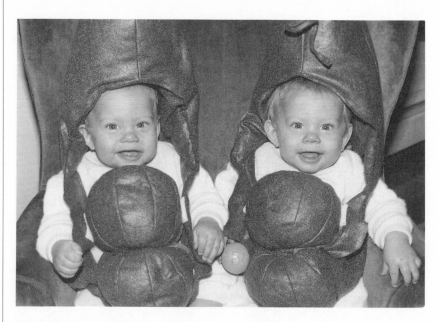

Identical twins in identical costumes look very cute.

Dressing

When buying clothes I always try something on my larger boy. It will surely fit his brother with less trying-on time.

While infants do not care if they are dressed alike or differently, new parents of twins receive many duplicate sets of clothing as gifts. Most parents are so proud of their multiples that they enjoy dressing the babies alike in the early years. Dizygotic twins may look very much alike at an early age and some parents may want to treat them as monozygotic. Other parents feel that unless the twins are dressed identically, their twinship will not be obvious. Twins appearing as a double act draw attention to the parents and make them feel special. Some parents even create father-son, mother-daughter outfits to wear with mixed-sex twins.

My twins choose their own clothes and sometimes will quite independently select the same outfit. I'm not going to start a fight just to get them to look different.

Nearly all parents, and certainly adult twins, feel that dressing alike, while fun on occasion, should stop when the multiples reach school age. The right time is when the children take an interest in choosing their own clothes (and they may always enjoy dressing alike on occasion). Not only does this clarify that establishing individuality at an early age is more important than twinship, but individual dress enables teachers and classmates to identify each twin without confusion. Identical clothing is usually associated with institutions that like to create anonymity and sameness, such as schools, hospitals, and prisons. However, because people in Western cultures do not usually dress identically, attention is drawn to multiples if their clothes are the same. This can make the other children in the family feel out of place. Parents usually do not dress siblings alike, although they may demand to be clothed like the twins to share some of the attention.

Dressing twins alike is not without its problems, even for those parents who fancy the idea. If one half of a set of clothing is stained, torn, or lost, the entire combination is no longer complete. Matching sets invite more scrutiny from passers-by. Twins themselves can be fussy and they often notice the slightest blemish on identical toys and clothes, which can lead to conflict. A psychological situation may develop when one twin demands the perfect item and the other accepts damaged goods. It can be boring to sew duplicate garments from the same fabric, although this may economize on patterns and leftover fabric. Remnants are usually cheaper but may not come in large enough quantity to make two outfits. Sale items are rarely duplicated. Secondhand clothing in sets of two is available only through Mothers of Twins Clubs. Stores do not always have identical garments in the right size. Both dizygotic and monozygotic twins can differ in height and weight, and they grow out of their clothes at different ages. Furthermore, as they get older they may not always agree on the outfit of the day.

Dressing the twins in the same outfits has a great advantage in a crowd or at a busy playground — it is easier to spot them.

Parents of twins who are trying to select different clothing frequently complain that it is easier to grab two of the same from rows of identical garments. Parents are often forced to do this if they cannot find two different and comparable outfits. One frequent solution is to buy two different colors. Of course, just because two identical outfits were purchased does not mean that both twins have to wear them simultaneously.

Treating twins as unique individuals does not depend so much on how they are dressed but rather on how closely the parents have bonded with each baby.

These issues are multiplied with triplets or quadruplets. The important point is not how the children are clothed but how they are treated. However, dressing them identically makes it obvious to society that they are treated primarily as twins rather than individuals.

Dealing with Prematurity and Multiples with Special Needs

THE EMPHASIS OF THIS BOOK has been on prevention of the difficulties that surround multiple pregnancy and birth. While excellent nutrition and prenatal care can alleviate many of the problems, fate is still outside human control. Some congenital anomalies, handicaps, and preterm births occur without any apparent reason. Of babies most at risk, 18 percent of very-low-birth-weight infants (less than 1,500 grams, or 3 pounds, 5 ounces) and 15 percent of infants born at less than thirty-one weeks are multiples.

At the International Society for Twin Studies 1989 Congress in Rome, French obstetrician Émile Papiernik calculated that for every thousand singletons, 36 days of neonatal intensive care unit (NICU) are needed, whereas for every thousand twins, 4,168 days are required. He also figured out that there are about 2 handicapped babies for every 1,000 single births, but 16 per 1,000 twins. The risk of handicap is related to birth weight. Babies weighing less than 1,000 grams (2 pounds, 3 ounces) have cerebral palsy or mental retardation at the rate of 200 per 1,000. Between 1,000 and 1,500 grams (2 pounds, 3 ounces to 3 pounds, 4 ounces) the incidence declines by half, and in newborns weighing more than 2,500 grams (5 pounds, 8 ounces) it is only 2 per 1,000.

Twins who are born early and are truly small-for-dates because of earlier lung maturation may be in better shape than singletons of the same size and age. Generally, the more babies, the smaller each individual member of the set. For example, if triplets arrive instead of twins, the babies may be smaller than expected. Parents may take heart from the smallest Dionne quintuplet (born in Canada in 1934), who weighed 2 pounds. These babies were born and cared for at home with simple measures such as warmth of the open oven. (Three of the quintuplets were still alive in 1990.)

The Mauss triplets, like the Dionne babies, weighed less than 3 pounds each at their birth in 1900 and were kept in a shoebox in the warming oven of a coal stove. Still going strong in 1990, Vinal, Valma, and Vilda are believed to be the oldest living triplets in the United States.

The Guinness Book of World Records lists the lowest birth weight for surviving twins as 2 pounds, 3 ounces combined weight. One twin weighed 1 pound and the other weighed 1 pound, 3 ounces. They were born in 1931 in England. The record for the smallest baby to survive is currently held by Ernestine Hudgins, who weighed 17 ounces when she was born eighteen weeks early in San Diego in 1983. The lowest birth weight recorded for a surviving infant is 10 ounces for a baby born in England six weeks premature in 1938. Measuring just 12¼ inches long, she was fed hourly for the first day with brandy, glucose, and water through a fountain pen filler. At three weeks she weighed 1 pound, 13 ounces and by her first birthday 13 pounds, 14 ounces. When she was twenty-one her weight was 106 pounds and she died at age forty-four. The most premature baby to survive is James Elgin Gill, who arrived 128 days early in 1987 and weighed 22 ounces.

At one hospital in Bogotá, Colombia, that can't afford high-tech medical care, mothers simply carry (low-risk) premature babies skin-to-skin, wrapped onto their bellies like a kangaroo pouch. (Premature twins are small enough to both fit in one pouch, and the father can create a kangaroo pouch also. This keeps the babies together as well.) It is not surprising to me that the babies do well with the benefits of mother's touch, smell, sound, and warmth and avoidance of the hazards of some high-tech equipment. Babies in the NICU may be exposed to inappropriate stimulation such as high-decibel mechanical noise and high-intensity fluorescent lights, both of which contribute to physical stress and are suspected of playing a role in hearing and vision impairment. By contrast, soft vocalization and sensitive touch — especially by the family — have a soothing, therapeutic effect.

Emotional Reactions of Parents to Premature Babies

Prematurity is a crisis in the parenting process as well as a disturbance in the development of the infant. The mother and father are deprived of the last few weeks of pregnancy, in which they would have furthered their psychological preparation. Parents require time and supportive discussion to adapt to this abrupt interruption of the normal process and to face the disappointment of their expectations.

The misfortune of prematurity is also relative. Women who repeatedly miscarry or have infertility problems may be overjoyed to

The first time I saw my twins after birth they were in their incubators. The staff wanted me to touch them, but for some reason I didn't want to; everything seemed too unreal. Pumping my breasts and reading kept me busy, but the next six weeks seemed like an eternity. Then one twin came home, followed by his sister three weeks later.

I found it helpful to keep a daily journal of events and my feelings. Knowing that we were visiting the babies, giving them expressed breast milk, plus the knowledge that they were receiving excellent care, made us feel that in time we could bring home two healthy babies, and we did.

Jim and I feel we developed a stronger sense of family togetherness because of our twins' prematurity. It made us more dependent on each other for moral and emotional support.

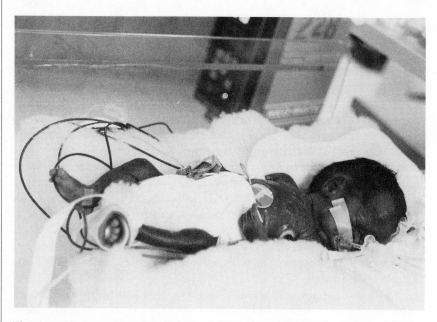

The size and appearance of a premature baby are very different from those of a baby born at term.

deliver living twins, even if they are premature. Other mothers of multiples may be warned so much about prematurity that if their babies are in the nursery for only a week or two, they consider themselves lucky.

It is difficult for parents to identify with one or more babies jerkily moving in an incubator, perhaps with a maze of tubes, wires, and electrodes covering their tiny bodies. What they see is so different from the "ideal" picture of a healthy baby. Premature babies are often very tiny and look thin and wrinkled, with disproportionately large, long heads. Sometimes they are still covered with fetal hair (lanugo).

Mothers often feel disappointment, guilt, or a sense of failure that they did not deliver a full-term baby with good weight, and they may wonder what they did wrong.

Many parents have a difficult time believing that the infants are real and will both survive, especially if one is very sick or has a potential* handicap. Society dictates that maternal love is instant and

---

* With premies, some handicaps may not be apparent until later — at least five years for cerebral palsy and eight years to detect intellectual deficits.

boundless, so the mother who finds it difficult to like babies who sleep most of the time, react very little, and never smile must also battle with diminished self-esteem. This pressure is very hard for a first-time mother who is attempting to create an image of herself as a parent.

Anxiety is a normal reaction and motivates parents to pursue information and seek support at this time. Regular interaction with the babies and the hospital staff helps the parents adapt to the particular characteristics of their premature infants' development. Some hospitals have parent support groups; others are listed in Resources.

The Neonatal Intensive Care Unit (NICU)

Not all hospitals have the technical equipment and trained personnel to provide advanced life support for premature infants. Level II nurseries are for infants requiring minimal oxygen support as well as intravenous therapy. Level III nurseries are neonatal intensive care; such units are often in a regional center to which high-risk expectant mothers and babies are brought by ambulance or helicopter, if necessary.

Although high-tech, most NICUs are no longer the cold fortresses against infectious outsiders they once were. Modern hospitals now have twenty-four-hour visiting and encourage as much parental contact with the babies as possible. Babies need their parents' care, feeding, and handling in order to thrive, just as the parents need to perform these nurturing activities to facilitate bonding. Love and warmth from the parents help to soften the environment of glass, metal, tubes, and machines, although the mother may find such contact difficult if she is recovering from a difficult labor, a Caesarean, or other complications. Mothers experience emotional anguish at seeing their tiny babies so helpless and sick, fear that they will not survive, and regret at missing the body contact that follows a normal delivery.

NICUs provide one-to-one nursing care in addition to neonatologists, who are pediatricians specializing in newborns, twenty-four hours a day. Sometimes each baby will be cared for by a different team.

Neonatology is a medical specialty that is about twenty-five years old. Technological developments in this field have dramatically affected the survival of very-low-birth-weight infants — babies born weighing less than 1,500 grams (3 pounds, 5 ounces). Twenty-five years ago only 40 percent of these babies survived. Today, the survival percentage has more than doubled, and most very-low-birth-

No one ever explained about NICU and it was a shock! I walked in and cried. Wayne was below his birth weight, lying face down with tubes, needles, and oxygen in and around him. If it wasn't for the last name on his bed, I wouldn't have known he was mine. Looking at him I felt I had delivered an alien. His ears were transparent, there were no eyelashes or brows or shape to his body. The monitors beeped but the babies didn't cry. They all looked lifeless yet alive.

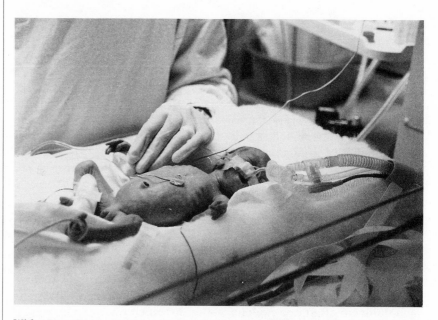

With 40 to 130 tests and procedures performed per baby per day, the cost of intensive care for twins may approach (and sometimes exceed) $4,000 per day.

weight survivors grow up without major handicaps. However, improvements in survival and outcome are largely concentrated among the bigger, more mature of these babies. For example, infants born weighing less than 750 grams (1 pound, 10 ounces) still have an overall mortality rate of 70 to 80 percent. Among the survivors, approximately one-third have handicaps serious enough to be diagnosed in babyhood. Because these infants require many months of intensive treatment at great human and financial cost and because the results are so often poor, some physicians and ethicists now suggest that intensive care for babies below 750 grams be carried out only on an experimental basis, if the parents give their fully informed consent.

Birth weight alone is not a reliable indicator of a baby's survival prospects. Equally important (though harder to determine accurately) is the baby's gestational age. At a gestational age of twenty-four to twenty-five weeks, twins in the fiftieth weight percentile have birth weights in the range of 600–750 grams at twenty-six to twenty-seven weeks, 800–850 grams; at twenty-nine weeks, 1,200 grams; and at thirty-two weeks, 1,600 grams. However, some babies are significantly bigger or smaller than average. Certain very small babies are much older and more mature than their birth weights would indicate.

Consequently, they have a better chance for survival than other babies of the same birth weight. Conversely, some relatively large babies are less mature than others of the same birth weight and are, therefore, at greater risk.

Premature babies usually stay in the hospital until close to their date of delivery, although babies with very complicated medical problems may need to remain for months longer. Neonatal care is often referred to as a "mixed blessing." To quote Helen Harrison, author of *The Premature Baby Book:* "It can sustain life, . . . but it does not always restore health. Used indiscriminately, it can inflict and perpetuate dreadful suffering." Neonatal therapies may also produce dangerous complications. One premature baby can be saved for a relatively normal life, while another with similar problems survives for a lifetime of illness and handicap. Unfortunately, it may be impossible at the outset of treatment to know what the outcome will be. Even if this information were known with certainty, doctors might be reluctant to act on it. Many physicians in the United States interpret the "Baby Doe" laws* as requiring them to treat all babies intensively, even if the prognosis is very poor and even if the parents wish care changed or stopped. Each day costs up to $2,000 per baby just for the NICU, and there may be up to 130 tests and procedures, including nursing care, performed daily.

Others argue that much of what is done in NICUs should be considered experimental and, Baby Doe laws notwithstanding,

* "Baby Doe" laws are amendments made in 1984 to the Child Abuse and Treatment Act that define the "withholding of medically indicated treatment" from newborns as child abuse.

Approximate Survival Rates

Weight	Age	Survival Rate (%)
700 grams (1½ lb)	24–25 weeks	25
850 grams (1 lb, 14 oz)	26 weeks	50
1,000 grams (2 lb, 3 oz)	27–28 weeks	75
1,200–1,500 grams (2 lb, 10 oz–3 lb, 5 oz)	29–30 weeks	90

Source: Roberta Ballard, M.D., *Pediatric Care of the ICN Graduate* (1988).

You see your baby suffering. You worry about lasting problems. You wonder if death might be better. You think you shouldn't feel this way when doctors and nurses with machines are working so hard to maintain your child's life. But the feelings of attachment were always there. The baby seemed like a part of myself, yet it was painful for me to be with him. I wanted to end his suffering.

We always made a tape recording of sessions with the doctors. It was helpful to replay the tape as needed and listen to the tone and implications of their voices.

While the boys were in respiratory distress, they were a mass of tubes, wires, tape, and patches. It was frightening to see them at first, but the nursing staff helped us understand what all the attachments were. As we understood what the equipment was doing, we began to see more of the babies and less of the gadgets.

should be carried out only with informed parental consent. They point out that neonatologists, eager to push back the limits of viability, have hastily introduced powerful drugs and therapies into the NICU without properly testing them for safety and efficacy. For example, the National Institute for Child Health and Human Development (NICHD) recently criticized neonatal practitioners for providing care "based on limited knowledge of new modalities not subjected to critical studies prior to introduction and acceptance" and for changing therapies "within months before adequate studies of safety and efficacy are initiated, much less completed." The poorly validated therapies listed by the NICHD include just about everything done to premature babies in the NICU. In the absence of consistent standards for validating neonatal therapies, caregiving practices may vary widely from doctor to doctor, hospital to hospital to hospital, and country to country.

The uncertainties of neonatal care and the lack of decision-making powers may be very discouraging to NICU parents. Nevertheless, it is important that they play an active role as members of their babies' health care teams. Parents should expect to be fully informed of the risks and benefits of proposed treatments, of alternative treatments, and of no treatment at all. They should feel free to question physicians about the quality of evidence supporting neonatal therapies, to consult the medical literature, or to seek second or third opinions. The family's regular pediatrician can often be a helpful ally and advocate.

Involved, informed parents can have an important influence not only on their own babies' care but also on the care of countless others. Activist parents have been at the forefront of campaigns to reform nursery policies, to humanize the NICU environment, and to alert the public and medical community to dangerous or inhumane medical practices. For examples, it was NICU parents who first called attention to the hazards of AIDS-infected blood transfusions, to the potential dangers of high-intensity fluorescent lighting, and to the cruelty of unanesthetized infant surgery. Currently parents and parent groups are becoming active in advocating stricter standards for the evaluation of neonatal therapies and the repeal or modification of laws that limit parental decision-making power in the NICU.

Equipment

Isolettes, also known as incubators, are closed, heated beds with transparent sides and top for observation and portholes for staff to tend the baby. Open warming beds heated with overhead infrared heat lamps give doctors and nurses easier access to a baby who requires frequent procedures. As the babies' skin color and appearance need to be monitored day and night, babies are usually naked or wear only diapers. Head caps help minimize loss of body heat. Proper positioning of the babies in bed is important. A flat-on-the-back, spread-eagle position can be highly stressful and cause problems with oxygenation. Premies are more comfortable and stable lying on their sides with arms and legs flexed close to the body. Blanket rolls provide support and a feeling of containment.

Monitors continuously record vital signs such as heart rate, oxygen levels, temperature, and blood pressure, and an alarm sounds if any of the signs deviate too far from normal. The leads are attached to the skin and may trigger the monitor if they are accidentally disturbed. Monitor alarms may be frightening at first to new parents. Such loud noises may also disturb the babies, causing the very disruptions of breathing (apnea) and heart rate (bradycardia) that they are intended to monitor. Parents should request that monitor alarms, telephone bells, radios, and conversations be as quiet as possible. In particular, isolette portholes should be closed gently and a blanket should cover the top before any objects are placed on it. This blanket will help blunt the noise as well as shield the baby from bright nursery lights, another potential source of stress.

Complications of Prematurity

With little body fat, immature sweat glands, and highly permeable skin, premature babies cannot easily regulate their body temperatures or hydration and therefore require care in a constantly heated, humid environment. With poorly coordinated sucking reflexes and digestive tract immaturities, they may need tube feeding or intravenous nourishment. Immaturities of the lungs, brain, liver, kidneys, and circulatory system can lead to other problems described later in this chapter.

Catheters (IVs) are inserted into the baby's blood vessels to bring in fluids, blood, medication, or nourishment. A central catheter may be placed in the artery of the umbilical cord stump, which allows the medical staff to withdraw blood and measure blood pressure. Venous catheters placed in an arm, leg, or the umbilicus can be used for antibiotics or nutrients.

Because of their immature immune systems, premature babies

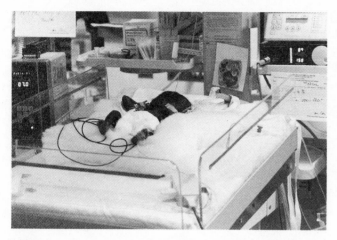

Your baby may seem dwarfed by all the high-tech equipment.

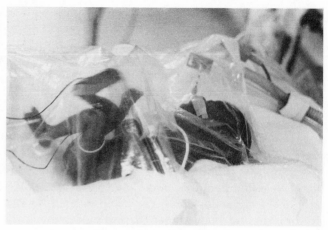

Plastic wrap keeps a premie free from drafts.

We kept our hopes up after the first few days, but were crestfallen with every weight loss or other setback. Most crushing were transfers back under the hood, from the intermediate nursery back to intensive care.

are especially vulnerable to infections. These infections are sometimes contracted in utero or during labor, especially after prolonged rupture of the membranes, or in the nursery. Careful hand washing by the staff and parents before handling the babies is important in preventing nursery infections. Antibiotic treatment is begun once an infection is identified or suspected.

Diuretics may be given for fluid buildup, but premature babies often have a problem staying sufficiently hydrated because of the heating of their environment and their inability to tolerate sufficient fluid intake.

Breathing difficulty is the most critical problem for premature babies because their lungs are not adequately developed or they do not function properly for oxygen exchange. The NICU staff can assist such babies' breathing until they can breathe on their own. This may take days, weeks, or months. Baby's respiratory status is monitored by taking chest x-rays, listening to the respiration, and analyzing the blood for relative amounts of oxygen and carbon dioxide. Mucous secretions in the lung passages are removed with a small plastic tube (suction catheter) connected to a vacuum machine.

Apnea spells, when the baby doesn't breathe for longer than 15 seconds, are very common. The heart rate may slow down (bradycardia) as well, so these episodes are known as "A and B spells." Gently touching the baby is usually enough to stimulate breathing again, and waterbeds are sometimes used for babies who intermittently stop breathing. An oxygen mask is used to resuscitate a baby who has

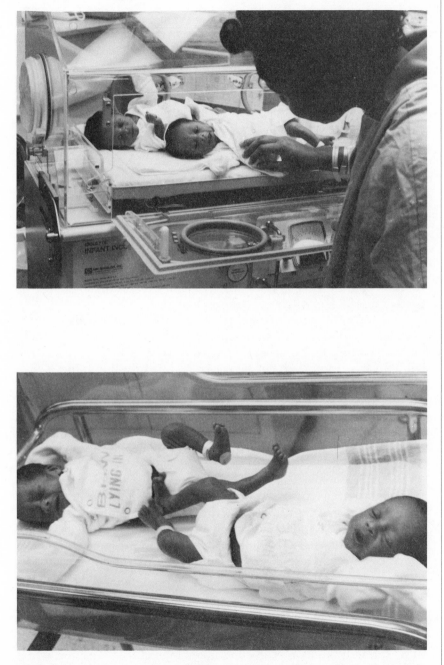

While there is usually one baby per incubator, it is important for twins to be together when possible.

stopped breathing. Premies who continue to have apnea at the time of discharge are often sent home with an apnea monitor; if apnea persists, medications such as caffeine or theophylline may be used to control it.

Circulatory problems are common in premature babies. The ductus arteriosus (the blood vessel that directs blood away from the lungs prenatally) often stays open in a premie after birth instead of closing as it would in a term baby. The condition sometimes requires a medication (indomethacin) or surgical closure if that drug is not successful or cannot be used because of bleeding or jaundice.

Jaundice is a condition in which the skin and the whites of the eyes turn yellow because of excessive bile pigment (bilirubin) in the circulation that the immature liver cannot break down. Some amount is normal after birth, but high levels can lead to brain damage. Jaundice is very common — occurring in about 80 percent of preterm babies — and it decreases as liver function improves. While breast-fed infants may show slightly higher levels of bilirubin than bottle-fed babies, the difference is not clinically significant and should not be used as a reason to discourage breast-feeding.

Phototherapy with "bililights" is the first treatment used when bilirubin rises to levels thought to be dangerous. It consists of shining blue and white fluorescent light on the baby's skin to convert the bilirubin to a form that can be easily excreted by the kidneys. Eye patches should be securely placed over the eyes of jaundiced babies during treatment. If a neighboring baby is being treated with bililights, make sure your babies are well protected from accidental exposure. If phototherapy doesn't succeed in lowering the bilirubin concentration, exchange transfusions may be needed to dilute it in the baby's blood.

Anemia is common in premature babies because their blood is so frequently removed for testing and because premies are born with insufficient stores of iron. Blood transfusions are sometimes required to correct this condition, and supplemental iron may be given. Breast milk has the most absorbable form of iron, and breast-feeding is encouraged throughout the first year of life to prevent or alleviate anemia.

Respiratory Distress Syndrome (RDS)

RDS, formerly known as hyaline membrane disease, gained widespread public attention when President John Kennedy's premature son died of the condition in 1963.

There is no requirement to test very powerful nondrug therapies such as respirators, spinal taps, phototherapy, or hyperalimination [intravenous feeding] for safety and effectiveness.
HELEN HARRISON

The syndrome develops if the baby's lung tissue is too immature to produce sufficient amounts of surfactant, a liquid that coats the lungs' tiny air sacs and prevents them from closing and sticking together after each breath. Without enough surfactant, the air sacs collapse every time the baby exhales, and breathing becomes progressively difficult. The situation may be worsened by the baby's low energy reserves and exhaustion after birth as well as by the premature baby's tendency to react to stress by failing to breathe (apnea).

RDS strikes 10 to 20 percent of all premature babies and close to 50 percent of very-low-birth-weight premies. After the twenty-eighth week of gestation, premature boys (who develop more slowly in utero) are more vulnerable to the disease than girls. Before that gestational age, both sexes are equally at risk. Second-born twins (who are more likely to have a stressful delivery) are more at risk than firstborns. Although nearly 80 percent of premies now survive this disease, it remains the leading cause of death among newborns, claiming about 12,000 lives each year.

RDS is treated by giving the baby supplemental oxygen and, if

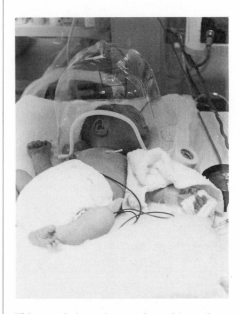

This premie is resting on sheepskin under an oxygen hood.

Treatment for Respiratory Distress Syndrome

Minor Breathing Problems

The babies may just need a face mask or oxygen hood (oxyhood or headbox) made of clear plastic to help them breathe. This brings humidified oxygen through a hose and tube to the baby's face.

Moderate Breathing Problems

Continuous positive airway pressure (CPAP) helps babies who have more difficulty breathing. A tube is inserted into the baby's nose with nasal prongs. Oxygen is delivered at a predetermined rate and pressure that will prevent the alveoli from collapsing.

Severe Breathing Problems

Ventilators are used when breathing difficulties are very serious. A deeper (endotracheal) tube goes all the way into the baby's windpipe, either through the back of the throat or directly with a surgical incision in the neck (tracheotomy). The ventilator mechanically controls the pressure and volume of air that is delivered directly to the lungs.

---

necessary, by placing the baby on a respirator, a machine that forces air in and out of the baby's lungs.

RDS may be complicated by such conditions as pneumonia, heart failure, pneumothorax (in which air leaks from the lung), broncho-pulmonary dysplasia (lung damage produced by respirator therapy), and brain hemorrhages.

The steroid drug betamethasone, if given to mothers forty-eight hours before a threatened preterm delivery, is sometimes successful in hastening the development of the unborn babies' lungs and pre-venting RDS. The drug does not usually work if the babies are less than twenty-seven weeks gestation.

New Developments

Jet ventilation gives respiratory rates of 100–600 per minute to infants who would otherwise be unable to take in sufficient oxygen. High-frequency oscillating ventilators give rates of up to 3,000 breaths per minute. As yet there is no evidence to show any improvement over conventional ventilators.

Another new development is surfactant made synthetically (the cheapest and most available form) or from animals (cow's lungs) or from human amniotic fluid (obtained at term Caesarean deliveries). This is put directly in the infant's windpipe after birth, and premature babies who respond to the surfactant do so quickly and can be rapidly weaned off oxygen. Because surfactant is not the only factor involved in RDS, some babies do not improve with this treatment.

Complications of RDS

One-third of the babies who survive RDS have some kind of residual deficit — physical, sensory, or intellectual. While eye and lung prob-lems are the most common, other side effects include damage to the vocal cords and trachea from prolonged use of tubes in the nose and throat, hearing loss (from use of diuretics, some antibiotics, viruses, and the noise from their NICU environment), liver damage from IV feedings, and infections and diseases from blood transfusions.

Retinopathy of Prematurity (ROP)

In the 1940s it was discovered that treating premature babies with excessive amounts of oxygen in the atmosphere can affect the blood vessels in the retina of the eye. This retinopathy is the most common cause of blindness in children today. In severe cases, there is abnor-

There is no requirement that drugs be specifically tested in neonates once they are proved safe and effective in older individuals, despite the fact that neonates metabolize drugs differently.
HELEN HARRISON

mal growth of blood vessels with excess fluid and scarring. In the worst cases, the retina detaches when the fluid and scar tissue build up enough pressure. Limited vision or blindness results.

Annually in the United States, retinopathy of prematurity causes 2,600 cases of vision loss, with total blindness occurring in 650 very-low-birth-weight babies. As many as one in six very-low-birth-weight infants born before thirty weeks develops ROP, and some of them will become blind.

When oxygen levels were reduced, the ROP epidemic of the 1940s and 1950s abated, but more premature babies died or were left brain-damaged. Today the disease is epidemic once more, owing in part to the increased survival rates of vulnerable very-low-birth-weight babies. Because ROP is on the rise despite sophisticated oxygen monitoring and because some victims never receive oxygen, the theory that oxygen is the primary or only cause is being challenged. Fluorescent lighting may play a role.

Attempts are being made with cryotherapy (freezing), lasers (light waves), and surgery to reattach the retina. The outcome, which takes time to assess, is successful so far in less than half of the cases. All premature babies who receive oxygen and all very-low-birth-weight babies, whether they receive oxygen or not, should be examined by an ophthalmologist at six to eight weeks of age and routinely until oxygen therapy is stopped. Examination of the condition of the blood vessels in the retina should be repeated at three, six, nine, and twelve months of age, and throughout childhood if indicated.

I regret not following my instincts as the mother of twins. I should have pursued the matter of Jason's eye problems when I first noticed the difference in their development. He seemed clumsy but had eye problems not recognized by doctors. I've learned not to be intimidated by strangers who may not recognize problems outside their field.

Bronchopulmonary Dysplasia

Although respirator treatment may be lifesaving for many babies, it can lead to permanent damage. Bronchopulmonary dysplasia is a condition in which the lungs lose their elasticity. Approximately 20 to 30 percent of babies treated with mechanical ventilation for RDS develop this damage to some degree and require respirator treatment for a month or longer. In a 1989 article, Gladstone stated that the incidence was 2–6 percent for all birth weights. In babies weighing 500 to 1,000 grams (1 pound, 2 ounces to 2 pounds, 3 ounces), the incidence is 14 percent; it is 6 percent in babies weighing up to 1,500 grams (3 pounds, 5 ounces) and 4 percent up to 2,000 grams (4 pounds, 6 ounces). There is about a 23 percent incidence of death, and survivors may have chronic respiratory problems because of lung scarring. For most babies with BPD, symptoms improve with age since the lungs can grow healthy new tissue up to the age of eight. Unfortunately, some BPD victims remain dependent on the respirator or oxygen for years, or even for life.

Brain Hemorrhages

In a premature baby's brain fluctuations in the baby's blood pressure may cause the fragile blood vessels to break, resulting in hemorrhages. Currently an estimated 40 to 60 percent of all premature infants in intensive care suffer from these hemorrhages. Major hemorrhages can lead to later developmental handicaps or a buildup of fluid on the brain (hydrocephalus). Many conditions of prematurity and many nursery treatments (some of which may interfere with blood-clotting factors) can produce the blood pressure fluctuations that may lead to hemorrhages. Ultrasound beamed through the fontanelle (the open area at the top of the skull), which involves a low dose of x-rays, is used to detect hemorrhage or hydrocephalus. If hydrocephalus develops, it is kept under control by a surgically implanted tube that drains fluid from the brain to the circulatory system or the abdominal area. This shunt usually must be kept in place for life.

Vitamin K is routinely given to premies until their intestines absorb it (when the baby begins to have food by mouth). This supplement enhances clotting factors in the blood and diminishes the likelihood of hemorrhage. In 1989, Dr. Walter Morales found that there were half the number of brain bleeds if a woman with threatening premature labor had one vitamin K injection every five days until delivery. It also helped to have one injection of vitamin K even just hours before the birth. Only 16 percent of mothers who took the preventive vitamin K had infants with brain bleeds, compared with 36 percent of those who did not receive the vitamin. While 11 percent of the control group had severe brain bleeds, not one of the experimental group did.

Feeding of Premature Babies

Make sure that your premie babies get your breast milk. Don't let the staff tell you it is not calorically right; on the contrary, it is better for the babies than the breast milk of a term mother.

Before thirty-two to thirty-four weeks gestational age, premature babies often have difficulty coordinating sucking, swallowing, and breathing. Until this coordination is developed, feeding via a tube into the nose or mouth is required. The tube may be removed between these gavage feedings. Sometimes the digestive system of a premature baby cannot handle milk, and a nutritional solution is given intravenously, often through a scalp tube (which is less likely to be dislodged) or via the navel.

After oral feedings are tolerated, a special bottle for premies with a very small, soft nipple is the next step, or the baby may begin nursing. Around thirty-two weeks, the sucking and swallowing pattern emerges and parents can take over more of the feeding. The mechanics of bottle-feeding and breast-feeding are very different, and recent studies show that even tiny premature infants suckle better at the breast than the bottle. During breast-feeding, the babies breathe better, absorb more oxygen, stay warmer, and remain physically more stable than during bottle feeding. However, since most mothers (in the United States, at least) are unable to be at the hospital for every feeding, some bottle feedings are almost always necessary. If you cannot breast-feed for every feeding, make sure that your babies are fed your breast milk, which you have expressed. Start to express colostrum from your breasts several times a day within twenty-four hours after the birth (the milk itself will be produced three days after the birth). Emptying both breasts at once is an efficient way to build supply.

The NICU usually has an electric breast pump (which is easier than a manual one if you're pumping for twins), or you can buy your own or rent one for home use from La Leche League, a pharmacy, or medical supply house. An electric breast pump can be adapted to pump both breasts at once if you do not receive the equipment with your pump. (Purchase a plastic T at the hardware store and buy additional tubing the same size as provided with the pump. Cut the additional tubing into two pieces and sterilize them and the T. Attach the pump's tube to the T and the two new tubes between your breasts and the double end of the T, hook up to the breast pump, and you can pump two breasts simultaneously.) You can also nurse one baby and pump milk for the other at the same time, which helps your letdown reflex. As discussed in Chapter 15, the breasts work on a supply and demand principle. The more you nurse, the more milk your breasts will produce and the more weight your babies will gain. You just need to eat very well, drink lots of fluid, sleep whenever possible, and pump.

In the hospital, check that the NICU breast pump is sterile, and use sterile collection bottles as it is important to avoid bacterial contamination for tiny babies. Refrigerated breast milk is best used within a day or so, but it can be frozen for a couple of weeks.

Whenever babies must be fed by tube or bottle, mother's milk remains the food of choice. Its special nutrients and disease-fighting properties are particularly important to premature babies. For ex-

One of my triplets was fed formula because the doctor thought my milk had too many calories. The two babies who received my milk thrived, but the one on artificial nourishment did poorly. Yet the doctor insisted that my milk would harm him. I insisted on breast-feeding him, and in a short time that baby's health turned around.

I had a really hard time producing or increasing my milk supply while I used the pump. I used massage, warm towels, pictures of my babies, and a tape recording of their hunger cries to stimulate my milk to let down. I was able to pump enough milk for half of the gavage feedings a day.

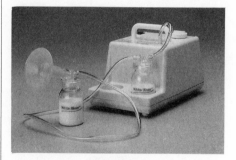

The White River® Electric Breast Pump. *Courtesy of NTI/White River.*

It took one look at my babies' tiny struggling bodies when they arrived ten weeks early to realize that if ever babies needed the benefit of their mother's milk, they did.

Every other day, I pumped my breasts to take the milk and drove three and a half hours to my surviving twin, for the two months he was in the NICU. Then I found out, like other mothers discovered, that the hospital staff just threw it away and gave her formula.

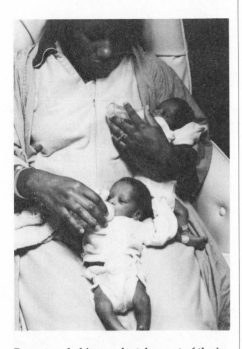

Premature babies can be taken out of the incubator for feeding (these twins are receiving breast milk in a bottle with a special nipple) . . .

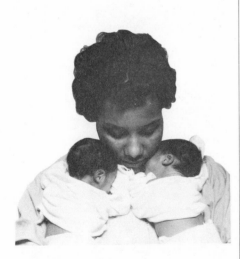

. . . or just cuddling.

ample, breast milk may play a role in preventing necrotizing enterocolitis (discussed under "Surgery" later in this chapter). Supplemental vitamins, minerals, protein, and calories may be added to meet the growth requirements of very sick or tiny babies.

As soon as possible after birth, state your intention to breast-feed to the neonatologist. Request the nursery's guidelines for expressing, storing, and transporting breast milk. Contact lactation consultants or nurse or physician breast-feeding specialists who work in the NICU. If none are available, call La Leche League or the International Lactation Consultants Association (see Resources).

Whether your babies are first fed by breast or bottle, early feedings may be frustrating for both mother and babies. Consider these first feedings as learning sessions and a time for closeness. A private room and an experienced nurse to assist with positioning the babies is helpful. Even if you cannot put the babies to your breast, give the bottle skin-to-skin and use the occasion for eye contact and voice stimulation. If possible, feed your babies when they are alert and hungry rather than according to a schedule.

A premie twin who is not good at sucking can be stimulated if the other twin nurses at the same time. The strong let-down reflex from the first twin's nursing will cause some milk to squirt into the other twin's mouth and stimulate a sucking reflex. Some babies will cough or sputter a bit at first.

If you have other children, it may be an incredible stress and burden for you to pump your breasts, transport the milk to the hospital, and be available for breast-feeding in the nursery. Your local Mothers of Twins Club or NICU parent support group may be able to help you handle these responsibilities. You are giving your child the gift of life, the "milk of human kindness." Expressing the milk helps to maintain your milk supply and is a valuable contribution to your infants' welfare that only you can make. If only one twin is receiving special nursery care, breast-feeding the other helps to keep up the supply. Donor breast milk can also be used, especially with triplets or quadruplets.

Mothers who breast-feed their premature babies also find that the emotional satisfactions go a long way toward compensating for the pain and separation of a premature birth.

Surgery

A very common surgical emergency in premies is caused by necrotizing enterocolitis (NEC), inflammation of tissues in the intestines and colon.

A baby with NEC is not fed by mouth and is treated with antibiotics. But if these measures fail, a portion of the damaged intestine is removed, often with the creation of a colostomy or ileostomy. These ostomies can usually be reversed and normal bowel function restored. However, some babies with severe NEC are maintained for months and years on intravenous nourishment, only to die eventually from liver damage caused by the IV feedings.

Sick newborns, both term and preterm, may require various kinds of surgery such as closure of the ductus arteriosus, repair of congenital heart or spinal cord defects, installation of shunts for hydrocephalus, or repair of hernias. In the NICU, arterial lines may be surgically installed or chest tubes may be surgically implanted to correct pneumothorax (collapsed lung).

Until very recently, these procedures were often performed without anesthesia because of doctors' mistaken assumptions that babies don't feel pain. Instead of anesthesia, babies were usually paralyzed for procedures with curare (Pavulon), a drug that left them unable to move or react in any way but able to feel everything that was done to them. In 1986 parents of premature babies, led by Jill Lawson, the mother of a baby who died after unanesthetized ductus surgery, called public attention to this barbaric state of affairs. Recent research has shown that unanesthetized surgery is not only cruel but also dangerous. Stress from unrelieved surgical pain has been found to lead to a high incidence of complications that can cause disability or death.

Nevertheless, the practice of unanesthetized surgery continues at some hospitals, and in many units adequate anesthesia and analgesia are still not given for excruciating nursery procedures or for postoperative pain. Clearly, parents have to supervise their babies' pain management and advocate for pain relief. Before any surgical procedure, parents should discuss their concerns with the surgeon and especially with the anesthesiologist. If anesthesia is not planned, parents may wish to withhold their consent for the procedure or seek another anesthesiologist with experience in properly anesthetizing premature babies.

Circumcision, practiced for centuries by Jews and Moslems around the world and declared for decades medically unnecessary by the American Academy of Pediatrics, is also routinely done without local anesthesia. At least in religious circumcision, the baby is given a taste of wine. According to Marilyn Milos, founder of NOCIRC, in Europe only Orthodox Jews practice circumcision. In the United States, almost all Jews and thousands of non-Jews continue this genital disfigurement. Adult men who have recalled the experience of circumcision through regression therapy report that it is excruciat-

We insisted that an order be written for pain medication for the twin in the NICU. I was amazed when a staff member told us that three-month-old babies don't feel pain. I know they do. I knew that the surgery, fever, IVs, diaper rash, and diarrhea had to make her feel uncomfortable. She rested much better once she had been given an analgesic.

ingly painful. (See Resources and Suggested Reading for information that will surely convince you to avoid this unnecessary and harmful surgery.)

Hospitalization of One Twin

It would have been helpful for us to have kept a copy of our doctor's order permitting all of us to stay in the baby's room. That way mix-ups in communication among shifts and part-time staff members could have been avoided.

The other twin wore hospital gowns and diapers too, which saved me a lot of trouble.

Sometimes one baby may be transferred to a high-risk center for additional special care, or one twin may need readmission after discharge. Dividing multiples between two locations means added stress and anxiety for the parents. Photographs of the baby help to keep the bond alive in cases where long distance is involved.

If you have other children, your parenting resources will be stretched even further. Visiting the nursery helps to make the baby or babies real for the siblings, who are sensing their parent's preoccupation and concern.

Andrew Wilkinson, director of neonatology at the John Radcliffe Hospital in Oxford, England, states that contact with and fondling of premature babies, not just by parents but by other family members and friends, has been an absolute priority in British nurseries for many years. Single mothers and couples whose extended families live elsewhere benefit greatly from having friends accompany them to the NICU.

Discharge of Premature Infants

An increasing number of hospital nursery units have facilities for the parent to live in or very close by, particularly prior to discharge, to ease the transition to taking care of the babies at home. Mothers may go home totally empty-handed or with only one multiple. When the day finally arrives to take the other baby or babies home, the parents may become quite apprehensive. Having depended on such advanced life support apparatus and techniques, the parents may panic at the thought of coping by themselves. Spend several full days in the nursery learning the routines until you feel quite comfortable providing total care yourself. Make notes about eating and sleeping patterns, medications, and so forth.

Discharge home is not based on achievement of a certain weight. Stability of the baby's vital signs and the ability to suck properly are more important parameters.

Developmental studies have shown that most premature babies catch up to normal milestones, but it may take up to five years. A Japanese study assessing twins who had jaundice, lack of oxygen, and other biological handicaps at birth found no difference at age one and twelve between those twins and the controls. In the beginning, however, parents need to subtract the prematurity interval to have a more realistic appreciation of the babies' age and abilities. That is, if the babies are two months old and they were born two months premature, they should be at the developmental level for a newborn. This is done up to two years of age, after which the gap between real age and the age corrected for prematurity become less significant. However, parents may still want to correct their children's ages for prematurity when considering readiness and placement in school.

Developmental delays, handicaps, and problems such as learning and behavior disabilities are more common among premature babies than among babies born at term. They are most likely to afflict babies who suffered such major neonatal problems as respiratory distress syndrome or brain hemorrhage. Very-low-birth-weight babies have a 20 to 30 percent incidence of handicaps serious enough to be detected in the first two to three years of life. These include cerebral palsy, retardation (IQ below 84), hydrocephalus, seizure disorders, and vision or hearing loss. By ages eight to eleven, an additional 40 to 50 percent of very-low-birth-weight children are diagnosed with milder problems such as borderline retardation, hyperactivity, coordination difficulties, or learning disabilities. Fortunately, these "milder" problems can be remediated to some degree and do not rule out an independent or productive life. Supportive parents can often be the factor that makes a crucial difference for these children and their eventual outcomes.

Be sure to discuss any developmental concerns you may have with your pediatrician. If you suspect that your child may have a problem, follow your instincts and have it fully investigated by a qualified specialist. Early diagnosis is often the key to a successful adjustment and remediation.

Problems related to prematurity may show up much later. Be aware of changes in muscle tone, erratic eye contact, or irritability. Trust your instincts, although often with premies parents know what is "usual" — you know your babies and their usual behavior better than anyone else.

As we have seen, very often a mother feels a sense of failure if her twins or supertwins were born premature. Bonding is difficult with premature and low-birth-weight infants, who spend most of their time sleeping or crying. Prematurity is a risk factor for child abuse, and so is multiple birth. Sheer exhaustion and feeding problems add to these factors to make for a very difficult situation.

I felt very isolated during my twins' first six months. It seemed no one could understand the difficulties of having premature twins. I suffered severe postpartum depression. I had really wanted a baby, but the arrival of two at one time and their marathon feedings were overwhelming. If my parents hadn't sacrificed by coming 1,200 miles to help me, I wouldn't have made it.

How to Help Your Premature Babies

1. Observe your babies carefully to learn the (often subtle) ways that they show distress and contentment. For example, falling blood oxygen rates (as observed on the monitors), apnea (disruptions in breathing), mottled or dusky coloring, sudden changes in muscle tone, grimaces, and gaze aversion can be signs that the baby is overwhelmed. Always respect a stressed baby's need to rest and suggest that the staff do likewise. Premature babies show contentment and physical stability by maintaining a steady normal rate of oxygenation, good color, and a calm, alert gaze (or a calm sleep). Take advantage of the times when your baby is stable and alert for caregiving and interaction.

2. If your babies respond favorably, touch or hold them as much as you can, even when the babies have arterial lines and oxygen hoses. Gentle rocking and swaying can be soothing for many babies and may help compensate for some of the uterine experiences they missed because of their early delivery. Premies are extremely sensitive to rough handling, noise, bright lights, and disturbances, and sometimes even gentle touching. Hold your hands a couple of inches away from their bodies and stroke their energy field, or aura. As soon as the babies are medically stable, cuddle them skin-to-skin to enhance their sense of touch and smell, all part of bonding. Physical and occupational therapists can help you with other ways to gently position, stretch, move, and stimulate your babies.

3. Explain everything to your babies. They understand and will benefit from explanations of their strange environment and procedures. It is normal and real for you to express your emotions about your baby's appearance, condition, and prognosis. Babies sense these things anyway.

4. Place a tape recorder inside each incubator or warming bed where the sound cannot become amplified or distorted. Tape your normal speech as well as singing so the baby can hear your voice.

5. Get a Stimobil to hang up for your babies to watch. Research on infant stimulation has shown that babies respond most to geometric shapes and to high-contrast colors such as black

and white, not soft pastels. For your babies' sensory, emotional, and intellectual stimulation, change the scenery, use different fabrics and assorted soft, colored toys. A "crib gallery" is now available that can be placed inside the isolette to display pictures and other items of visual stimulation. Always offer such stimulation carefully and assess and reassess your babies' reactions. Don't be discouraged if your babies seem uninterested in or stressed by novel sounds, sights, or sensations. Some babies find even eye contact stressful at first. Be patient. What a baby may find overwhelming one day, he or she may find fascinating the next.

How to Help Yourself

Many hospitals now link new parents of premature babies with a "graduate parent" who has been through the ordeal and understands their anger, confusion, and depression. Such volunteers provide support, babysit for older siblings so that the parents can visit the hospital together, and may accompany them to NICU to help explain babies' progress reports.

Keeping a diary helps not only to document reports given by hospital staff but to preserve a record of your feelings and observations. A diary gives some structure to what seems a disoriented time and makes an important keepsake for the twins.

Complications and problems related to multiple birth and prematurity in particular put tremendous stress on a marital relationship as well as interfering with the development of parental attachment. Films, books, and studies are now available for members of the obstetric and pediatric team so they can help a couple work through their anger, guilt, and grief in a sensitive and caring way. Some units have a full-time nurse for parent communication.

Subscribe to *Parenting Premies*, a quarterly newsletter published by parents for parents faced with the consequences of a premature birth. Parent Care, Inc., offers information, referrals, and other services to parent support groups, families, and professionals concerned with infants who require special care at birth. These organizations support families with critically ill newborns, help parents create and maintain local groups, and encourage communication between perinatal professional and health care organizations. (See Resources.)

Resources lists organizations that provide education, support,

For a while the twin with Down's syndrome and the normal twin were developing similarly. But as they get older the gap is widening. One prints letters and the other can't even hold a pencil. I feel bad about comparing them, but I get trapped in it.

The joys have far outnumbered the sorrows, and the love our family has for these two little girls, handicapped or not, has bound us closely together and given us increased realization of those things in life that are truly important.

and assistance for various handicaps, such as cerebral palsy, cystic fibrosis, Down's syndrome, and other genetic diseases.

Infants with Special Needs

I'll never stop wishing that my son with Down's syndrome could be as bright and active as his twin sister, but we're doing all we can by providing a preschool experience and stimulation at home. I know he'll do the best he can. Besides, he's really cute.

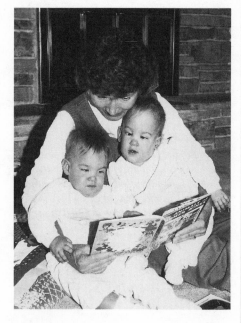

Grandparents can play a vital supporting role in the face of pain and uncertainty; a child with disability helps adults learn strength, endurance, and intense love.

A child with a congenital defect or a handicap can be a tremendous shock to a mother and father. Sometimes the anomaly can be observed prior to birth with ultrasound, but seeing it in the flesh may still be traumatic. Some defects, such as heart anomalies and cleft palate, can be surgically corrected. Others, such as Down's syndrome, are irreversible, but with appropriate stimulation learning can be facilitated more successfully than previously expected. Much has to do with parental expectations and enthusiasm.

Well-intentioned friends and professionals may advise parents of a twin with a handicap not to compare the two or even to think of them as twins. This is very difficult to do after all the preparation and anticipation with twin cribs, paired clothing, and other double gifts. These people expect the mother to act as if the babies had been born a couple of years apart. Avoid dressing them alike as this will draw attention — and possibly callous remarks when people see that one twin has a problem.

Parents of children with handicaps, like parents of premature infants, need to adjust their expectations, especially with regard to the time required to reach developmental milestones. The risk of mental illness, particularly to the mother of a handicapped twin, is higher than with a singleton. Life is more difficult with multiples because of the pressure to balance parental attention between children of the same age but of different mental and physical needs. The siblings, especially the normal twin, may also have feelings of responsibility and perhaps guilt that they are healthy.

Parents need to see and hold a baby with anomalies from the very beginning, in the delivery room. This makes adjustment to the situation easier in the long run. If a twin is whisked away while the parents are told that "something is not quite right," the parents usually envision far more serious defects than are actually present. It is very important to have your questions answered by the doctors; sometimes they may try to protect you from details. Also, doctors and nurses may perceive a problem to be more serious than the parents see it, especially if the normal attributes and good features are emphasized to the parents.

If both twins are affected, the parents have the burden of raising two disabled children. More commonly, however, one infant is affected (even in a monozygotic pair); this imbalance creates complex family dynamics.

The social situation when a child has a handicap creates added stress. Parents typically go through the same stages with the loss of the idealized child as they do with a death. Shock, denial, anger, and guilt can drive the parents to isolation. Friends and relatives do not know what to say, so they may avoid calling or visiting.

Comments like ''Well, at least you've got one normal baby'' are insensitive and let you know that this individual cannot support your grief. The writings of Albert Solnit and Mary Star, as well as Marshall Klaus and John Kennell, stress the sequence of events that help prepare parents to organize their adjustment to a child with special needs. The parents' first grief must be for the loss of the ideal infant whom they visualized before birth. Then they can take the next step of becoming attached to the real child. Sometimes a healthy twin becomes jealous of the attention his handicapped twin receives and he may have difficulty handling his twin's disability, feeling that it could have been he. (The story of a set of twins, one of whom had hydrocephalus, is described in Chapter 6.)

If the parents can accept the disability, then other children in the family will too. Young siblings of a disabled child are generally completely accepting and calm with outsiders who have trouble dealing with the situation. Adolescents may feel shame and embarrassment. Dr. Martin Levison, who has a son with a developmental disability, recommends holding family meetings in which each child talks about the things he likes and doesn't like about all his siblings, including the sibling with a disability.

Of course, accidents and illnesses in later life can also cause mental and physical impairment to children. Mothers Against Drunk Driving (MADD) gives statistics of death and destruction from drunk driving accidents that are worse than those caused by preterm delivery or birth defects. But birth is a unique experience accompanied by powerful emotions, and this makes congenital anomalies or birth-related handicaps usually harder to accept.

Many support services are available today for children with special needs. A team may include a physical therapist or occupational therapist to improve self-help skills and activities of daily living. The March of Dimes, United Cerebral Palsy Foundation, organizations for parents of children with Down's syndrome, cystic fibrosis, and so on, a state or local human services department, and hospitals and clinics in your area can be approached for assistance with early intervention.

I discovered that I compared them less and thought of their twinship less as their second birthday approached. I know they're twins and I always will, but the comparisons have finished and the pain of adjusting to the one twin's handicap is easier now.

We rejoice at every new accomplishment each little boy achieves! They continue to surprise us with their ever-increasing capacity to grow and learn.

I was emotionally isolated in those early months. The concerns of other mothers seemed so inconsequential to me. I couldn't relate to one teething baby when I was coping with two, and with one baby having cerebral palsy. Other mothers didn't know how to respond to my problems either.

When I realized that my beautiful girls were "extraordinary" instead of "normal," my entire attitude changed. Other children simply do things automatically; everything that ours have accomplished is a miracle.

A special program to stimulate and educate children with special needs will maximize their learning potential and minimize developmental delays.

The Pre and Perinatal Psychology Association of North America can provide names of therapists who can assist with helping individuals of any age, especially infants, to relive and release early trauma. This psychological healing is an often overlooked but very important dimension of recovery.

17 | Emotional Consequences of Twin Loss

LOSS AND DEATH are painful, challenging dimensions of life to acknowledge and accept, especially during the childbearing year. However, bereavement and disability are more common in families with multiple births, and the problems may be more complex for the parents and surviving children. This chapter explores the death of a twin from conception through early childhood and the impact of this loss on parents, siblings, and the surviving twin.

Whereas pregnancy is considered the beginning of life, death and birth are two sides of the same coin. The emotional denial of this paradox, among couples and the maternity care providers who serve them, is common: no adult cares to consider the death of an infant.

Expectant parents who confront the unthinkable by reading this chapter — without undue worry or preoccupation — will be at a tremendous advantage should they experience a loss. Despite being in shock following the death of a baby, they will be better prepared to create memories while the opportunity is there to do so and to avoid regretting things left undone. It is also very important that the partner be aware of the mother's wishes in case she is anesthetized or otherwise unable to act at the time. Parents of multiples will inevitably meet other parents who have suffered the loss of a multiple. Reading this chapter will educate you to respond appropriately and provide support.

The heightened awareness that accompanies the miracle of the childbearing experience invariably stirs up questions about the purpose of life, what happens after death, why a certain child is conceived at a certain time, and so forth. For parents expecting singletons, these questions are interesting to ponder but usually remain philosophical. But despite advances in obstetrics and neonatal care for various types of high-risk pregnancies, the risk of loss in twin pregnancy remains about four times that for singletons.

How could I make sense of something that made no sense to me? How could I explain that we had been given two very special gifts and now one had been taken back before we could even know her?

The Double Bind of the Double Bond

The initial shock leaves you totally exposed to the people around you and without confidence to deal with them. I found myself unable to focus my thoughts in any form. In fact, in the first few days one wonders if one's sanity and equilibrium have gone forever.

The technician blurted out, "I think one baby is dead."

The death of one twin presents a totally different situation than the death of both twins or the death of a singleton. A mother of twins, who went through several months proudly pregnant with two babies, is suddenly thrown into the bizarre situation of having one living baby and one dead baby, or perhaps one who is struggling to live. Flooded with conflicting feelings, she must face the daunting task of nurturing and bonding with the living baby while grieving for the baby who died. These feelings, which polarize her reaction to each baby, are in direct conflict: bonding and separation, attachment and detachment, pride and guilt, joy and regret, excitement and disappointment, happiness and grief.

Unfortunately, the rest of the world often acts as if nothing happened, since unborn and small babies are not given much value for their brief existence. Hurtful comments may be made, such as "Maybe it is for the best — two would have been a handful" or "She wouldn't have had a normal life." Parents may even be told that they are "lucky" as they still have one baby. Just as the survivor in any loss never replaces those who are gone, the tragedy in this case is not lessened because the mother has another baby of the same age. The shock and confusion not only are devastating for parents but often bring out the worst in those who should be there to help.

When one twin dies after an illness of several months or a prenatal diagnosis of a fatal problem, parents experience the grieving process differently from a sudden and unexpected death. The shock may be less sudden, but the parents have invested more time in the baby's life as well as hope in his recovery. Mourning can be delayed by the total involvement with the survivor and the often grueling demands of his or her care.

A Multitude of Losses

I became very angry at the baby who stayed. I felt it was not fair that this one got to stay when the other couldn't. I spent three days in a rage unlike anything else I'd ever experienced. Then numbness set in again.

In addition to experiencing the loss of one or more children, parents experience the loss of a special kind of parenting and a new personal and social identity. The great majority of women who conceive twins feel blessed, "chosen by God," "special, because not everyone can have twins." Expectant parents of multiples have enjoyed a wonderful new status and also often have begun friendships with other parents of multiples. The more they have been the center of attention in their family, community, or physician's practice, the greater their loss of status following an unexpected death.

Another type of loss is sustained by the surviving infant. He or she has lost a twin and a future twin relationship, with all its special status and unique features. Fetal grieving does exist, memories do last, and children and adults who were twins carry their losses forever.

It is important to know if the cause of death was intrinsic to one of the twins, such as a genetic disease or an anomaly with the cord, or some condition of the mother affecting the intrauterine environment, such as diabetes or high blood pressure. Occasionally, the cause of death cannot be determined.

The Stages at Which Loss Can Occur

The triple loss of baby, identity, and twin relationship may occur at different stages of the childbearing year, each with its own particular experiences. The medical aspects are described in Chapter 7 in the section "Loss in the Childbearing Year."

Loss in Pregnancy

"Vanishing Twin"
Since ultrasound is becoming more widely used (although the long-term side effects are not known), more women will be informed about a "vanishing twin" after a second ultrasound examination. This may be a relatively benign situation medically, but emotionally it can be very difficult to grieve for the lost baby and "twins" while carrying on through the rest of the pregnancy and birth.

Miscarriage
The later a miscarriage comes in the pregnancy, the more chance the mother has had for prenatal bonding, but miscarriage at any time brings with it a profound sense of loss. Parents may find it helpful to name the lost child and to have a funeral or memorial service, although this is not required by law in some states unless the baby weighs 500 grams (1 pound, 2 ounces) or more or the pregnancy is at least twenty-eight weeks.

Selective Reduction
Selective reduction does not result in the formation of a singleton pregnancy. Although the body will gradually adjust to one baby, the hormonal and physical changes in the uterus have been those of a

So many people want a reason for the loss of a baby — such as being poor, not eating a good diet, or not going to the doctor. When an infant dies, it's easy to think that you must have done something wrong — not eaten quite enough vegetables, gotten too much exercise or too little, not had sufficient "positive thoughts," lain on one side too much, not been "really ready" emotionally for twins, not accepted all the tests, etc., etc., etc. — not realizing that you may have nothing to do with it.

When I saw the ultrasound of my dead baby, curled up in a little dark ball, I felt like half of me had also died.

The doctor said very matter-of factly: "What we have here is one live baby and a dead fetus."

The doctor told me that ultrasound was inconclusive and began to list possible causes of my bleeding. When he said it could be the miscarriage of one twin, I stopped listening. I knew.

The Anguish of Loss, **from the book** *The Anguish of Loss,* **by Julie Fritsch with Sherokee Ilse.** *Photo reprinted with permission from Wintergreen Press, 3630 Eileen Street, Maple Plain, MN 55359.*

twin pregnancy throughout the initial months. Many mothers will find carrying a dead baby for the remainder of the pregnancy very distressing. Several studies report successful removal of the dead twin through an incision in the uterus, but this is a serious intervention and carries a high risk of preterm labor.

As Elizabeth Bryan points out, "Couples who undergo selective fetocide must cope not only with their bereavement but also with the stress of carrying a dead fetus for many weeks and later explaining to the surviving twin what has happened." Mothers who have undergone this experience frequently feel that the staff did not show enough respect for the dead baby and did not acknowledge the mothers' feelings of real loss. Clearly, much counseling and support are necessary when this procedure is performed — before and after.

Counseling becomes even more essential and complex when selective reduction is recommended for healthy babies because there are simply "too many." The procedure has sometimes been suggested because the prematurity rate is almost 100 percent for quadruplets and quintuplets. As everyone knows from the media, higher-order multiples occur more commonly today as a result of advanced reproductive technology. But the questions are sticky. Who decides which babies are to be sacrificed? If you are carrying quadruplets, do you decide to carry triplets or twins? What if there are problems with the survivors and you regret the choices?

One solution is preconception counseling, more careful monitoring of hormonal stimulation, and not transplanting more than three embryos.

Intrauterine Death of One or More Fetuses

A number of women are faced with the death of one twin or triplet at twenty-six to thirty weeks and (if delivery is not immediate) of trying to carry the other baby until thirty-four to thirty-six weeks to avoid prematurity for the survivor while hoping to avoid the same fatal condition in the survivor.

Mourning is very difficult during pregnancy, whether for an unborn baby, a sister, a friend, or other family member. Yet unresolved grief can interfere with mothering skills and may even predispose to child abuse. Suppressing feelings about the loss for the sake of the baby inside can cause the mother to become emotionally isolated. This affects her interaction with the baby so that bonding becomes a challenge, both prenatally and postpartum.

Loss During Labor (Stillbirth)

The shock of a stillborn baby surely shakes our basic trust in nature, and superstitious fears, negative or destructive thoughts, and consequent feelings of responsibility and guilt may result. It is especially hard for a mother who thought she had finally "made it" to term. As British psychiatrist Emanuel Lewis has correctly observed, birth involves a transition from the "inner" to the "outer" worlds, with many accompanying changes. With a stillbirth, both an outer and inner void remain, and even though a birth has occurred the normal transition never takes place. This leads to a deep emotional confusion that

Even though I am a nurse, I didn't realize that I would have to carry my dead baby inside of me until the living baby was born.

I wanted to dress the baby for the funeral but they advised me against it because of the autopsy. I was saddened not to be able to make this small motherly gesture.

We were very upset when Anthony died and the nursery removed the sign that said Twin A, as if he wasn't a twin anymore and there was no need to make a distinction.

Seeing the milk drip out of my breasts several days after the birth was like having an open wound. I wanted so badly to take to my breast a baby whose mother had died.

is greatly underestimated by outsiders and that is all the more confusing when there is also a living baby.

Stillborns may be perceived as having ghostlike qualities. Lewis describes how a resident in obstetrics, asked to photograph a stillborn baby said, "What is the point, it will come out fuzzy." Another case is mentioned by Lewis where a vicar reluctantly allowed a stillborn infant to be buried in his church's graveyard but insisted that the gravestone be left blank. Likewise, stillbirth to many people means no history, no known cause of death, and no name. (See Appendix 3 for advice about how parents can retain decision-making power at this vulnerable time and avoid additional losses.)

SIDS: Sudden Infant Death Syndrome

The SIDS group was a place I could go to once a week and feel rotten without feeling guilty about myself. I didn't have to put up a strong front like I did at work. These people understood.

Parents may use an apnea monitor for surviving multiples (see Chapter 16), although the benefits are not entirely conclusive. Some parents feel the monitor introduces an added stress; for others it is a reassurance. The monitor is not a treatment but simply an alarm that is triggered if the baby stops breathing, and all who care for the baby must learn infant cardiopulmonary resuscitation (CPR) to respond effectively. One mother of trizygotic triplets had a haunting fear for four months: "What if more than one monitor goes off at the same time? How will I choose which baby to save?"

SIDS support groups have been formed, and some offer support groups for siblings as well as parents. In Minnesota a group has been started for child care providers who experience a SIDS death.

Emotional Consequences of Loss

Saying Good-bye

The worst thing was going in the front door empty-handed and going out the door again to face the world.

The few days between the death of the baby or babies and the burial or cremation are critical because this is the only time to be shared with that child or children and it is the time to say good-bye. This period is especially significant where one premature baby has died and the other is struggling to live, and indeed may die also. Holding and viewing the dead infant are important so that the mother, especially, can concretely recognize which baby lived and which one died. Parents need to feel that they did enough for the baby who died. This in turn makes it easier for celebrating the life of the survivor and attending to his or her care.

In the absence of adequate and timely grieving, serious psychological difficulties can develop. It is easier for parents and siblings to grieve and talk about the dead baby later if they have formed a strong memory and clear image of that child. Because time is usually short, every tangible experience and item of contact counts. Photographs or videotapes if possible, especially of the babies together, are particularly significant. (See Appendix 3 for a list of other mementos.)

Grieving

Autopsies cannot always determine why one baby died and the other lived, and this uncertainty can remain a source of frustration for the family. Sometimes a boy may die and a girl will live, for example, and parents may feel guilty as they wonder about their unconscious desires. Furthermore, the living baby may have a permanent disability or medical problem needing immediate intervention. Even if this twin is perfectly healthy, parents may have trouble bonding for fear that they will lose this baby too. Sometimes parents will even avoid naming the surviving baby or taking photos in the first few weeks. However, these proofs of identity will be even more important in the event of loss as bonding actually facilitates letting go.

If the parents focus on the loss of twinship, this may eclipse their grief for the individual who was lost. Often the grieving will resume at a later time when the mother or father realizes the impact of the event. If grief and joy can be experienced separately, this can help the healing. Parents need guidance to grieve the loss of the individual baby first and worry over the loss of the twinship later. Jean Kollantai, who began *Our Newsletter*, a network for parents who lose a multiple, points out that it is crucial for parents to take time from the physical and emotional demands of the surviving baby to focus totally on the twin who died and discuss their feelings about the loss. She warns that the surviving baby offers a tempting escape from the painful business of grieving but that this avoidance backfires in the long run. Later the parents may fall prey to the pitfalls of postponed grieving and have problems caring for the living twin, endangering his or her safety as well as their own.

The hardest thing I ever did in my life was to hand our dead baby back to the doctor knowing we would never see him again.

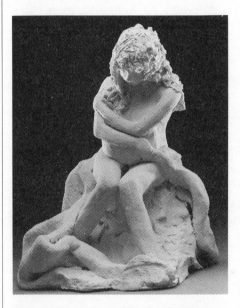

Stay Within, from the book *The Anguish of Loss*, by Julie Fritsch with Sherokee Ilse. *Photo reprinted with permission from Wintergreen Press, 3630 Eileen Street, Maple Plain, MN 55359.*

I regret that I didn't love her more, hold her, tell her I love her.

Many times the doctors told us to go home and take care of Corey and forget about Katie. They said they would let us know when she died and not to really love her. That's hard. How do you not love your own baby?

There were two aspects to the shock — physical and mental — and both can be briefly described as total exhaustion and complete turmoil. Hormone changes and raw emotions become so mixed up that it becomes impossible to separate the two, and one is carried along on a tidal wave of numb recognition of the awful facts, topped with the feeling that this can't be happening to me.

I haven't been too good about celebrating my twin daughter's birthday. It's still too painful.

It helps to have the other baby who has to be taken care of, despite inner heartbreak.

For the first six months I was totally preoccupied with ignoring what had happened, and then in the next six months I was totally preoccupied with it.

If the surviving baby is very sick, the loss of the other twin may seem more "acceptable." But once the surviving child recovers and begins to develop normally, mothers often find the death of the twin more and more painful. For a long time mothers may look at the living baby and "see two." While watching their child talk and play, they often can't help thinking that there should be two little ones talking and playing together. Sometimes parents question why the living one escaped death. Depending on the circumstances of loss, some parents come to terms with the loss by acknowledging that it wasn't a question of one twin dying, but more a miracle that the other twin lived. For other people, who suddenly lost a baby after a normal pregnancy and who have a healthy survivor, the feeling may be "This one is here, where is the other one?"

Preoccupation with grieving may cause parents to delay attachment to the living baby. In such cases, the mother is functional but may be so emotionally distant that it can affect the behavior of the survivor as he or she develops. Bryan rightly observes that it is easier to refer to the dead baby by name to differentiate between the twins and to confirm that the dead baby was real.

Grieving is a long-term process that can go on two years or more, and crises and events may trigger emotional responses linked to the death years later. Postponed grief can emerge at any time, and parents often feel that they are sitting on a time bomb that makes earlier resolution of their feelings an important goal. This is a much greater challenge for parents of multiples than of singletons because of the greater physical and emotional burdens of recovering from multiple pregnancy and looking after the survivor (as well as additional siblings, if any). Plans to breast-feed may become disrupted after the death, which becomes another loss. Nursing can be difficult to establish and maintain at this particularly painful time, and nursing mothers need much support so that despite the circumstances the experience can be rewarding and comforting.

Many of the excellent books in Suggested Reading deal with the stages of grieving — shock, denial, anger, guilt, and resolution. In this chapter I focus on the special aspects of twin loss. Parents need to talk about the loss, express their feelings regardless of whether they are rational, judge, blame, and go over the "if only's." These normal components of recovery may be directed inward and can lead to depression. Many of the mothers I interviewed who had lost a twin did experience depression. They had no one to whom they could turn for sympathy and support, no one who understood their unique predicament, and they felt alone, isolated, and "crazy."

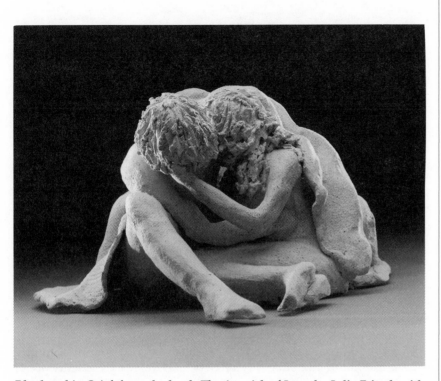

Blanketed in Grief, **from the book** *The Anguish of Loss,* **by Julie Fritsch with Sherokee Ilse.** *Photo reprinted with permission from Wintergreen Press, 3630 Eileen Street, Maple Plain, MN 55359.*

The death of a child creates the ultimate stress on the marital relationship, and its impact varies with each couple. Sometimes tragedy and the way that it is handled strengthens a marriage, but often it shatters it. Partners often experience the stages of grief at different times, and this can cause conflict and misunderstanding. One partner may be at the shock stage, while the other is experiencing anger or guilt, for example, and the next day or week the roles may be reversed. Society tends to expect the father to remain composed and deal with the formalities — death certificate, burial, support for the mother — so his private grief is the more likely to be misunderstood. The father needs to express and explore his feelings so that the mother doesn't perceive his lack of emotional expression as a sign of not caring. Mothers, in contrast, tend to seek out people with whom to discuss the loss, a healthy part of the grieving process.

In our society, many people find it difficult to discuss death and

I can't honestly say it passes. The intensity of it fades, the unfulfillment remains. It is just not possible to replace one child with another . . . and it is this irrevocability that is so hard to accept, even to realize at first. As with a scar, the lividness slowly fades, and so does the intensity of grief, anger, and guilt. But the scar remains and nothing can eradicate it.

It is too bad that people think a man doesn't get really upset at the loss of a baby. We all pay heavily for this assumption. A few weeks after the birth I found I was obsessed with thoughts of death, filled with anxiety, and pretty well convinced that I was losing my mind. The sheer agony of losing a child still overwhelms me.

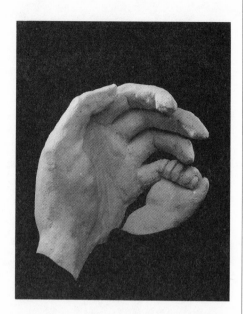

Your Hand, My Hand, from the book The Anguish of Loss, by Julie Fritsch with Sherokee Ilse. *Photo reprinted with permission from Wintergreen Press, 3630 Eileen Street, Maple Plain, MN 55359.*

At the funeral not one person mentioned my baby who had died, they only talked about my surviving twin.

The possibilities for insensitivity are so much greater in multiple birth losses; we parents have to be ready to stand up for our rights at a very devastating time.

Recently at a family gathering they took a photo of all the family twins — three sets. But they didn't include my daughter because her twin had died.

share grief, sometimes even with other members of the family. It is easy for people to ignore the death and fuss over the surviving baby — and to assume that the parents are doing the same. Relatives, friends, and neighbors may be reluctant to call and may avoid contact or discussion of the tragedy. This only encourages the parents to avoid confronting the painful reality. Silence about the death can haunt the family for years. Parents experiencing loss need to set the example for timid relatives by remembering and talking about the dead child and by asking for the kind of support they need. One woman complained that at family get-togethers two cousins each with twins would talk nonstop about "the twins" and totally ignore her and her surviving twin.

Sometimes a mother recalls how she had a strange feeling that something was not quite right or an intuition that one twin was doomed. Several women have related to me that while their husband jumped up and down with excitement in the delivery room or the technician went out to get the doctor, a thought flashed through their minds that one twin was dead or wouldn't live. One expectant mother heard herself telling her husband to wait and hear all that the doctor had to say before celebrating.

Mothers sometimes idealize the dead baby as a spirit strengthening the life of the survivor, or they may resent comments about their "angel in heaven." Outsiders often encourage the idea that the other baby was an "extra who didn't work out." If the mother has other young children, other people seem encouraged to say that it "didn't matter" or was "just as well." Yet it is because these mothers really love children that they feel strongly that their lost baby was really supposed to be part of their family and was not just an odd happening.

Therapy, counseling, support groups, and making connections with family anniversaries all ease the adjustment. Very often in families with twins, as in ordinary families, amazing coincidences occur with regard to anniversaries of conceptions, births, and deaths (see "Family Time" in Chapter 6). The greatest help are other parents who have suffered the same experience, whether they lost a member of twin, triplet, or other multiple. (A list of such individuals and support groups can be found in Resources.) In contrast, mothers of living twins are often reported as lacking in sympathy. Women whom I interviewed for this chapter who had experienced a loss described being ignored or whispered about if they attended club meetings for mothers of twins. This attitude is changing, however, as such groups develop their resources for bereavement support. Some clubs have taken the initiative to present mothers who lost one or both twins with honorary membership, and most mothers deeply appreciate the gesture.

While talking is helpful, it may not be enough to release the deeper anguish. The intense anger, rage, and grief also may need to be expressed physically — by punching pillows, screaming in a private place, or undergoing a type of body-oriented psychotherapy.

YOU'VE PROBABLY SEEN ME

You've probably seen me out with my boys
I'm a painful reminder of your stolen joys
The joy of twins is something you should have had
I know when you see me, you turn away sad
But I share in your tears when you see me
Because for us there should have been three.

Terri Koelling

Ongoing Challenges

Even after the initial grieving, parents still face the challenge and heartbreak of having to parent the survivor through birthdays, anniversaries, and developmental milestones with the presence of the survivor as a constant reminder of the death of the other. Knowing so poignantly that life offers no guarantees, these parents have a heightened awareness of all the risks and hazards that threaten the living twin and a strong need to protect him or her.

Another issue is the question of identity and group participation. For example, does the mother feel more comfortable joining a group of mothers of singletons or of mothers who have lost a baby (many of whom do not yet have a living child and desperately want one)? How much does a mother say to others about the lost twin? Can people recognize the living baby without acknowledging the dead twin? Does the survivor consider himself a twin or triplet even though his or her present status may be single or part of a pair? Almost all mothers continue to consider the survivor as a twin or triplet.

Parenting a twin on these terms is more than sheer challenge and heartbreak — it is high-risk parenting. This is especially true for first-time parents, after all the excitement of a twin pregnancy, often after many years of infertility.

It is a challenge for parents to let the survivor grow up feeling

Losing a triplet meant I was cut down a notch, because in others' eyes now I just have "twins." The hospital put on wrist bands that said Twin A, Twin B, and Baby C. What was I supposed to make of that?

Mothers who have a surviving twin, like everyone else, never think that a woman with two babies may have lost a triplet. With higher-order multiples, loss of one or more of the babies is common.

The dreams of having two little babies are gone. That second bassinet and all the matching clothes will never serve their purpose. The twin stroller is now useless. I want my little baby back and there is nothing I can do about it.

If only I had known something was wrong. All of a sudden I lost her and I never was able to help.

It's not like pulling and tugging, it's more like ripping and tearing and they are two violently different pulls.

that he or she is enough, all that they ever wanted, without experiencing life as "half of a broken set."

The Twin Bond

The twin bond has invariably been described as the closest of all bonds, especially between monozygotic twins. The loss of a twin is thus a devastating tragedy. One study found that 49 percent of monozygotic twins said they would miss their twin most of all family members in the event of death. In contrast, 25 percent of same-sex dizygotic twins and 13 percent of mixed-sex twins said they would miss their twin most. The rest of the dizygotic twins said that they would miss their mother most. Another study found that 90 percent of monozygotic twins and 61 percent of dizygotic twins felt closer to their twins than to their mothers. Ninety-eight percent of monozygotic twins are intensely satisfied with being a monozygotic twin compared with 72 percent of same-sex dizygotic twins. Ninety percent of same-sex twins were satisfied with their relationship.

In a 1988 Michigan trial for the death of one twin, the dead twin's sister was awarded the same amount as the dead twin's husband for "past and future loss of society." Research psychologist Nancy Segal interviewed some of the 157 twin children released in 1945 from Auschwitz. They confirmed that the twin relationship was the key factor in their physical and psychological survival. Simply knowing that if one twin died the other could be killed steeled their determination to survive and to think up ingenious strategies to protect each other. Perhaps twins fared better because they had the presence of their twin to keep human bonds intact and thus diminish their dehumanized existence.

Segal has also interviewed more than one hundred twins who were reared apart. In her fascinating work the impact of genes and strong bonds of twinship can be appreciated. Studies of twins who became bereaved in adult life found that the bond of twinship strengthens with time. In fact, especially with monozygotic twins, the death of one may soon be followed by the death of the other, from similar or unrelated causes.

Acknowledgment of the Death to the Surviving Twin

Parents are naturally concerned about the effects of the death on the surviving twin. This chapter focuses on the prenatal and perinatal periods, before twins develop as separate individuals. Even at this time, however, the twins and their parents are aware of the twins as a unit. Parents need to present the living twin with evidence of the reality and identity of the dead twin, even though the emergence of feelings of loss, guilt, and anger in the survivor may make it difficult for parents to deal with their private feelings about the loss. Elizabeth Bryan suggests that twins from whom information about a twin's death is hidden or who are not allowed to express their feelings about the loss suffer most. The child will sense a family secret, if he or she does not already unconsciously know its content, and family secrets are potentially lethal because they violate the child's sense of trust. If the survivor is not included in the funeral, he or she may wonder why later.

It is important for parents to avoid speaking of death as "going to sleep," because this may lead to nightmares or the child may become afraid to sleep alone. If parents are not comfortable explaining death to the survivor, then they should seek assistance from counselors or avail themselves of some of the books and materials recommended in Suggested Reading and Resources.

Just as parents who lost a twin like to meet other couples in the same situation, it is helpful for the twin to make contact with other survivors. The Multiple Births Foundation in London has set up a Lone Twin Register to offer support and networking to survivors who lose a twin at any stage of their lives. Subgroups are formed according to the time of loss (birth, childhood, or adult life), whether the twin was a sister or a brother, or whether the twin died in exceptionally traumatic circumstances. The Minnesota Center for Twin and Adoption Research has a Twin Loss Project that studies responses by survivors to the loss of the twin. Segal has also investigated cases where one twin commits suicide and found that the response of the surviving twin may be one of deep anger as well as grief.

Reactions of the Surviving Twin

Psychotherapy that enables adults to access early memories has demonstrated that twins in utero are, like all fetuses, conscious and aware, most significantly aware of each other. Adults who are unaware that they were part of a twin pregnancy have relived experiences they shared with their twin in utero and at birth (see Chapter 6). Therefore, it makes no sense to withhold information from a child until he or she can supposedly "understand." A surviving twin actually "knows" more than anyone else because of organic memories stored in the body.

A 1986 article in *Pediatrics* discussed the results of a questionnaire sent to parents who joined SIDS support groups about siblings' grief reactions. Parents believed firmly that their children had been deeply affected by the tragedy and had responded appropriately, even in cases of preverbal children. Parents have observed unusual behavior and restlessness, nightmares, other sleep disturbances, and loss of speech in the baby who survives. Of course, some of these comments may be projections of the parents' feelings or may even result from the survivor experiencing the parents' overt or covert grief.

However, as I pointed out in Chapter 6, unborn babies receive a lifelong imprint of traumatic events. Even in the hospital, the survivor may act upset at the time when the twin is dying. Bryan writes about a baby who could not be consoled for forty-eight hours after the death of her sister. One mother described her infant's cry as "pitiful, a cry of sorrow." Sometimes survivors are fussy babies who calm down only when swaddled, held firmly, or have a stuffed animal close by. After months of close contact within the uterus, the loss of a twin is keenly felt.

Toddlers who have lost a twin at birth or soon after may later appear to have totally forgotten. The memory, however, is not gone but is simply buried, and it is better to keep it alive as recommended in the anecdotes at the end of this chapter. One mother described her surviving twin, at the age of eighteen months, "standing up in her crib and staring into space," and the mother felt intuitively that the baby was remembering her dead twin sister.

Survivors may later demonstrate feelings about the twin when looking at themselves in a mirror, an especially common reaction among monozygotic twins. They may ask the mother if they were born alone or may search for their missing sibling in various ways. Even in an unaware twin survivor, it is not uncommon for the child to sense that someone is missing, to draw pictures of people and objects with parts missing, or to portray two people in self-portraits. Chapter 6 discusses some of the creative outlets explored by twin survivors.

Emanuel Lewis quotes a case of a three-year-old survivor who would habitually point out two of his animals and blocks. One day "he held up a toy car with a split windscreen, half of which was missing, and said 'Why? Who broke the window?'" Then he picked up a car with one front tire missing: "Why? Puncture?" Then to his mother, "How?" His mother then told him about his dead twin, to which he responded, "I am one."

Preschool children may want to set the lost twin's place at the

I can never decide whether it is harder, in a way, to have Tim as a constant reminder of Oliver's absence or whether we are luckier to have, so to speak, half left. . . . I think it's perhaps an unanswerable question. A loss is a loss, and it has to be sustained; there are no replacements.

dinner table, to talk to the twin, to draw him or her, to put out clothes for him or her, and so on. Some twins even talk about dying as a way to be together. Occasionally the survivor feels angry at the twin for dying or at the parents for not "making" him or her stay alive.

The child may choose to grieve in ways that upset the parents, but the process resolves more smoothly if the child can express both negative and positive feelings without criticism. The survivor may become withdrawn or rambunctious. Sometimes he or she exhibits unusual behavior that continues for months. At other times, the living twin develops a psychosomatic illness that may require psychotherapy (hysterical paralysis on one side is not uncommon).

Although some twin survivors are held back by their grief, others experience a great acceleration in development, speech, and social skills when on their own.

Adults who lost a twin at birth and earlier have reported experiences of loss as "something missing" that pervaded their life since that time, affecting relationships, fertility, and self-confidence. Bryan, in a 1987 article on grieving, agrees that "there is evidence that at least some lone twins have personality problems which could be related to the loss of their twin partner."

Survivor Guilt

Survivor guilt is observed when a person escapes a situation of death, be it a concentration camp, plane crash, or a multiple pregnancy, while others, often loved ones, die. New knowledge of prenatal psychology provides evidence that survivors from loss at birth or in pregnancy may be haunted throughout life by memories of the loss and by guilt feelings. It is always important to reassure the survivor that he or she did not cause the death.

In childhood, death of a twin may cause the survivor to become fearful and dependent. Sometimes the survivor puts himself or herself into difficult and dangerous situations, risking death perhaps as a way to rejoin the dead twin. The survivor may react with complete denial, fantasizing that the twin is still alive.

Parents have to guard against their expectations that the surviving twin be a combination of himself and the dead twin. Such expectations pressure the survivor into living a double life. Psychologists have noticed that the surviving twin may take on mannerisms or skills of the twin, unconsciously or deliberately to please his parents.

Researchers at the Maudsley Psychiatric Hospital in London

found in 1981 that 26 percent of twin patients had lost a twin. Almost twice as many patients diagnosed as psychotic had a dead twin than those with a living twin. (The nonsurviving twins were more often male and of a lower socioeconomic class and with other demographic features associated with infant mortality in general.) However, there is no clear evidence that twins as a whole suffer psychosis more than singletons. Certainly, parents today can help prevent such mental illness by handling the situation at all times with complete openness.

Dealing with the Feelings of Siblings

It is hard to try to love and care for a survivor and other children while wanting to be alone to grieve. In retrospect, I think I was extra hard on my children, resenting their needs and their wanting my attention.

Other children in the family with twins may have wished that one or both of the babies would disappear (jealous young children usually do), and after the loss of a twin they may feel responsible and guilty. Parents feel guilty that they are not emotionally available for the other children, who may also be grieving or figuring out what happened to the baby. Children will often express, verbally or behaviorally, what their parents repress. Young children are so perceptive that it is essential to be honest with them at all times, even on such a seemingly difficult subject as death. Also, when parents express emotion, this reassures the children that adults have feelings too and that it is safe to show them.

Sometimes an older child predicts the twin pregnancies or seems to know intuitively the sexes of the unborn children. If the lost baby was not named, the older child or children will appreciate being consulted on the choice of a name. Often an older sibling has a name ready without hesitation.

It is helpful to facilitate as much discussion as possible of facts, dreams, sandbox play — whatever helps the subject to be explored and explained. When most of today's adults were children, deaths in the family tended to be surrounded with unresolved tension and issues involved with death were evaded. Consequently, many adults avoid contact with bereaved families. Today, in contrast, people have a greater awareness of the benefits to expressing openly all feelings involved in the grieving process, and much more information and support are available through specialized networks to facilitate that process.

Subsequent Pregnancies

Unlike single pregnancies, the opportunity to do it again and try to get it right almost never occurs. Only mothers of twins, insensitive as they sometimes are, can understand better than anyone else — if and when they care enough to put themselves in my shoes — what a loss it is to have "just one."

Mothers of twins are often apprehensive of becoming pregnant again, wondering about their chance of having another set of twins with problems. Some do conceive a second set, and the extent to which they worry depends on whether the prior loss related to some random problem with the baby or a maternal condition. Some are disappointed to be pregnant with just a single baby the next time. Other mothers conceive twins again and experience ambivalent feelings, more pronounced when they have undergone fertility treatments. Some, of course, are thrilled to have twins again but realize that it could never be the same as it was supposed to be with the original twins.

It is hard for a surviving twin or a subsequent sibling to be a "replacement." He or she may suffer a vague sense of guilt and experience the pressure of having to live up to certain expectations or the feeling of walking in another's shoes. Unresolved mourning on the part of the parents can cause problems in the children, according to Lewis, such as confused identity, gender uncertainty, sexual problems, and disturbed ambition and achievement drive. Ideally, any pregnancy loss should be fully grieved before another conception is attempted. A new conception three months after a loss is not recommended, as the baby will be due around the anniversary of the death. It is a difficult task for the mother to work through mixed feelings toward the dead child, whom she may still picture inside herself, while coping with hopes and thoughts about a new baby. The mother who has lost one twin is not free to fully grieve at the time of birth, and she may need more time and self-searching before she is ready for the next baby. In fact, Bryan has suggested that a mother who loses one twin is in a similar situation to a mother who has a quick replacement pregnancy after a singleton loss.

Loss of Both Twins

I do not intend to imply by the focus in this chapter that parents will come out of a twin pregnancy with at least one twin and have to deal with the problems of having only one survivor. The experience of both twins dying is much less common, but the loss is twice as great and doubly devastating. Parents who experience the death of two or more multiples often feel that their loss is so horrible that people don't want to acknowledge it or the parents' grief at all.

While parents who lose one twin are reminded by outsiders to feel grateful that they have one baby, parents who lose both may receive worse "commiserations" such as "Well, at least you didn't know them" or "Just think of it as a miscarriage, you'll get over it faster." Recovering in the maternity ward (if no other beds are avail-

I wanted twins again, but as soon as I found out I was pregnant I became terrified that I'd have twins.

Next time I was pregnant, I kept thinking how the baby must be lonely, that there should be two inside.

I was really glad to have another baby two years later. My surviving twin had a lot of problems and his body developed contractures because he lay so long in intensive care. He wasn't cuddly, so this baby has made up for that.

I always thought that somehow my two babies were guaranteed, and I would casually see how much I could cheat on bed rest and the other limitations my doctor described. Going to a funeral of a friend's twin changed all of that, and I see that the outcome of multiple pregnancy can't be taken for granted.

able) can be extremely painful. Insist on a transfer if you wish.

Sometimes both babies die with no apparent cause and the parents are left empty-handed without a clue as to why. The mother who undergoes labor and delivery of babies already dead takes on an awesome task; others may not feel they can handle this and choose anesthesia and a Caesarean. (If it is too late for surgical delivery to benefit one or both twins, I feel the mother should have support for a vaginal delivery because her physical recovery will be much easier and the risk to her for a subsequent pregnancy and birth will be lower.) Again, the mother should be open to the paradox that the more freely she experiences the death and grief, the more she can bond, let go, and heal.

The challenges of carrying on after the loss of both babies are immense. As one mother wrote, "The stillness is deafening." Another described how the period of holding the babies, taking photos, planning a funeral, buying a casket, and burying them was such an unnatural experience that she felt completely isolated from society. Parents are left without babies and often with huge bills. One family's debt of $75,000 to the hospital was forgiven but they had to pay off $20,000 to the doctors.

All the recommendations in this chapter and in Appendix 3 for the loss of one twin apply, of course, to the loss of both. The best support is from other parents who have experienced the same situation, whether the twins died together or at different times and whether the loss occurred in pregnancy, labor, after birth, through SIDS, or in childhood.

Research and Self-Help in Bereavement

Jean Kollantai in Palmer, Alaska, lost one of her twin sons at thirty-nine weeks of unknown cause and as a result began a support network for parents who have experienced the death of one twin before birth, at birth, or in early infancy, including from SIDS. Recognizing that about 70 percent of all marriages break up after a loss, "not because of this fact, but because of not understanding and accepting it," she emphasizes how important it is for parents to talk about their loss. She edits *Our Newsletter*, which was an extensive source of material for this chapter. (See Resources.) Through her network, parents can receive the names and addresses of others who have experienced a similar loss, self-help and informational materials, as well as assistance in locating specialized information and resources. Resources are also available for parents who have lost both twins or who have lost a twin in childhood or adolescence. The support activities are not intended to take the place of counseling or bereavement groups but to help meet the special needs of parents of multiples as outlined in this chapter.

There are three groups: parents who have lost one twin, parents who have lost both twins, and parents who have one twin who has died and another who is struggling to live. This struggle can go on for weeks, months, or even years. Jean and her colleagues are researching the effect on the surviving children in these groups and would appreciate being contacted by parents who have suffered such experiences.

Segal and her staff at the Minnesota Center are currently carrying out a study of twin loss initiated in response to requests for information and assistance by twins who had lost twin siblings and parents who had lost twin children. A proposal is under way to establish a network of singleton twins.

I still get depressed near his birthday, but most of all because I have never been told what actually happened to my baby. The doctor convinced my husband to let the hospital "take care" of everything.

Coming to Terms with the Loss: Two Families' Stories

Nobody wants to concede that life has no meaning. Untimely death brings about new levels of understanding of the human condition and deeper experiences of awareness and compassion. The Australian film *Some Babies Die* is a deeply moving account of neonatologist Peter Barr's support for an entire family's grief. The dead baby is dressed and brought to the mother and siblings frequently through the hospital stay. Photos are taken and put with the medical records in case parents who refuse them at the time want them later (as they generally will). The children's acceptance and comfort with the process is impressive. This exceptional documentary can contribute to much greater authenticity around the bereavement experience.

It's not easier because you have one left; it's different. You're not lucky, but the time will come when you can rejoice in your surviving child.

Teddy's Story

Lisa Fleischer and Doug Blankensop's son Teddy was a gorgeous 8½-pound baby who suffered a prolapsed cord on his due date and was born with severe brain damage due to asphyxia. His twin sister, Sophie, survived. Teddy lived on a respirator for ten days and then his parents made the decision to remove it. During that interval, largely because of the support and information provided by the local twins

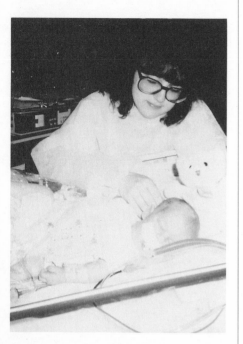

Teddy on the respirator.

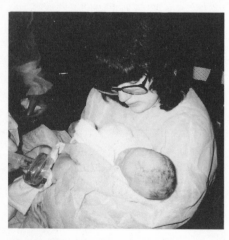

Lisa holding Teddy after the respirator was removed.

club bereavement group, the parents were able to create a ceremony to honor Teddy and baptize Sophie and hold a wakelike event at home. Their five-year-old daughter and Sophie were present when Teddy died and his older sister was involved in his care and burial, just like the children in Barr's film. Lisa wrote the following moving account:

> We learned the folly of believing we have control over what happens in our lives and the wisdom of letting go when the time comes. We found depths of hurt and strength in ourselves we'd never known and watched the boundaries drawn between birth, life, and death blur until they ceased to exist or matter. We became aware that there is an essence, a life-force beyond what we call ''personality'' and that this is what we came to know in our son and how he communicated so much to us. He was a quiet teacher. In the first few moments after his life ended, an amazing change came over his face. We watched as all the pain and struggle faded and his features become more and more lovely. It was a kind of most perfect beauty we had never seen before — he looked like what we imagine an angel should be. We were seeing his original face, the face of his soul before it returned home. There was no ordeal or sadness or fear, only victory and peace. This is how we will always remember Teddy's face.

We should recognize the fine line between acknowledging the twinship and making a shrine of the twin that will become a perpetual shadow throughout the survivor's life. The following story is one example of how this dilemma can be handled in an honest, caring, and practical way.

Lisa's Story

Barb Schaack Kaminski of Bloomington, Minnesota, shares some of the ways her family kept alive the memory of monozygotic twin Lisa, who died at six and a half months of congenital problems. Her twin, Amy, seemed to sense what had happened. The day after Lisa's funeral, Amy woke up from her nap and dramatically leaned toward Lisa's crib. When she was taken to it, she surveyed every corner for five minutes, clearly aware that her sister had gone.

The parents were especially concerned to keep Lisa special for Amy. Each time Barb passed a photo of Lisa, she pointed to it and said, ''Lisa.'' Gradually Amy learned to say Lisa's name and to ask questions and express herself about Lisa in many ways. As she grew

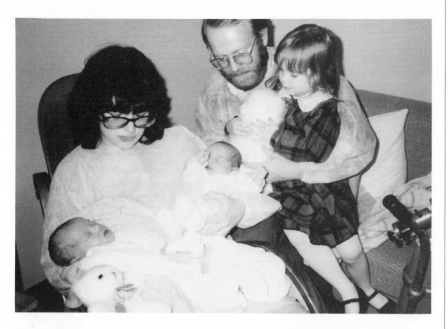

After Teddy died: Holding both twins together with the whole family.

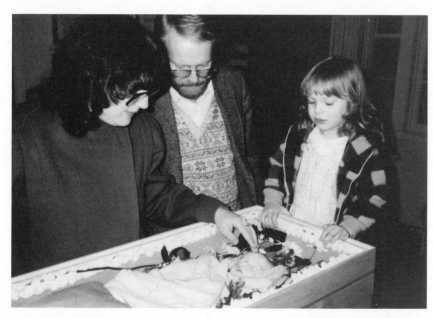

Saying good-bye: Including siblings in the wake and funeral helps them understand and resolve the loss.

Celebrating
The birth, life and leaving of
Teddy Blankensop
September 13, 1987 to September 23, 1987
and
The naming and baptism of his twin sister
Sophie Blankensop
on
September 27, 1987
Our Lady of Providence Chapel
Providence, Hospital
Anchorage, Alaska

A time of new beginnings

older, Amy made graves with clay and when she saw an "L," she would say, "That is the letter of Lisa's name." Lisa is remembered in some way when the twin birthday is celebrated, and Amy visits Lisa's grave, always with photos taken. The parents expect that Amy may decide not to go to Lisa's grave at some time. During the first Christmas after the birth/death, the Kaminskis designed a simple Christmas card with an outline of an angel on it which said, "Our angel in heaven, Lisa, and Brett and Amy, Barb and Dave wish you happy holidays." They also keep a candle lit through the holidays for Lisa. Another valuable treasure for Amy will be the book in which her parents wrote about the day the twins were born.

As noted childbirth author (and mother of living twins) Sheila Kitzinger wrote: "Gradually the space between the pain will get longer and the death of a baby becomes woven as one vivid strand in the whole texture of life."

18 | Some Special Features of Twinship

As we saw in Chapter 1, twinship has been the subject of various myths, taboos, and social customs since time began. Public interest in multiple birth is always great. Twin cities, twin peaks, twin beds — the idea of a matching set is appealing. As with twin objects, both twin persons must be present to make a set. Therefore, while twins are paid much attention as a twosome, especially if they are of the same sex and look alike, twins by themselves are individuals like the rest of us.

Boy-Girl Twins

In 1986–87 Theroux and Tingley surveyed 119 mothers of boy-girl twins ranging from five years to early teens. Boy-girl pairs are often not perceived as twins but generally are considered as a pair and may be called "the babies" rather than "the twins." Almost all the mothers described their twins as having a close relationship, helping and supporting one another. Only 20 percent of mothers reported that their twins had primarily a mutual set of friends. About one-third said that each twin had unique friends and 43 percent reported a combination of separate and mutual friends. Girls tended to be ahead of their boy twins with toilet training, fine motor skills, speech, and reading. Eighty-four percent of these mixed-sex pairs had been in school together at some point. Ninety-five percent had separate bedrooms by age six. The challenge with these twins is the different developmental levels between the sexes rather than their twinship.

Monozygotic Twins

Monozygotic twins tend to cooperate more, whereas dizygotic twins are more competitive. In a study done by Nancy Segal, 94 percent of

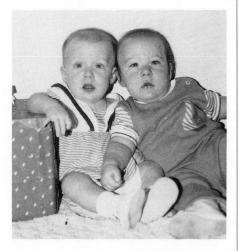

Most twins don't look like twins.

I often feel furious when someone says, "Oh how easy it must be because twins keep each other company." Mothers push themselves to limits to give their best to the huge demand for time and attention.

I was trying on coats once and a customer came up and asked which twin was the duller.

Two of our triplets are identical twins and one is fraternal. The fraternal triplet looks quite different from her sisters. When people ask why they are triplets, she replies: "Jesus wanted me to have curly hair."

monozygotic twins solved a puzzle together within the time frame, compared with 46 percent of dizygotic twins.

Twins may become defensive about their closeness because all their life they have been told they must be different and be individuals. It is fun for them sometimes to dress alike or emphasize their twinship, which may make outsiders jealous.

Jane Greer, a psychologist and consultant on twins, found that twins do not have a lower degree of success with separation-individuation than nontwins, but they do experience greater difficulty in their overall marital adjustment than singletons. Twins have to integrate the exclusivity of the marital bond with the existing bond to their twin. As a result, some twins look for another set of twins at twin gatherings for a dual marriage, and Greer recommends this.

The Challenges of Twinship

Both parents and twins readily become adjusted to all kinds of questions and other disadvantages of being special. Many of the questions and comments about twins carry a negative component because of the implication of superiority and inferiority in contrasting characteristics. That is, if one twin is quick, it follows in people's minds that the other twin is slow. Typical queries include "Is the first-born heavier?" "Which twin is the passive one?" Parents have thought up some good answers, such as "The smaller twin kicked the bigger one out" or "Susan was born at 2:05 and Irene was born at 2:45."

The Louisville Twin Study demonstrated that temperament is genetically influenced but its expression in the newborn period is affected by health at birth (such as weight, Apgar score, and the like).

Twins remain amazingly congenial to the tiresome questions about their differences and similarities. They may even have to tolerate the skepticism of people who, not understanding the nature of dizygotic twinning, may insist that children cannot be twins if their hair is a different color. On the other hand, they sometimes really do look exactly alike (particularly when they are small) although they are biologically dizygotic. Such twins may be under pressure to carry out a "double act" even though they are not monozygotic. Higher-order multiples, such as triplets, are usually assumed by people to be twins plus another sibling, especially if there are differences in size and sex. The average person doesn't expect to see triplets or quadruplets.

Each member of a twin pair grows up accustomed to the unique twin relationship. In childhood twins may ask their parents why other children are not twins and may speculate on what it would be like to be a singleton. Similarly, single children may have difficulty grasping the concept of twinning and may wonder what it is like to be a twin. If twins are dressed alike, other children may isolate clothing as the key to being twins. Some singletons wonder which twin celebrates the birthday.

It must be a bewildering experience for monozygotic toddlers to look at two identical faces in the mirror and wonder who is who. All of child development involves separating oneself first from the mother and later from a mirror image. Parents should be careful not to confess in the presence of twins that they cannot tell them apart; the idea may be alarming for the twins who are trying to differentiate each other. Even twins who are the image of each other will not be psychologically identical. There will always be people who prefer one twin to the other, as with any family members.

Twins are not simply two duplicates but share and interact with each other and society as part of a couple. Their personality development is shaped from the beginning by their parents as well as by the unique bonds they share with each other. Singletons do not have to compete with another baby at the same level of development for the attention of the world, so formation of self-image is less compli-

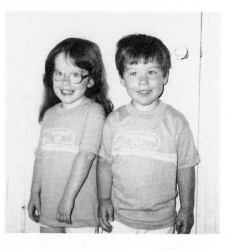

Mixed twins may look very different.

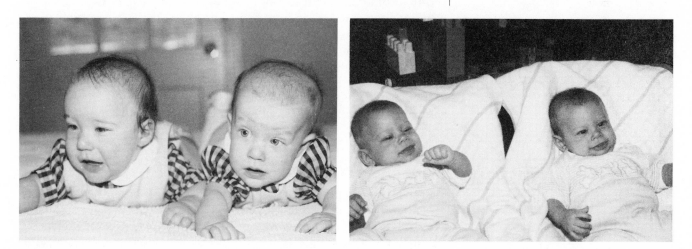

Twinfants are never lonely.

"What must it be like to never have your mother to yourself?" I asked an experienced mother of twins. "They won't know any different," she replied, "and each of them has someone special that few others have — a twin!"

Twin girls live next door to us. One day my little boy put on one of their coats and asked, "Am I a twin now?"

Our twins once crossed the street at a time when that was forbidden. "But we held each other's hand," they said. And so they often venture off, holding hands, giving security to each other in new and strange situations.

YES!! We're Twins

I'M A SINGLETON

cated. Boy and girl twin pairs develop at a different rate. As in any family, the girl usually matures first. Mixed sets and twins who do not look alike — "invisible twins" — are more easily considered as separate individuals.

Parental attitudes, always the major influence in the formation of a child's personality and self-image, may cause additional repercussions in the case of multiples. This is because of the built-in tendency for comparison and certain beliefs about how twins should be raised. Even during pregnancy the mother differentiates between the twins and unconsciously assembles a set of expectations for each child. After the twins are born, such expectations may be astute and appropriate responses to cues from the child, but sometimes they arise out of stereotyping. Parents may project themselves onto each twin: "A boy for Dad and a girl for Mom." The mother often takes the weaker, less competent twin under her wing, regardless of sex, while the father romps with the more robust member of the pair. Sometimes in mixed-sex twins, sex role models are reversed, attracting unkind comments about "switched genes." Happily, society is growing out of its gender stereotypes, which will make life easier for assertive females and retiring males. Schoolteachers often notice that parents claim that one twin is superior in a subject, whereas tests show the twins' abilities to be the same. Parents may even be concerned if the twins are not the same.

Roles between the twins invariably shift and may even be reversed. Mothers of triplets observe that different members pair off at certain times and that it is not always the same triplet who is happy to be alone and amuse himself or herself. There is more imbalance, however, when the triplets comprise a monozygotic pair and one singleton. Sometimes a quiet member of the set who rarely gets into mischief may suffer from benign neglect. Of course, twins have confessed to their parents that they hate being twins. These feelings should be explored, never denied. Most multiples, however, enjoy their special relationship and remain close throughout their lives.

Emphasizing Individuality

Proper use of a person's name is important in his or her development of identity and individuality. No one likes to be mistaken for someone else. Each of us believes we are unique. We resent being called by somebody else's name or having likenesses sought between us and other family members, especially if the comparisons are unfavorable.

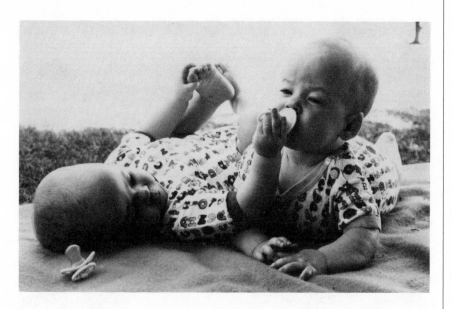

We dressed our twins alike. One day we heard one say to the other, "Stand over there so I can see how I look."

I was so relieved to learn at our twins club meeting that I was not the only mother who felt more for one twin than the other. We all felt that by expressing this we were able to make a conscious effort to get closer to the other child.

The bedrooms in our house were too small for triplets. So they were split into twosomes and rotated each month, with the other triplet sharing the big brother's room.

Twins enjoy each other as playmates . . .

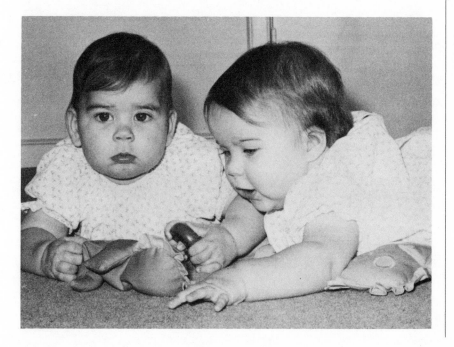

I like the attention at the mall. It makes me feel I am very special on days when I feel harried and frustrated.

It is hard for parents of twins not to compare them and make comparisons with the "average" baby in the books as well as with your friends' babies.

We encourage everyone to use the twins' names or to refer to "your brother" or "your sister" rather than "your twin."

I think a lot of parents are so zealous about how to treat the twins. They look so hard for problems that they often create the problems they find. When you grow a plant, you give it light and water, but you let it be a plant.

Jeremy is as loose as a goose, but Christopher is a real go-getter — a winner.

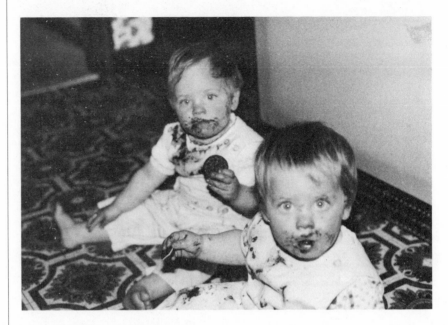

. . . **making a mess together** . . .

One of our twin boys is very good in school, but the other is the swimming star in the family.

Twins can understand if one is ready to go ahead and the other is not ready, without guilt or stigma.

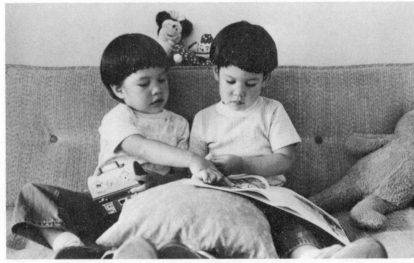

. . . **reading stories together** . . .

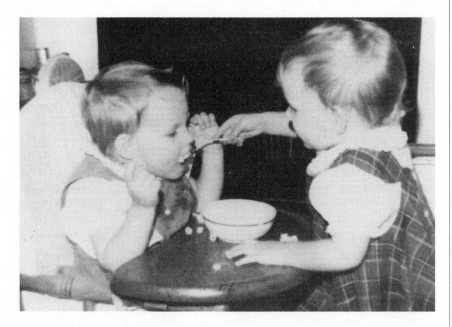

. . . **feeding each other.**

It is important that parents are aware of problems that can arise with twins but are not alarmed by them.

The other kids in the class didn't understand about twins at first. They thought each girl was called AnnieMichelle.

When visitors ask after "the triplets," we keep reinforcing the names, such as "Julie and Andrea are fine, but Eleanor has a cold today."

Multiples in particular need to be appreciated as individuals, separate from their membership in a set. It is more polite to ask the name of a twin member rather than repeat the tiresome question "Which one are you?" Group references such as "the twins" and "the quads" should be avoided. Dizygotic twins experience more frequent use of their names since they usually do not look alike. People retain the names of unlike twins, while monozygotic twins tend to be called "the twins" more often. Twins may also confuse their own identity at first and may both respond if one name is called. Symbiotic names like BoJo for Bobby and Joseph are confusing to other children who have not yet comprehended what makes two persons twins.

Twins will generally correct their peers but not their teachers or other adults. It is important for parents to help each twin be recognized individually so that the use of "the twins" or the avoidance of names is not necessary.

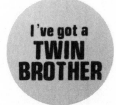

I've got a
TWIN BROTHER

Separation and Independence

Twins have one great advantage over singletons: they always have each other for company and understanding and rarely need a security

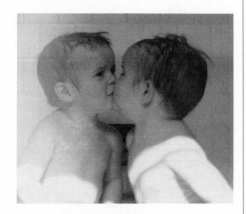

Twins enjoy their special bond.

Make sure that you take plenty of photos of each twin separately, so you're not always emphasizing their twinship.

There is never any trouble getting the twins to bed. They always have each other for company.

blanket. Socializing is also easy for multiples, especially if they are alike in appearance. They attract attention, and people notice and remember them. Multiples enjoy very close mental and physical contact from infancy on. Twinfants play and cuddle together and may even sleep interlocked. As they learn to crawl and walk, multiples follow each other around. Later one may read stories to the other. Twins often learn skills in dressing and feeding each other before they can manage for themselves. Parents often comment that multiples play together better than other siblings do.

Brief separations should start from the very beginning. Twins do not always have to be nursed, rocked, or played with together. Certainly triplets have to take turns. One of the multiples can spend time at home while the other child can go shopping. Friends and relatives should be encouraged to invite one twin for day trips or overnight stays. In fact, it may be easier for some families to include one extra child than two. Social relationships vary greatly with the environment: twins who live on a farm may be thrown together much more than twins who live in a city. Sometimes one receives an important invitation and the parents may provide a special treat for the excluded twin. The often-excluded singleton siblings must not be forgotten either.

Schooling of Multiples

Paradoxically, mandatory school policies can deny multiples the individuality that schools try to promote by separating the twins. Schooling is one of the big problems that parents of twins face. Teachers prefer to separate twins because it is easier for them than struggling to tell them apart and comparing their work. Only 25 percent of parents in an Australian study of more than 1,200 teachers found that separation became more common over the first three years of school, but 20 to 25 percent of the twins separated after one year were back together the next.

In contrast to the Australian experience, a 1987 study of 638 mothers through the National Organization of Mothers of Twins Clubs found that most mothers were satisfied with the school situation, whether the multiples were separated or together. Rarely did mothers request a change in their twins' placement, but there was general agreement that any policy should be flexible and each set of multiples be considered separately.

Teachers receive no special training for multiples, and they need

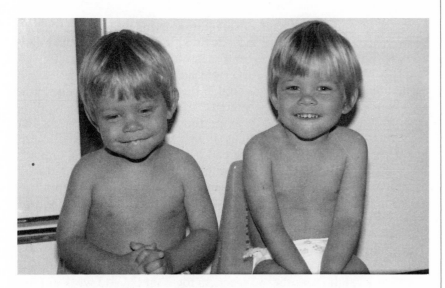

Twins may look identical but can have different body language.

Parents of multiples are lucky because of the constant companionship the children give each other. But some twins still complain once in a while that they have no one to play with!

When we took anniversary photos of our twins, we always had them in the same position in the photo. This is a big help for recording the subtle differences in identical twins.

to have resources, workshops, and videos to educate them (such as *More than One*, made by the Australian Multiple Birth Association). As it has never been proved that separation is essential to individual development, the only question is how each child can learn best, and solutions will vary.

Short separations, from each other and from the mother, may be begun well before playschool, kindergarten, or school commences. However, cautions Patricia Malmstrom, founder and director of Twin Services, twins forced apart into separate classrooms before they are ready can suffer disabling levels of anxiety and loss of self-esteem. "We get many calls and letters each year from parents all over the country who are distressed because a school put their twins in different classrooms and one or sometimes both children are having serious behavior and learning problems," says Malmstrom. "Policies which require separation of multiples seem to be based on assumptions that separation will promote individuality and independence. But no school administrator has ever been able to cite to us a study or reference which supports this notion, and we find no research which validates routine separation. On the contrary, research findings and our observations support routine placement together. We feel separation should be the exception, not the rule, and that parents' opinions and twins' own desires about placement should be respected."

Because I had so many infertility treatments to conceive, we made the mistake of overprotecting our twins.

Our identical twins often get the same marks on a test. The first time it happened the teacher suspected cheating. But even in separate rooms they get the same answers and make the same errors.

My twin sister and I never had any problems being in the same classroom. We are each other's best friend and it was easy to do our homework together.

I think starting school is such a trauma for twins that they need each other for security until each can make other friends. After that, I think separation helps with their individuality since twins are compared so much.

Malmstrom and others have observed that twins who are allowed to be together when they need to be during the early school years easily accept, and often request, separate classes in later grades.

In a 1989 Twin Services survey of California school psychologists, respondents unanimously agreed that there should be no blanket policy about twin classroom placement. Arbitrarily imposed separation gives multiples a disturbing message about their relationship. As one six-year-old girl said to the principal who was insisting that she and her sister be separated, ''Are we bad because we're twins?'' Individuality and independence from parents and siblings develop gradually over many years — forced separations at age four or five are unnecessary and often counterproductive, according to Malmstrom and other Twin Services staff.

School personnel generally complain if parents of multiples want to keep the children together. Many Mothers of Twins Club meetings focus on the topic of gaining more cooperation and understanding from school staff. Parents and teachers together have to work out the best educational environment for each member of a multiple set. There is no best way for everyone, so there should never be a blanket policy.

Occasionally twins are involved in an unplanned separation when the school suggests that one moves up to the next grade while the other has to repeat. Experts advise that this dilemma may be avoided by picking up learning problems early enough so that special tutoring can keep multiples at the same grade level. Usually schools, even some nursery schools, provide testing at the outset so that learning discrepancies between multiples can be ameliorated. If there is a very large difference, separate classes are invariably recommended. The IQ of monozygotic twins varies only by about five points. Dizygotic twins' IQ scores vary by less than ten points, and those of other siblings range between a ten- and fifteen-point difference.

Parents who can afford it may seek out private schools with flexible programs for their multiples because they disagree with the policy of separating twins at the local school. Camp Adventure School, a private school in Tucson, had several sets of twins among its students when I visited it. In addition to providing extensive testing and evaluation of each twin's abilities, the school personnel encourage the children to work at their own pace.

Parents of twins, and of supertwins especially, may want to consider home schooling. State laws require that you provide your children with an education — it doesn't have to be within a school — but you need approval from your school district to educate your children at home. As a writer, I am well aware that by the time a book

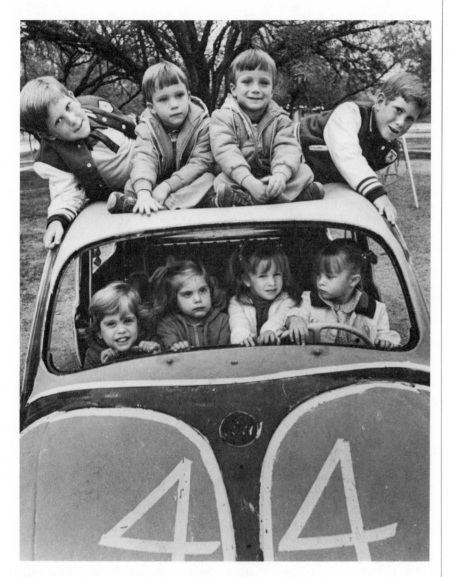

We put our twins in separate classes after we found out that Elaine was doing all the work for Paul. Even in school, he'd send papers to the back of the room where she was sitting.

We both hated sharing the same class. Our teacher used to embarrass us by asking us to stand side by side and get people to try and see differences.

There were four sets of twins at Camp Adventure School.

gets into print, much of the information is outdated. Textbooks in this computer age will soon go the way of the dinosaur; besides, it never made much sense to me that each child in the class had to open his or her book at Chapter X, when some are far behind and others far ahead. Putting the quality of knowledge aside, there remains the is-

I decided that once a week I would keep one of my twins at home with me. This gave me some special time with each and allowed them to develop relationships with other children without a twin looking on. Far from being detrimental to their education, the two half-days each one missed per month enabled them to become very independent and easily establish friendships, together and separately. I would recommend this to anyone.

sue of whether learning is best achieved by filling kids up with knowledge, as if they were bottles, in an institution divorced from the mainstream of life.

Some mothers of multiples may well look forward to school because the kids will be out of the house for most of the day, after the rush to get them all out the door. But so many parents of twins have problems with school — with forced separations, comparisons, ranking of different abilities, problems telling them apart if they look identical, teasing, to name a few — that home schooling makes even more sense for them. Multiples, like other children in the family, can learn and play happily together without developing problems with dependency and competition.

We now home-school our children; I only wish we'd done it sooner. I have subscribed for years to the newsletter from Growing Without Schooling, a Boston organization founded by the late author and educator John Holt. However, my daughter did not decide that she was fed up with the school until third grade, and I wanted a decision to remain at home to be her free choice. Obviously, the process of home schooling needs supervision by a parent or other adult, but the parent does not have to "teach class." An extensive array of resources exists for home learning; it is truly exciting to be able to choose the form and content of your child's curriculum. The flexibility of home schooling and the possibilities for travel outside of crowded vacation periods have been important for our schedules. The children have plenty of opportunities for socialization with other home schooling families and extracurricular activities. I particularly appreciate the way the children get involved in their own projects and rarely watch TV, which used to be a major attraction at the end of the school day. At home, learning is continuous!

Parents who are themselves twins often make an exaggerated effort to treat their twins separately and differently. This can be carried to an extreme. Dina and Melanie both like ballet, but a coin will be flipped to see which of the twins will be allowed to take classes. Brian may be given violin lessons and Sandy piano lessons. This may be unkind to Brian if both share a talent for piano. Twins also enjoy shared activities. Homework is less of a chore when multiples assist each other (with parents checking occasionally to see that assistance is really mutual).

Like the rest of us, twins must learn that life is not fair. It is not always possible for parents and teachers to treat twins equally. One child may excel in sports and the other in schoolwork. Certain personalities attract other personalities. Positive parental response will reinforce a particular pattern of behavior in a child. Each twin will find his or her own compensations in the world. Certainly singleton siblings do not get equal treatment. Praising one twin, however, may automatically make the other feel inferior and diminish his or her motivation. Private attention and praise are preferable.

The duty of all parents is to help their children develop independence. The special attachments between multiples make this an interesting challenge. These children have to define their concept of selfhood not only from their parents but from the others in the set. Three aspects of identity need to be integrated: that of the individual, that of his or her twin, and the shared identity as a multiple. Whether the personal or twin identity is emphasized depends on the expectations of the family and society and whether the twins were raised to be a unit or to be a mix as individuals.

Twin Talk

Language is essential not only for us to communicate with others but also to define thoughts and concepts for ourselves. As children we learn to speak by imitating with correction the sounds we hear. First-born singletons usually do better with language acquisition because parents are the models for speech rather than siblings.

The development of language usually follows a given sequence, beginning with babbling and cooing sounds, recognition of parents' voices, and turning toward sound at age six weeks to six months. Babies at this phase also enjoy getting a parent's attention from mimicking sounds. From nine to twelve months infants will understand simple commands, and at about a year they will use true speech and speak simple words like "mama," "papa," "dog," "apple." True speech for twins may not be noted until fifteen to eighteen months.

Consonants near the front of the mouth (*m, d, b, t, p, n*) are the easiest to make. The year-old child responds appropriately to different sounds and some instructions and enjoys imitating. By eighteen months the child is usually speaking about ten words. Infant girls speak earlier, and a first-born girl twin born at term reaches the same standard as a singleton. Monozygotic twin boys have taken as long as eighteen months before saying their first word.

Toward the second year, the child will use two-word combinations (such as "all gone") and will begin to attach adjectives to nouns: "big apple," "nice ball." At this age the child enjoys identifying pictures in books and the parts of his body. Twins may combine their names.

Between the second and third years, the child can use about

Nobody had a clue what any of their language meant. The twins clearly understood it all. They even had special names for each other — Ter and Tar.

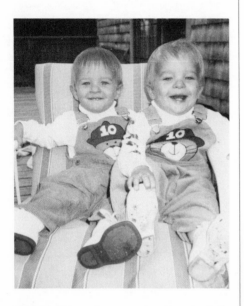

Twins always have each other to talk to.

three to six words in a sentence. He or she asks questions and uses negatives. Some sounds, such as *ch, sh,* and *th* may be difficult to pronounce. From the third to fourth year, the sentence length increases, with more questions. The child can invert verbs and use plural nouns. By the age of four, according the Cincinnati Speech and Hearing Center, the child can use all possible sentence types and has correct grammar, if not articulation, and can recount experiences and follow directions.

Speech development is a fascinating aspect of twinship and is being studied by many researchers. Twins enjoy a special social situation. They have each other as the most frequent speech model, chattering away and amusing each other. Twins are often so in tune with each other that they comprehend all kinds of sounds and noises. Some parents are too busy to devote much time to encouraging and correcting the multiples' attempts at speech, and they are slower than singletons to develop language skills. Singletons, on the other hand, have to make themselves understood. With twins, there is a limited use of words, and mistakes and mispronunciations are prolonged. Stuttering, stammering, and lisping are reinforced unless the parents take time to work on such problems. Pointing may also persist as a substitute for speech.

Sometimes twins develop their own special form of communication, especially if left alone to play together without much interaction with others. This twin talk may consist of private abbreviations, unique body language, and made-up words.

Patricia Malmstrom, founder of Twin Services, made a survey of twin language and found that almost half of parents of twins reported observing "twin effects" such as nonverbal communication in place of spoken words, using a "team name" and singular verbs to refer to themselves together, and using the pronoun "me" when they meant the unit. Twenty percent of parents did not allow twin language. It is important that parents with concerns about language delay have their twins checked for physical problems such as hearing loss. However, Malmstrom warns against undue anxiety and suggests that parents relax and enjoy their twins' language idiosyncrasies. She also points out that their environment, which requires twins to take turns even in infancy, gives twins an edge over singletons in learning the art of conversation.

The medical terms for this invented twin speech are *idioglossia* and *idiolalia.* Sometimes it is called *cryptophasia,* which means "not communicable to others." In fact, twins are aware of this phenomenon and do not use their special language with others.

The literature describes one case of four-year-old twins who were unable to speak at all. Their IQs were estimated to be in the low 60s. Their mother was given extensive education to help develop the twins' individuality by learning to call them by their own names and dressing them differently. One year later the twins were speaking fluently and their IQ had doubled. This was clearly a case of environmental deprivation rather than congenital retardation.

Family Health printed an article in September 1978 on the speech patterns of a particular set of twins. A sample of the twins' private language was the title: "Cabendo padem manibadu peetu." The history of these twins was unfortunate. They survived seizures in early childhood, but the parents were warned that the twins might be mentally retarded. Both parents of these twins had to work to make ends meet, so the children had little encouragement at home to speak. By seventeen months they knew only a few English words, such as "Mommy" and "Daddy." However, by themselves they chattered all the time in their special dialect. After their sixth birthday, these little girls could not be enrolled in school because of their severe communication problems. Fortunately, they were referred for treatment and underwent speech therapy. As they learned English, their twin talk was deciphered phonetically. In one fifteen-minute session, twenty-six different pronunciations for the word *potato* were counted, ranging from "puhted" to "pancahydooz." Even though that type of sample takes hours to decipher, linguists feel that such research provides insights into the origin and learning of language.

They don't really have a twin language, but they copy each other's baby talk. They clearly understand each other better than we do.

A study in France on language development found that twins performed less well on verbal tests (an average delay of six months, with lowest scores achieved by monozygotic twins). This was compensated for by better scores on perception and performance. The fact that twins scored in the normal range on motor and postural tests showed that there was no neurological deficit. The low performance on social relationships and language points to environmental factors. This was confirmed by the fact that twins with deceased partners scored very high on verbal and reasoning tests. Development of audio-vocal skills depends very much on the home situation and the parents' social and economic levels.

They were like alien beings when they talked to each other in their own weird sounds.

Talking and reading to your twins is the best way to improve their language skills. Encourage the less vocal twin to talk, and converse simply and clearly to each one separately, using his or her own name, as often as you can. Parents need to keep modeling correct pronunciation. There is no need to imitate the twins or repeat errors when correcting a child, and never ridicule. Dr. Burton White feels that it is more important to monitor early understanding and that a child should understand at least three dozen words by fourteen

Why shouldn't we be alike? We are identical twins; we share the same career; we think alike about most things. My brother may have done a bit better at school, but then he worked harder!

months. He advises that there is no need to be concerned about speech unless a child isn't saying any words by eighteen or twenty months.

Intelligence tests are slanted toward language skill, which probably explains why twins score a few points below the average singleton (apart from prenatal factors such as maternal malnutrition and low birth weight). The late Ronald Wilson of the Louisville Twin Study found that while twins lagged below singletons on intelligence tests at age four, by age six they caught up.

The Cincinnati Speech and Hearing Center suggests that parents seek professional help in the following situations:

Anytime you suspect a child isn't hearing properly.

If the child does not use two-word combinations by age two and a half.

If by three and a half years, the child doesn't have intelligible speech.

If the child has persistent articulation problems past age five with *p/f*, *b/v*, distortions of *l*, *r*, *s*, *ch*, *sh*, and *j*.

If the child has had a difficult birth or illness in early infancy and you suspect any problem later.

Speech difficulties can be evaluated by a speech therapist; therapy is most effective the sooner it is begun. A child may also have a mechanical problem with the tongue or palate. (See Resources under "Special Needs.") Hearing loss may also be involved. Approximately 25 percent of children will have untreated repeated illnesses leading to fluid in the middle ear, which can result in hearing loss, and subsequent problems with language development, by age two. (Milk can be the culprit; see the discussion on dairy products in Chapter 9.) The National Association for Hearing and Speech Action has a toll-free number (see Resources).

The Twin Bond

Twins share their age, uterine environment, and family life. This bond is often closer than that of marriage or of mother and child. Twinship is especially strong in monozygotic pairs, who usually remain very close throughout their adult life. Dependency on each other, rather than jealousy, may be a problem. Genetically the same and more attached than friends, monozygotic twins may choose the same career and lifestyle. If they share an apartment or a car, much of their social life may be shared. Many teenagers and adults really enjoy their twinship and resent pressures on them to be different or separate. Monozygotic twins who are reared together find their own ways to become different. If reared apart, without such pressure, their likenesses are often greater, as Bouchard's work at the Minnesota Center for Adoption and Twin Research has shown.

You can never tell a lie to your twin.

Almost all the twins I interviewed went on dates alone. (One pair, coincidentally, had boyfriends with the same last name.) Members of twin pairs marry less frequently than singletons. Some twins date twins and even marry twins, as did La Vona and La Velda Rowe, who married Arthur and Alwyn Richmond. All four published a newsletter, *Twincerely Yours*. Marriage between twins can be ideal because only they truly understand the twin bond.

The "Invisible" Twins

Dizygotic twins are less affected by twinship than monozygotic twins, although if they look alike they may be treated as if they were monozygotic. Boy-girl combinations are little different from other siblings apart from their shared birthday. Differential development oc-

All our lives we search for our soulmates. When you are a twin, you are born with and begin life with a soulmate. What security, what joy!

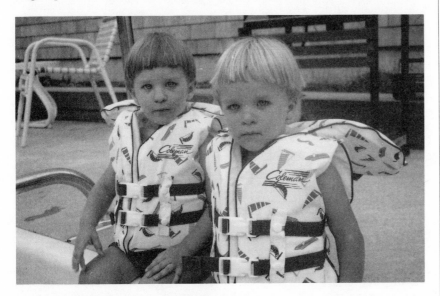

Alike, yet different: "twindividuality."

curs between the two sexes. The girl matures first, leaping ahead in weight, height, and sometimes school grades. The balance may alter in adolescence, when parents often have a different set of social or moral standards for their sons than for their daughters. Tommy may be allowed to take the car and go off with friends, while his parents feel that twin Jeannie needs more protection. Jim may get tired of having to escort Suzanne to parties and make sure she has a good time. Fortunately, sex roles are changing and so is the assignment of family tasks. Experts advise that the more responsible twin should never be held back because of a less mature twin.

Cooperation is more the norm with monozygotic twins and competition is common between dizygotic twins of opposite or the same sex. Life can be hard if one twin is much more attractive or more brilliant, as also happens in families with singleton siblings.

Parents of twins, after the hard work of the first couple of years, express joy and satisfaction in the experience of raising twins. The overwhelming feeling about twinship is positive. It is a rare twin pair who would deny that the fun of being a twin outweighs any conflicts. People form a variety of family and friendship ties in life, but few are as close or as long-lasting as the bond between twins and other multiples.

19 Thrice as Nice:
Having Supertwins

AS WE HAVE SEEN, higher multiples have become common because of the increasing use of hormone treatments and the introduction of reproductive technologies, such as in vitro fertilization, GIFT, and embryo transfer, to assist infertile women. At present, about half of all supertwins (triplets and higher-order multiples) result from assisted conceptions. When they request such assistance, many infertile couples are unaware of the possibility of twins, let alone larger multiples, and the risks associated with bearing them. One mother conceived two singletons, triplets, and then quads, all on progressively lower doses of ovarian stimulants.

When embryos are transplanted, three or more seem to be necessary for implantation and survival with the current state of the technology. Because of the increased risks of higher-order multiple pregnancy and birth, many specialists are recommending that the limit be set at three embryos.

Influences on the natural occurrence of supertwins are similar to those for twins, as discussed in Chapter 3. However, statistics today are confused with the data from assisted conceptions. There are some exceptions: Japan has the lowest twinning rate in the world, but the highest rate of identical triplets and quadruplets reported outside of Nigeria. In central India between 1960 and 1965, the frequency of triplets was as high as 1 in 880 births, but the rate declined in the 1980s to 1 in 1,700, which is still higher than the rate in Indian cities (1 in 4,000).

With triplets, there are, of course, more combinations of zygosity than with twins. For example, triplets can be three fraternals, which are called trizygotic (from three different eggs) or a "pair and a spare," which are monozygotic (identical: from one egg) and one singleton. (Boklage suggests the possibility of the extra triplet being half of a monozygotic twin pair whose other member vanished in early pregnancy. This seems logical to my mind, too.)

The Triplet Connection's research survey in 1988 of 3,300 infants comprised 6 percent monozygotic, 28 percent trizygotic, and 66 percent singleton plus monozygotic. One boy and two girls was the most likely combination. More triplets are born in April and May than in any other months. Weight gain and increasing maternal age predicted longer duration of pregnancy and higher infant birth weight.

The diagnosis of triplets and higher-order multiples may be missed. Sometimes the babies are very active during sonograms, or one body shadows another and they look like twins. One Danish study of 73 triplet pregnancies from 1980 to 1989 found that the prenatal diagnosis of twins was not corrected before delivery of the third triplet in 11 cases, despite at least one ultrasound being obtained in each pregnancy. One woman who had several ultrasounds that indicated quintuplets ended up with quadruplets, so the error can be in either direction.

Most of the advice and information in this book pertains to twins, but this chapter will examine the medical facts about pregnancy and birth with supertwins and explore some special dimensions of this experience.

Prenatal Care

Although some obstetricians may never deliver triplets or quads, make sure you have a competent physician who at least has experience with the natural childbirth of twins. If you deliver in a high-risk hospital (level III) with a neonatal intensive care unit (NICU), you can avoid a transfer to another hospital if any of the babies require level III nursery care (explained in Chapter 16). Babies less than thirty-six weeks should be delivered in a center with a level III nursery.

If you are not satisfied with your doctor, call the neonatology department at the nearest NICU and ask for a recommendation. Visit the NICU during your pregnancy and take a Caesarean birth class, but hope that you won't need either. Educate yourself about the risks involved in carrying and delivering supertwins and find out what you can do to prevent problems. In the United States, the likelihood of a Caesarean section is extremely high. Some other countries have a lower Caesarean rate for supertwins than the United States does for singletons, but in general Caesarean rates are rising everywhere. One study reported a Caesarean rate of 80 percent for quads and 72 percent for triplets in England and Wales if the mothers had conceived with medical intervention. For those women who conceived their su-

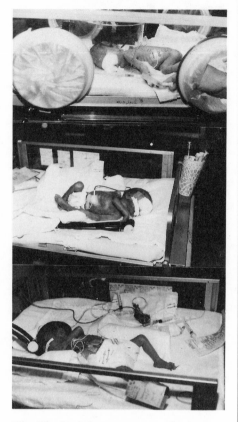

The Bleyl triplets at two weeks . . .

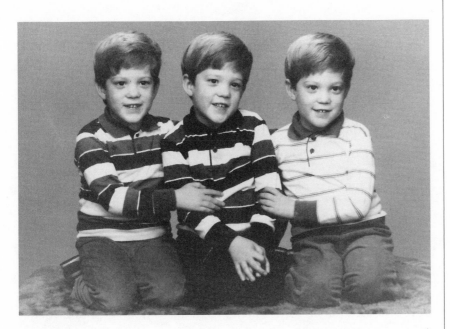

. . . and at four years.

pertwins naturally, the Caesarean rates were lower — 67 percent for quads and 59 percent for triplets. There is always an unexplained higher Caesarean rate when technology has been used, perhaps from an attitude that the babies are "premium babies"; and doctors who put the babies inside like to bring them out.

Also keep in mind that many mothers have carried triplets uneventfully, and sometimes unknowingly, to term, and some have delivered triplets at home with no medical intervention.

Nutrition, Hydration, Weight Gain, and Education

The cardinal rules for a healthy pregnancy (discussed in full in Chapter 9) are three times more important for supertwins. *Nutrition is the single most important factor in outcome* and, fortunately, something over which you have complete control. Mothers expecting triplets need to eat for four, and mothers expecting quadruplets need to eat for five. This means about 400–500 extra calories and 20–25 grams of extra protein per baby. That is, 1,200–1,500 extra calories and 60–75 extra grams of protein per day for triplets. Well-nourished mothers of singletons who attend my Maternal and Child Health Center in Cambridge gain 40 pounds on the average — about a pound a week. Mothers of twins gain at least 60 pounds. Mothers of triplets should gain even more — at least 60–70 pounds. The problem is never too much weight gain (unless it is from junk food) but rather not enough. Eating as much as you require is certainly difficult when there is greater need but less room inside the mother's stomach because of crowding from the uterus. The mother's decreased levels of activity mean less appetite too. Of course, prepregnancy weight is significant, and many mothers of higher multiples are below normal weight at conception (which also plays a role in conception difficulties that may have led to the hormonal treatments that resulted in a multiple pregnancy). The evidence is quite clear: mothers who had the larger, healthier babies and carried them longer had better nutrition than mothers with smaller, less healthy babies and gained at least 50–75 pounds. A medical questionnaire by the Triplet Connection with more than six hundred responses indicated that, with rare exceptions, mothers of supertwins who gained less than 35 pounds delivered very prematurely.

This is one time in your life when you have the best possible reason to gain weight. In a society where there is so much obesity, don't let weight gain bother you! You will lose most of it very quickly after the birth. One expectant mother of triplets was hospitalized for observation because she had gained 50 pounds at thirty weeks. The hospital wanted to put her on a restrictive diet, but she had educated herself about good nutrition and threatened to sue the hospital. It is up to the expectant parents of supertwins to be highly informed and to educate those around them, even health care providers. You may be referred to a dietician if you have a condition such as gestational diabetes (discussed in Chapter 7). Some dieticians are rather academic, so be careful not to be put on a diet that is too low in calories to sustain a multiple pregnancy.

As Janet Bleyl of the Triplet Connection says, "Eat like a horse and drink like a whale." Eating small amounts constantly makes the task of maintaining good nutrition and good weight gain easier and also helps prevent you from feeling low in energy. Remind yourself every day how much your babies need the food to grow. Keep nibbling nutritious snacks even if you don't feel hungry. Many mothers of multiples have said, "If I'd known then what I know now, I'd have made myself eat more."

Adequate fluids are also essential, up to 20 glasses per day depending on individual factors such as climate and activity level. The research of Dr. Tom Brewer shows that the importance of maintaining an adequate blood volume to prevent premature labor, and fluids contribute directly to blood volume. If you experience preterm contractions, you will most likely be asked to drink several glasses of water while you rest.

Getting Off Your Feet

Rest is extremely important in such a challenging pregnancy. The greater hormonal changes in the first trimester cause you to feel very tired, and then the extra weight and pressure in the last two trimesters bring added fatigue. However, lying flat can be uncomfortable with larger multiples, and mothers find it nearly impossible to stay in bed. Recliners, adjustable chairs, or electric hospital beds may be better than a bed. An overhead pull bar is a great help, and plenty of pillows or a wedge are needed to support your overextended belly.

Comfort Measures

Avoid using mineral oil for the severe itching and often painful stretching of abdominal skin. Use cocoa butter, any vegetable or nut oil, and add baking soda to your bath. Regular massage for the extra fluid and muscle strain and a swimming program should not only be required for mothers of multiples but should be paid for by health insurance, even if the woman has to be transported to the masseuse and pool in a wheelchair! Hospitalized expectant mothers should seek a daily float with mild exercise in the physical therapy department, if available. Hydrotherapy pools or tanks are used for serious burn cases and other patients, so there is no reason why an expectant mother of higher multiples should not enjoy the same resources. And there is every reason why she should. In water, she will be relieved to experience only one-tenth of her body weight. This relaxation is extremely beneficial for an "irritable uterus" and can diminish or stop preterm contractions. This pleasurable exercise demands very little effort but it reduces swelling and maintains healthy joints, muscles, and cardiovascular system. Today many hospitals are installing large whirlpool baths in the labor suites, which you could ask to use if a pool is not available.

Sonograms tend to be long and rigorous with three or more babies. This strain can trigger premature contractions. Make sure that you lie on your side for ultrasounds to avoid a drop in blood pressure

I just loved to soak in the bath, even when I could hardly fit anymore. During the months of my bed rest in the hospital, I asked if there was a deep tub somewhere that I could soak in. Unfortunately, the doctors were so irate at the nurse who inquired on my behalf that she was removed from her position.

My doctor did an ultrasound and remarked: "They're stacked in there like cord wood, with no room to turn!"

that can occur on your back from the weight of the uterus compressing the major vein returning blood to your heart. If the ultrasound exam becomes an ordeal, ask the technician to stop and reschedule it.

Medical Studies

Supertwins, despite their increasing rate of occurrence, are still uncommon, and parents may have difficulty finding specific information. The following recent studies are presented in detail so that expectant couples can have some "hard data." These perinatal outcomes were presented at the 1989 Congress of the International Society for Twin Studies Congress, held in Rome. The single most important factor influencing the health and survival of supertwins is their degree of maturity. According to Drs. Papiernik and Pons in France, nearly 50 percent of triplets need advanced technological support.

Pons and his colleagues followed 32 triplet pregnancies from 1977 to 1988. The mothers were not systematically hospitalized, nor was bed rest routinely prescribed. However, expectant mothers of

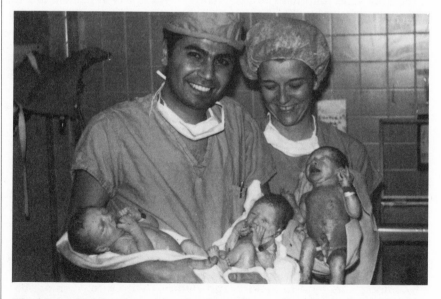

The birth of triplets is exciting for the staff as well as for the parents.
Courtesy of Labib Habashy, M.D.

multiples were seen in a special clinic, had home visits from a midwife, and took leave from work at twenty-four weeks. Even so, the
prematurity rate for this group of triplets was over 90 percent and the
mean age at delivery was thirty-four weeks. Mean birth weight was
1,717 grams (approximately 3 pounds, 12 ounces), with a range from
780 to 2,580 grams (1 pound, 11 ounces, to 5 pounds, 10 ounces).
Nine children died out of 96, yielding a perinatal mortality rate of less
than 10 percent. Corticosteroids were used from the twenty-sixth to
the thirty-fourth week to speed lung maturity. Less than 5 percent of
the children whose mothers received corticosteroids had respiratory
distress syndrome, compared with 20 percent of children of untreated
mothers. Almost all infants were delivered by elective Caesarean section.

Pons also reported on six sets of quadruplets born at the Antoine
Beclère Hospital in Clamart, France, between 1977 and 1988. Three
sets were conceived as a result of using Clomid and three after HMG
(human menopausal gonadotropin) therapy. All babies were born
prematurely and averaged fifty days in the hospital after birth. The
average duration of the pregnancies was thirty-two weeks. All deliveries were Caesarean and the mortality rate was 29 percent. Birth
weight ranged from 900 to 1,900 grams (just under 2 pounds to 4
pounds, 3 ounces).

In a Danish study by Borlum, 50 percent of the triplet pregnancies resulted from in vitro fertilization. The mean length of pregnancy
was thirty-three weeks, one week less than in the French study. Only
18 percent had vaginal births. Eleven women experienced intrauterine death of one or two of the triplets. Fifteen children died during
the first week of life, making the perinatal mortality rate 13 percent.
The 70 pregnancies of twenty-eight weeks or longer had a perinatal
mortality rate of 8 percent. The average weight for the triplets, in
order of their births, were 1,827 grams (just under 4 pounds), 1,811
grams (3 pounds, 15 ounces), and 1,777 grams (4 pounds, 14 ounces).

A 1988 study by Thiery, Derom, and colleagues in Belgium reported an 81 percent vaginal delivery rate for 16 triplet and higher-
order deliveries. Sixty-eight percent of the infants were born before
the thirty-sixth week. The perinatal and neonatal mortality rates for
infants weighing at least 1,000 grams (2 pounds, 3 ounces) and born
after twenty-eight weeks were 7 percent and 3 percent, respectively.
Caesarean section resulted in more complications for the mother than
for the mothers who delivered vaginally. The authors doubted that
the outcome for the babies could have been markedly improved by
performing more Caesareans.

In 8 of the 10 triplet births and 5 of the 6 larger multiples, the

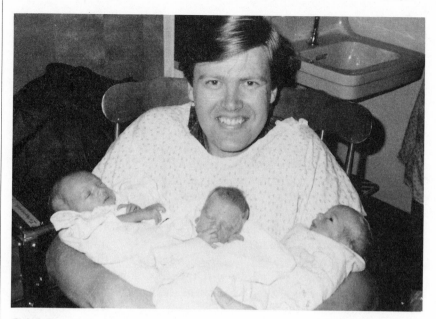

Triple joy.

length of pregnancy was extended by an average of seven weeks by bed rest and tocolytic drugs in Thiery's study. Itzkowic (1979) found that bed rest was of no value of prolonging triplet pregnancies.

In Japan the incidence of triplets is increasing, as it is elsewhere, with ovulation-inducing hormones. Eleven sets of triplets had been delivered at the Tokyo Medical College Hospital by 1989. Three sets of triplets delivered before twenty-nine weeks of gestation were all stillborn. Another set, delivered between thirty-four and thirty-six weeks, did well except that one had anecephalus (absence of brain and skull). Six sets were delivered after thirty-seven weeks, with one fetus papyraceus (an undeveloped fetus compressed into the placenta); all infants were well but most of the babies were small for their dates. *In no case was a Caesarean section performed*. When I questioned Dr. Yoshida about this, he replied, "Triplets are usually smaller, they don't need surgical delivery!" I learned that the Caesarean rate for twins (who are also usually smaller) at 5 percent was half what it is for singletons (which at 10 percent is still two and a half time less than the U.S. rate). I was pleased that the Japanese trust in the natural process of birth extends not only to twins but to higher-order multiples as well.

Outcome for Higher-Order Multiples

Year	Number of Cases	Weeks of Pregnancy	Median Birth Weight (grams)*
TRIPLETS			
1922–79	44	34.6	2,020
1980–83	48	34.4	1,920
1984–87	135	33.9	1,810
1988–89	70	33.4	1,760
QUADRUPLETS			
1912–83	15	34	1,550
1984–88	40	31.1	1,210
QUINTUPLETS			
1972–88	17	29.4	1,050
SEXTUPLETS			
1981–88	5	29.1	970

Combined Birth Weight per Multiple Set

	Number	Median Birth Weight (grams)*
Triplets	297	5,510
Quadruplets	55	5,390
Quintuplets	17	5,310
Sextuplets	5	5,720

*1,000 grams equals 2 pounds, 3 ounces.

Death Rates Before First Year†

	1978–83 (%)	1984–89 (%)
Triplets	1.8	4.3
Quadruplets	13.6	15.8
Quintuplets	28.0	22.5
Sextuplets	33.0	27.8

†In this context, "death" is defined as the death of an infant before his or her first birthday. The two groups with a six-year span are not fully comparable. The ABC Club was founded only in 1982. Mothers who had lost their children before 1983 never reported the deaths. This explains the seemingly higher death rate in the latter six years. On the other hand, ever smaller babies are surviving the first few weeks of life.

Helga Grützner, founder of the ABC club (discussed later in this chapter) compiled the data in the chart about supertwins in German-speaking Europe, showing that the numbers are increasing but the outcome is less favorable than formerly. This is because advanced technology is used to keep alive very premature babies who previously would not have survived. I also believe that the increased obstetric intervention these days, especially with twins and supertwins, does not always improve outcome.

The Triplet Connection surveyed 1,330 families with higher-order multiples in 1989. Of those, 1,250 had triplets, 76 had quads, and 11 had quintuplets. The data are presented in the second table, with the percentages rounded off. The average age of the mothers was thirty, and 31 percent had incomes of $50,000 or more (and were probably the couples who could afford to pay for expensive infertility treatments). At the other end of the scale are single mothers of triplets, who have a support network (see Resources).

Preventing Preterm Labor

The overwhelming challenge with supertwins, as with twins, is to avoid premature, low-birth-weight infants. (Chapter 11 contains a complete discussion on ways to avoid prematurity.) Women pregnant with larger multiples rarely feel contractions because the uterus is already stretched so taut that they don't feel it getting any harder. Yet it is important to be in touch with your body and to recognize any early warning signs of premature labor. Unfortunately, many women ignore discomfort, backache, or other worrying signs because they don't want to bother the doctor or they want to carry on as usual and not make an issue of their special status.

Janet Bleyl contacted more than 3,000 mothers who had delivered larger multiples, and very few had been able to detect preterm labor. Bleyl warns expectant mothers that preterm labor contractions will be painless and recommends careful home monitoring. She cautions that doctors may wait until the mother reports contractions, and by then it may be too late. Some women will begin to have contractions from eighteen weeks and it is important to stop contractions before the cervix starts to thin out and dilate. Bleyl advises mothers to contact companies that make home monitors, such as Tokos Medical Corporation or HealthDyne Perinatal Services (see Resources). These organizations will also help you find a home monitoring nurse near you who can explain home monitoring in detail and advise you about health insurance coverage.

I don't think the term "Braxton-Hicks contractions" should be used at all in pregnancies with higher multiples. With my first child, I felt these intermittent tightenings, but I didn't notice them with my triplets. With supertwins, contractions are contractions and more than four an hour is scary.

Conception, Zygosity, and Gestation of Higher-Order Multiples

	Triplets (%)	Quadruplets (%)	Quintuplets (%)
METHOD OF CONCEPTION			
Spontaneous	39	8	10
Pergonal	19	49	55
HCG (human chorionic gonadotropin)	11	27	28
Clomid	40	34	19
IVF (in vitro fertilization)	7	9	19
GIFT (gametes intra-Fallopian transfer)	1	12	10
Other methods	3	8	—
ZYGOSITY			
Monozygotic	6	3	0
All trizygotic	28	36	11
Mixed (monozygotic and a spare)	66	62	89
All male	18	5	4
All female	21	10	4
Mixed	61	87	9
WEEKS OF GESTATION* OF LIVING BABIES			
	34	32	30

*This rate was lowered by some very low gestations; excluding these the average length of gestation was still low:

35	33	30+

Monitoring contractions at home to avoid preterm labor gives mothers more freedom from bed rest. With the home monitor mothers need to resort to strict bed rest only when their uterus is more active. Bleyl recommends that home monitoring be done twice a day beginning at twenty weeks and that biophysical profiles should start at thirty-two weeks and continue twice weekly after that, even if labor has been controlled. (See Chapter 11 for more details on home monitoring.) Many stillborns occur after thirty-five weeks, perhaps as a result of a placenta that can no longer function adequately. Bleyl knows of many cases when one of the babies died within days or even hours of a labor that started after thirty-seven weeks, and she believes strongly that supertwins should be delivered around thirty-six weeks by Caesarean section. Mothers of multiples who experience loss at the end of their pregnancy also favor intervention. As a happy contrast, others go to term uneventfully, and Mary (see Chapter 12) went to forty-one weeks and had her triplets at home after a prior Caesarean! Another woman I know birthed her babies vaginally, with an interval of one hour and forty-five minutes between the births of the second and third triplet!

Breast-Feeding

Just decide that you are going to breast-feed and see what works best. Some babies will only nurse, some won't take the breast, and some will take anything.

I really didn't like expressing milk and I felt a little like a cow doing it, but I just kept thinking of the babies, that I wouldn't have to do it for too long and that it was just one of those things that has to be done.

*There once was a young gal who begat
Three babes named Nat, Pat, and Tat
'Twas fun in the breeding, but hell in the
    feeding
When she found there was no tit for Tat!*
AUTHOR UNKNOWN

Breast-feeding triplets or quads can be a challenge even for mothers who have nursed previously. While it is certainly possible to breast-feed higher multiples, it may not always be easy. Sometimes the mother nurses two babies while the father gives a bottle of breast milk to the other or others.

Breast-feeding a premature infant is difficult enough. With triplets the problem is multiplied times three. The first problem is getting the premature baby to stay awake to feed. The second is getting the infant to suck strongly enough to get the milk to let down. If the mother has other children at home, she might be able to go to the hospital only once a day. The electric pump can be used on leaving

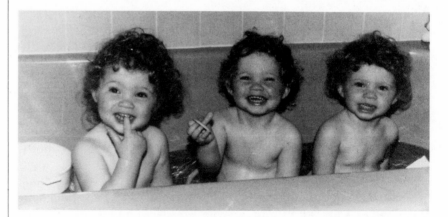

Triple fun.

and arriving, as well as every three hours or so at home. Electric pumps can empty the breasts in less than 10 minutes. (See Chapter 16 for a complete discussion of breast-feeding, including using an electric pump to express milk.)

Many mothers try to get the infants on a schedule where they wake and feed together. Others feel that because it takes so long to feed three or more, it is better not to disturb the sleeping baby or babies. They also hope that the babies will sleep a little longer between feedings, which they eventually do. Other mothers decide that they need sleep themselves more than spending the time expressing milk, so the father gives the babies supplementary feedings with a bottle of formula. It is a common experience that bottles are more likely to be accepted by babies if given by someone other than the nursing mother.

Triplets may need 36 bottles and nipples a day — breast-feeding in many ways is much less hassle. However, take bottles and nipples from the hospital so that you can sterilize them and keep them for storing breast milk or formula.

Some mothers of triplets have breast-fed their babies until they wean, often for as long as one or two years. Another mother of quads exclusively breast-fed her babies for the first six months (and that was about all she did!).

Coping Postpartum . . . Organize Help, Help, and More Help

Along with rewarding and joyful experiences with supertwins is the reality of physical and emotional round-the-clock care. This total commitment doesn't begin only at birth; many mothers expecting higher multiples need help before and after. Mountains of laundry, the needs of other children, food preparation, cleaning, and shopping are all added burdens. The birth of multiples changes the family's living standard and can drag middle-class families down to near poverty. The loss of the mother's income is an added financial strain, and the father may need to work extra jobs to pay the bills (frequently feeling guilty that he is not helping more at home).

Sometimes mothers of triplets end up with a baby at home, one in a local hospital to gain weight, and one or more in a distant NICU waiting to mature. Commuting, which can involve two or three hours a day, has to fit in with feeding schedules that are both frequent and time-consuming.

It didn't seem fair that my triplets should be bottle-fed just because they arrived at the same time.

Nursing three babies wasn't easy, but I'm sure it had to be easier than bottle-feeding three babies. Having to prepare just three clean bottles and nipples a day was hard enough. I can't imagine doing it all day, every day.

I never kept track of nursing or had a schedule. I always had enough milk. Time, not supply, was the problem. I always seemed to have a baby at the breast, enjoying the closeness but always feeling tired.

When they came home we were quite unprepared for the never-ending marathon of meeting the needs of these tiny, still-sick infants who required feeding every two hours (each feeding taking more than an hour to accomplish) around the clock.

Live not just a day at a time but an hour at a time.

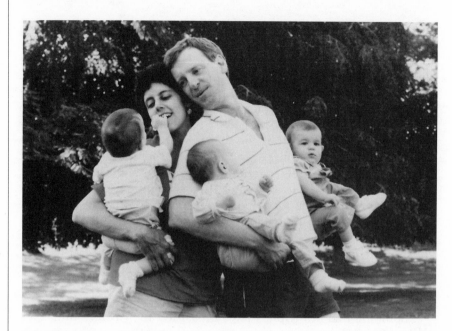

A family outing with triplets.

A significant factor in the ability of mothers of multiples to cope is their expectation of help from the father. But even that is not enough. In a study conducted at Antoine Beclère Hospital in France, 14 mothers of triplets said they felt that having multiples was a real source of psychological stress. Almost half of them did not have adequate help, which is a serious problem because the mother's reactions to the triplets depends greatly on how she perceives her support.

Unfortunately, few insurance companies today are willing to pay for home help. A letter from the obstetrician may help, if it convinces the company of the substantial amount saved on hospitalization and intensive medical care. Parents need to lobby for these measures. Home help may include housework and meal preparation during pregnancy and a nurse on duty from 7:00 P.M. to 7:00 A.M. postpartum. Nursing care postpartum can mean earlier discharge home for babies who need monitoring, oxygen, and so forth. This helps to bring all the infants together as soon as possible and saves traveling time and costs.

Mothers need a lot of help for themselves, too, especially if in addition to the challenge of carrying supertwins they have undergone a Caesarean delivery or have had any complications. Such factors may make it even harder for the mother to have direct contact with her babies in the NICU, and she may have other children at home for whom she is concerned, too. The mother needs peace and quiet to breast-feed one or more multiples while someone takes care of the rest of the household and family chores.

Set up a schedule for postpartum help as offers begin to come in during pregnancy, and organize it so that it continues for the first year at a minimum. Most people would rather help others than ask for help themselves, but mothers of supertwins invariably wish they had let themselves ask for and receive more help. As Karen Gromada, author of *Mothering Multiples*, said, "Never deprive another person of the chance to do a good deed!" It's handy if one friend assumes the job of scheduling other friends for cleaning, meals, babysitting, bathing the babies and so forth. This kind of gesture is worth more to the parents than expensive gifts. (See Chapter 15 for general advice on postpartum assistance.)

Hints for Home

Before you leave the hospital, ask for extra name bands if you need help to tell your babies apart. Higher-order multiples often need pacifiers because they don't have as much time to satisfy their need to suck. (Binky makes a smaller than usual pacifier with a very soft nipple for babies who won't take a Nuk.)

The multiples are happiest if they sleep together, but remember that three or more babies generate plenty of body heat; don't dress and cover them too warmly. It is simplest to put a mattress on the floor: there is nothing to fall out of. (The same is true of a changing area; make sure you kneel or sit.) Some parents use dresser drawers as cribs. Later you can put the children in separate beds; it is easier to change a single bed occasionally than a queen-size bed every day.

About 60 cloth diapers per day are needed, for burping as well as for bottoms. Five dozen usually are sufficient, because you will be doing laundry every day. Diaper service is less costly than disposables, without the ecological hazards, although there is still a lot of work in the rinsing. Disposable diapers are handy for traveling.

A triplet stroller is absolutely essential so that you can get out of the house. From the babies' point of view it is nice if you can go with someone and use baby carriers (on the back; don't create a load in front that is the equivalent of being twelve to eighteen months preg-

I didn't feel like those three little babies were mine; instead I felt like I was watching three tiny strangers struggling for their lives, but feeling no maternal instinct whatever. I've come to understand since then that it is normal for parents of critically ill newborns to delay bonding — a barrier against the possible pain of their loss. Nevertheless, it is upsetting and difficult to experience that vacuum of feeling for babies you've waited so long to love.

It's okay to say that things are not fine and that you are not coping and that you desperately need help. If you ever felt like a squeaking wheel needing grease, now is the time to speak up loud and clear.

nant!). Converted twin strollers don't always stand up to the extra wear and tear of three babies. (See Resources for different types of strollers, which can also be bought used through Mothers of Twins Clubs.)

Mothers of higher multiples generally advise new mothers to stick to priorities, do what works, don't count diapers and bottles (which is a reminder of the less pleasant part of parenting), and just enjoy the babies as much as you can.

Organizations for Higher-Order Multiples

Triplets will experience different issues than twins as they live the dynamics of a group rather than a pair. Triads are less stable than dyads, and the intragroup pairs change from time to time, just as twins may flip-flop with their behavior. Support groups for parents of higher-order multiples can be found through the self-help associations such as TAMBA in the Great Britain, POMBA in Canada, SAMBA in South Africa, and AMBA in Australia. In the United States, the Triplet Connection in California was founded by Janet Bleyl, a mother of ten including triplets. Since it was founded in 1983, this organization has helped guide more than three thousand families

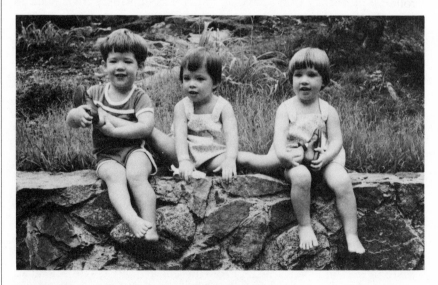

Triplets like to help each other with their shoes.

of multiples worldwide. The network has more than two hundred expectant mothers and families at any time. There is a quarterly newsletter with extensive listings of expectant and new parents as well as ads for triplet equipment. An information packet is sent to expectant parents; it can mean the difference between life and death in explaining how to minimize the risks of supertwins. A telephone hotline for consulting and an annual convention are offered to members. Send for and complete the group's medical questionnaire as this is a crucial source of information for you and other parents of multiples. (See Resources for the addresses of all these groups.)

The ABC Club is an international organization serving triplets and higher multiples primarily in German-speaking countries. More than a thousand families with higher-order multiples are in contact with the ABC Club. The group is organized in a network concentrated in Germany and reaching into Switzerland, Austria, and Liechtenstein. Expectant parents and new parents learn from the experiences of others, while adult multiples enjoy sports and social activities. The club is also committed to educating the public, making long-term observations about premature infants and family dynamics, and lobbying for the health interests of premature infants. Volunteers collect data, provide phone counseling and contacts for parents, send brochures, translate articles, write a quarterly newsletter, organize conferences, and mediate the buying, selling, or renting of strollers.

Free Baby Products

Several corporations that manufacture diapers and other baby products will give free selections to families of higher multiples.

Although some families have found certain companies to be very generous, usually the gifts don't last long. In 1989, some examples were the following: Kimberly-Clark gave Huggies coupons worth $10. Procter and Gamble sent three large cases of Pampers or Loves. Gerber provided sample foods and spoons worth about $10. Johnson & Johnson offered large sizes of their products, worth about $25, and sent gift packs. Evenflo provided a gift pack, Newborne Co. sent three bibs, and Carter's provided some baby clothes. Wyeth, Mead Johnson, and Ross Laboratories sent formula. Monterey Laboratories offered three Infafeeders, Ross Laboratories sent a gift pack, International Playtex provided nursing products, and Beech-Nut Foods sent coupons and free baby food. Dundee Mills offered clothing, sheets,

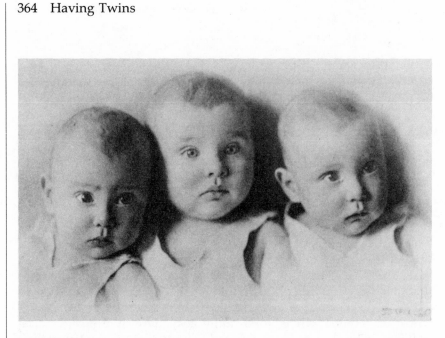

Age 8 months

The Narva triplets have been a happy trio since birth. (Each newborn baby weighed over 6 pounds.) The triplets continue to meet monthly for a TLC Club luncheon. God chose the members of this special group who share "tender loving care."

and blankets. Lehn and Fink Products and Glenbrook Laboratories offered baby wipes. In addition, Twin Services in Berkeley, California, has free used infant and children's clothing for anyone in need. For families with quadruplets and higher multiples, Gerber supplies all the baby food free of charge. Addresses are listed in the Resources; address your inquiries to the Consumer Service Director or Public Relations Department.

The Joy of Supertwins

Most passers-by are speechless at the sight of three or more babies or may make comments like "You poor woman" or "I certainly don't envy you." Kathie Nogushi relates how one little girl came up and asked if all the babies were hers. On learning that they were, she rushed back to her mother and exclaimed, "Oh Mommy, that woman has three babies — isn't she lucky!"

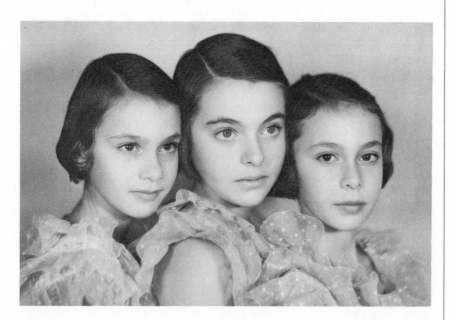

Age 17

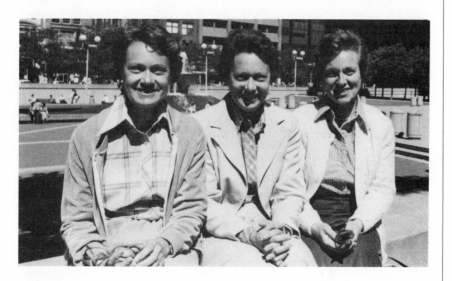

Age 54

Our triplets are wonderful. They have been a great experience and joy. Luckily, they are happy and healthy — and we love them all.

One mother had triplets after a stillbirth and two miscarriages and felt that God had given her back all that she had lost. Another woman had triplets first and then quads. In both pregnancies she gained 42 pounds and both sets of multiples went to thirty-eight weeks. However, she gained 20 pounds before conceiving the quads and lost the total 62 pounds by six weeks postpartum. The triplets weighed 6 pounds; 5 pounds, 9 ounces; and 5 pounds. The quads weighed 6 pounds, 1 ounce; 5 pounds, 10 ounces; 5 pounds, 8 ounces; and 5 pounds, 1 ounce. The mother had no problems during pregnancy; she was always able to get in and out of bed by herself and could walk a little right to the end. She attributes her good outcome to encouragement and support, a positive attitude, good food, rest, an air bed, and confidence in her doctor. This mother breast-fed all her children but limited nursing the quads to a few weeks because she felt she needed to use her energy for her other five children! If they had been her first pregnancy, she would have breast-fed them for much longer, she said.

Expectant parents need to remember, as they read about all the risks and possible complications, that it is certainly possible to carry triplets and quadruplets to term and deliver healthy babies of good birth weight. Look for mothers who have done so, and maintain contact with them during your pregnancy for inspiration. Birth, like life, means risks, and the best you can do is to be well informed and choose the path of action that feels right for you.

Appendices

Glossary

Resources for Multiple Pregnancy

Bibliography and Suggested Reading

Resources

Index

Appendix 1
The Pregnant Patient's Rights and Responsibilities

The Pregnant Patient's Bill of Rights

American parents are becoming increasingly aware that well-intentioned health professionals do not always have scientific data to support common American obstetrical practices and that many of these practices are carried out primarily because they are part of medical and hospital tradition. In the last forty years many artificial practices have been introduced which have changed childbirth from a physiological event to a very complicated medical procedure in which all kinds of drugs are used and procedures carried out, sometimes unnecessarily, and many of them potentially damaging for the baby and even for the mother. A growing body of research makes it alarmingly clear that every aspect of traditional American hospital care during labor and delivery must now be questioned as to its possible effect on the future well-being of both the obstetric patient and her unborn child.

One in every 35 children born in the United States today will eventually be diagnosed as retarded; in 75% of these cases there is no familial or genetic predisposing factor. One in every 10 to 17 children has been found to have some form of brain dysfunction or learning disability requiring special treatment. Such statistics are not confined to the lower socioeconomic group but cut across all segments of American society.

New concerns are being raised by childbearing women because no one knows what degree oxygen depletion, head compression, or traction by forceps the unborn or newborn infant can tolerate before that child sustains permanent brain damage or dysfunction. The recent findings regarding the cancer-related drug diethylstilbestrol have alerted the public to the fact that neither the approval of a drug by the U.S. Food and Drug Administration nor the fact that a drug is prescribed by a physician serves as a guarantee that a drug or medication is safe for the mother or her unborn child. In fact, the American Academy of Pediatrics' Committee on Drugs has recently stated that there is no drug, whether prescription or over-the-counter remedy, which has been proven safe for the unborn child.

Prepared by Doris Haire, Chairperson of Committee on Health Law and Regulations, International Childbirth Education Association, Inc. Reprinted by permission of Doris Haire.

The Pregnant Patient has the right to participate in decisions involving her well-being and that of her unborn child, unless there is a clear-cut medical emergency that prevents her participation. In addition to the rights set forth in the American Hospital Association's "Patient's Bill of Rights" (which has also been adopted by the New York City Department of Health), the Pregnant Patient, because she represents *two* patients rather than one, should be recognized as having the additional rights listed below.

The Pregnant Patient's Rights

1. The Pregnant Patient has the right, prior to the administration of any drug or procedure, to be informed by the health professional caring for her of any potential direct or indirect effects, risks, or hazards to herself or her unborn or newborn infant which may result from the use of a drug or procedure prescribed for or administered to her during pregnancy, labor, birth, or lactation.

2. The Pregnant Patient has the right, prior to the proposed therapy, to be informed not only of the benefits, risks and hazards of the proposed therapy but also of known alternative therapy, such as available childbirth education classes which could help to prepare the Pregnant Patient physically and mentally to cope with the discomfort or stress of pregnancy and the experience of childbirth, thereby reducing or eliminating her need for drugs and obstetric intervention. She should be offered such information early in her pregnancy in order that she may make a reasoned decision.

3. The Pregnant Patient has the right, prior to the administration of any drug, to be informed by the health professional who is prescribing or administering the drug to her that any drug which she receives during pregnancy, labor, and birth, no matter how or when the drug is taken or administered, may adversely affect her unborn baby, directly or indirectly, and that there is no drug or chemical which has been proven safe for the unborn child.

4. The Pregnant Patient has the right, if Caesarean birth is anticipated, to be informed prior to the administration of any drug, and preferably prior to her hospitalization, that minimizing her and, in turn, her baby's intake of nonessential preoperative medicine will benefit her baby.

5. The Pregnant Patient has the right, prior to the administration of a drug or procedure, to be informed of the areas of uncertainty if there is *no* properly controlled follow-up research which has established the safety of the drug or procedure with regard to its direct and/or indirect effects on the physiological, mental, and neurological development of the child exposed, via the mother, to the drug or proce-

dure during pregnancy, labor, birth, or lactation (this would apply to virtually all drugs and the majority of obstetric procedures).

6. The Pregnant Patient has the right, prior to the administration of any drug, to be informed of the brand name and generic name of the drug in order that she may advise the health professional of any past adverse reaction to the drug.

7. The Pregnant Patient has the right to determine for herself, without pressure from her attendant, whether she will accept the risks inherent in the proposed therapy or refuse a drug or procedure.

8. The Pregnant Patient has the right to know the name and qualifications of the individual administering a medication or procedure to her during labor or birth.

9. The Pregnant Patient has the right to be informed, prior to the administration of any procedure, whether that procedure is being administered to her for her or her baby's benefit (medically indicated) or as an elective procedure (for convenience, teaching purposes, or research).

10. The Pregnant Patient has the right to be accompanied during the stress of labor and birth by someone she cares for and to whom she looks for emotional comfort and encouragement.

11. The Pregnant Patient has the right, after appropriate medical consultation, to choose a position for labor and for birth which is least stressful to her baby and to herself.

12. The Obstetric Patient has the right to have her baby cared for at her bedside if her baby is normal, and to feed her baby according to her baby's needs rather than according to the hospital regimen.

13. The Obstetric Patient has the right to be informed in writing of the name of the person who actually delivered her baby and the professional qualifications of that person. This information should also be on the birth certificate.

14. The Obstetric Patient has the right to be informed if there is any known or indicated aspect of her or her baby's care or condition which may cause her or her baby difficulty or problems.

15. The Obstetric Patient has the right to have her and her baby's hospital medical records complete, accurate, and legible and to have their records, including Nurses' Notes, retained by the hospital until the child reaches at least the age of majority or, alternatively, to have the records offered to her before they are destroyed.

16. The Obstetric Patient, both during and after her hospital stay, has the right to have access to her complete hospital medical records, including Nurses' Notes, and to receive a copy upon payment of a

reasonable fee and without incurring the expense of retaining an attorney.

It is the obstetric patient and her baby, not the health professional, who must sustain any trauma or injury resulting from the use of a drug or obstetric procedure. The observation of the rights listed above will not only permit the obstetric patient to participate in the decisions involving her and her baby's health care but will help to protect the health professional and the hospital against litigation arising from resentment or misunderstanding on the part of the mother.

The Pregnant Patient's Responsibilities

In addition to understanding her rights, the Pregnant Patient should also understand that she too has certain responsibilities. The Pregnant Patient's responsibilities include the following:

1. The Pregnant Patient is responsible for learning about the physical and psychological process of labor, birth, and postpartum recovery. The better informed expectant parents are, the better they will be able to participate in decisions concerning the planning of their care.

2. The Pregnant Patient is responsible for learning what comprises good prenatal and intranatal care and for making an effort to obtain the best care possible.

3. Expectant parents are responsible for knowing about those hospital policies and regulations which will affect their birth and postpartum experience.

4. The Pregnant Patient is responsible for arranging for a companion or support person (husband, mother, sister, friend, etc.) who will share in her plans for birth and who will accompany her during her labor and birth experience.

5. The Pregnant Patient is responsible for making her preferences known clearly to the health professionals involved in her case in a courteous and cooperative manner and for making mutually agreed-upon arrangements regarding maternity care alternatives with her physician and hospital in advance of labor.

6. Expectant parents are responsible for listening to their chosen physician or midwife with an open mind, just as they expect him or her to listen openly to them.

7. Once they have agreed to a course of health care, expectant parents are responsible, to the best of their ability, for seeing that the pro-

gram is carried out in consultation with others with whom they have made the agreement.

8. The Pregnant Patient is responsible for obtaining information in advance regarding the appoximate cost of her obstetric and hospital care.

9. The Pregnant Patient who intends to change her physician or hospital is responsible for notifying all concerned, well in advance of the birth if possible, and for informing both of her reasons for changing.

10. In all their interactions with medical and nursing personnel, the expectant parents should behave toward those caring for them with the same respect and consideration they themselves would like.

11. During the mother's hospital stay the mother is responsible for learning about her and her baby's continuing care after discharge from the hospital.

12. After birth, the parents should put into writing constructive comments and feelings of satisfaction and/or dissatisfaction with the care (nursing, medical, and personal) they received. Good service to families in the future will be facilitated by those parents who take the time and responsibility to write letters expressing their feelings about the maternity care they received.

All the previous statements assume a normal birth and postpartum experience. Expectant parents should realize that, if complications develop in their cases, there will be an increased need to trust the expertise of the physician and hospital staff they have chosen. However, if problems occur, the childbearing woman still retains her responsibility for making informed decisions about her care or treatment and that of her baby. If she is incapable of assuming that responsibility because of her physical condition, her previously authorized companion or support person should assume responsibility for making informed decisions on her behalf.

Appendix 2

Model for an Alternative Birth Experience of Twins in a Hospital

Marge and Jon Saphier, of Carlisle, Massachusetts, successfully pursued their own style of giving birth to twins. Here is Marge's explanation of how they did it. Other expectant couples may not have the same concerns, but the Saphiers' request letter serves as a useful checklist of options that should be available to those who are committed to natural childbirth.

On October 22, 1977, Graeme and Gregory were born to Jon and me at a Boston hospital. I would like to share with you the preparation that we did to ensure the occurrence of this beautiful birth experience.

I started preparation early for the hospital birth experience so I would have as much time as possible for my negotiations. I picked a hospital with which my obstetrician was affiliated and where he felt that Jon and I could have the birth experience we wanted. When I was five months pregnant, Jon and I went to the postpartum unit of the hospital to discuss with the nurses our desire that there be no separation of the babies from us if we were all healthy. Because twins are often born prematurely, I was very concerned about Jon's and my being involved in their care. As it turned out, all my requests regarding care of the premature baby were routine policy.

In my seventh month I wrote to my obstetrician, itemizing my requests for labor and delivery, and I wrote to my pediatrician with regard to the twins' care. Jon and I then set up appointments to discuss these requests with each doctor. Both my obstetrician and my pediatrician were enthusiastic from the beginning, but I put my requests in writing to be sure that I had communicated everything to them.

A local organization, Homebirth, Inc., and the book *Maternal-Infant Bonding* by Marshall Klaus, M.D., and John Kennell, M.D., were the main references I used to write the following letter to my obstetrician.

Dear Doctor:

I would like to explain to you what Jon and I want at the hospital during labor, delivery, and the immediate postpartum period. Jon and I feel strongly that maternal/paternal-infant bonding during the immediate postpartum period will enhance the relationship between our babies and

Reprinted with permission from the Children in Hospitals, Inc., *Newsletter*, Winter 1978.

ourselves as it develops over the years. We feel the bonding will be facilitated if there is as little medical intervention as possible during labor and delivery so that there will be fewer distractions for Jon and me, enabling us to focus our attention more readily on our babies. Let me say that Jon and I are not naive and that we are well aware of the complications of twin births. We trust your medical judgment and feel confident that you will support our requests as long as they are medically feasible. Our requests include those for a "normal" birth and those for one with complications.

In this letter I include my requests to the pediatrician so that you will have an overall picture of what we want.

Requests in the Event of a Normal Birth

1. To have Jon present throughout the labor, delivery, and immediate postpartum period.

2. To have my birth attendant with me throughout the birth.

3. To go to the hospital at the beginning of active labor.

4. To have you as the only doctor attending me during labor and delivery unless, for medical reasons, you decide to call in another obstetrician. This physician should be aware of and in agreement with Jon's and my wishes. We would also like the attending nurses to be supportive of our requests.

5. To have no interns or residents observing the birth, so that a quiet, intimate atmosphere can be maintained.

6. To have no routine prep (shaving and enema).

7. To have no sedatives, tranquilizers, pain medication, or anesthesia.

8. To have no routine stimulants to start or speed up labor.

9. To have no routine rupture of the membranes.

10. To have no routine intravenous.

11. To have no routine electronic fetal-heart monitoring.

12. To bring and use during labor: our own pillows; lollipops to suck for energy; ice chips or damp washcloths to quench my thirst; a hot water bottle to relieve back pain during labor; and chamomile tea to make compresses to relax my perineum while the baby is crowning.

13. To wear my own bedclothes during labor and delivery.

14. To be free to walk around during labor — no routine confinement to bed and/or the labor room.

15. To be taken to the delivery room before "the last minute," if possible. It is also important to me to continue labor and delivery *in bed*, not on the table.

16. To have the option to modify delivery positions; for example, not to use stirrups or cuffs; to deliver on my side, on hands and knees, squatting, or in whatever position feels best at the time. I realize that in the case of a breech birth you may prefer me to be in the traditional supine position on the delivery table. If this is necessary, I prefer no stirrups and no handcuffs.

17. To have the lights in the room dimmed and the temperature warm.

18. To avoid a routine episiotomy. Instead, for you to judge during the crowning of the baby's head whether that is necessary and to use massage, hot compresses, and alternative positions to facilitate the stretching of the perineum.

19. To delay cutting of the cord to allow the baby to obtain the maximum blood before the cord stops pulsating.

20. To use local anesthetic for the episiotomy repair.

21. If possible, to have Jon receive the first baby immediately after s/he is born. We do not want the baby to be put in a warmer. Likewise, Jon or I should receive the second baby. If possible, I would like to nurse one or both immediately.

22. To allow adequate time for the placenta — no routine pitocin stimulant or manual removal.

23. To have no routine separation of either mother or father from the babies any time following the birth.

24. After the birth of both twins, to have the delivery room cleared of all but those people essential for observation of vital signs, so that Jon and I may have a quiet period together with our babies.

25. To have early discharge for the three of us, barring complications, six to twelve hours after delivery, as I feel I can rest better at home. If you are concerned about my getting adequate rest at home, I am more than willing to discuss with you the arrangements I have made to ensure that I will get enough rest.

Requests in the Event of Complications During Labor and Delivery

1. For the obstetrician to meet the above requests if medically feasible.

2. If I should have to have a Caesarean birth, to have Jon present so that he can hold the babies, to begin the bonding process.

3. To have Genevieve, our 3½-year-old daughter, visit me daily in my room if I stay longer than twenty-four hours. This is very important to me.

4. To have a private room.

Requests to the Pediatrician with regard to the Care of the Babies under Normal Circumstances

1. To have Jon catch the first baby, if possible, or to hold the first baby immediately after s/he is born. Neither baby is to be put in a warmer.

2. To have no routine separation of the babies from Jon and me.

3. To have an early pediatric examination so that we all may be discharged six to twelve hours after the delivery.

4. To have no bathing to remove the vernix from the babies' skin.

5. To have no silver nitrate drops administered to the babies' eyes until three hours after delivery. We would prefer a less irritating medication, such as Ilotycin.

6. If feasible, to nurse the babies on the delivery table, or soon thereafter.

7. To have only essential medical staff present during the birth and to have them be supportive of our requests.

8. To have all but essential medical staff leave after the birth of both babies and to have the lights dimmed so that Jon and I can enjoy our babies without distractions. Ideally, essential medical staff would consist of one or two people.

9. To have our babies wear clothing that we bring from home.

Requests to the Pediatrician if One or Both Babies Require Care in the Neonatal Intensive Care Unit

1. To be able to hold the babies, if medically feasible, or at least touch them, before they go to the NICU.

2. To have unlimited visiting privileges at the NICU for Jon and me.

3. To be able to touch and care for the babies as much as possible.

4. To allow our daughter Genevieve, aged 3½, to see the babies by looking through the window, if we decide this is desirable.

5. To have the babies receive breast milk that I pump for them and to nurse as soon as they are able. My strong feelings about this are based on a study by Barbara Barlow, M.D., and on "Acute Necrotizing Enterocolitis."

6. If one or both babies are well enough to be with me — twenty-four hour rooming-in.

7. The baby that is well should receive only breast milk and should be fed according to demand, not schedule.

8. If one baby is in the NICU, the other baby and myself should be on the same floor as the NICU.

9. To have both babies discharged at the same time unless one is considerably sicker than the other.

10. If the twins are ill, to call in our private pediatrician for a consulting opinion.

Thank you for taking the time to review these requests and for discussing them with Jon and me.
Sincerely,

It needs to be stressed that I was directed to my supportive obstetrician by Homebirth, Inc., and we got to know the doctor well, so I felt assured he would support our requests if feasible. I made sure I wrote in the letter that I trusted his medical judgment and that I was well aware of the complications of twin births. He felt reassured by that, but he knew that we expected to have everything (why, what, and how) explained if intervention proved necessary. The pediatrician facilitated our request for the care of the babies. I met him only once, but his enthusiasm for what Jon and I requested was overwhelming and reassuring. He was not convinced of the advisability of withholding silver nitrate drops for three hours until I quoted Drs. Klaus and Kennell in *Maternal-Infant Bonding*. I highly recommend being familiar with references to support requests, because this gives added clout.

I did not ask the physicians to co-sign my requests and place them in my chart as orders because I felt confident that they would abide by my requests, but we did a few things to ensure this. When I was admitted to the hospital, I had to sign a consent form that covers any need for a Caesarean. I noted on the form that I would have to be consulted before any medical intervention was introduced other than a normal vaginal delivery. (With twins, when membranes rupture prior to labor, as mine did, the incidence of Caesarean birth increases.)

Graeme and Gregory did not come prematurely. They came at forty-one weeks, weighing 8 pounds and 8 pounds, 9 ounces. The babies were born vaginally, with no medication or intervention. The medical staff — one nurse, one obstetrician, and one pediatric resident — rejoiced with us in our very quiet, intimate birth.

The steps I took to ensure our positive natural birth experience were:

1. Early preparation.

2. Location of a supportive obstetrician, pediatrician, and hospital.

3. Written requests, with footnotes citing supportive medical literature, and use of the word "routine" to give the doctors the option to use these procedures if medically necessary.

4. Review of our requests with each doctor at his office and providing background information about Jon and me that supported a request. This enabled any differences and questions to be ironed out. Our private pediatrician was also included as he was to be available as a consultant.

5. Having a birth attendant who knew our requests and who was familiar with the birthing process present at the birth to remind us and, when appropriate, to remind the medical staff of our request. This proved to be of great importance since Jon and I were working hard on the labor and it was easy to miss what was happening around us. Our birth attendant would tell us and ask, "Is this what you want?" If it was not, Jon directed the staff accordingly.

Appendix 3

Plans for Parents and Hospital Personnel in the Event of Loss

Parents' Action Plan in the Event of Loss

1. I/we would like to hold the baby/ies for as long as I/we wish and as often as I/we wish.

   It is now well accepted that parents need to see and hold their baby in the event of a death, unlike some years ago when well-meaning professionals thought they were "sparing" the parents by whisking a baby away unseen. When one member of a multiple set dies, it is even more important to see the baby in order that a concrete reality may be grieved and to resolve this grief alongside the presence of the living twin/s.

2. I/we would like _____ (siblings, relatives) also to see/hold the baby/ies as often as I/we wish.

   Reality is never as grim as fantasy, and death can be comprehended by small children and provides important closure. It is important for family and friends to see that this person had a body and an existence.

3. I/we want to name the infant/s _____.

   Naming the infant(s) provides identity and by acknowledging the reality of that existence makes it much easier to talk about him/her/them later on and reduces the illusory aspects of the experience. If a particular name has been chosen for the infant(s), experts recommend that it still be used in the event of death. Reserving it for the next baby may confuse that baby's identity and s/he may feel that s/he has to walk in the shoes of the deceased sibling.

4. The following mementos would be especially significant for us to keep:

   For example, lock of hair; footprints; photographs,* regardless of condition, of the baby who died, including photograph of the baby washed and dressed; photographs of both babies together; ultrasound scan or x-ray; crib blanket; medical record; birth certificate; fetal monitor tracing; identification bracelet; cord clamp.

* Have a friend or relative take good-quality photos. Hospital Polaroids — often the only photos the parents may have — can be disappointing.

5. I/we would/would not like to have a baptism.

6. I/we would like details about zygosity.

   This is important for medical and genetic reasons as well as natural parent curiosity (and that of the surviving twin) to know as much as possible about the offspring.

7. I/we would like to know the cause of death if it can be determined.

8. I/we do/do not wish to have an autopsy.

9. I/we would like to have a burial/cremation/ or to donate the body/ies.

   For example, if a baby is less than 20 weeks or 500 grams (approximately a pound) and you do not express your wishes, the hospital will dispose of the body after sending it to the pathology department. A grave is an important symbol and an act of closure for the bereaved. Otherwise the dead baby is experienced like someone missing in action. Psychiatrist Emanuel Lewis at the Tavistock Clinic in England points out the existence of the Tomb of the Unknown Soldier is likewise an important symbol. However, a common grave is vague and confusing to the siblings, who can benefit from attending a burial. An open casket (which requires embalming) allows all who attend the funeral to register the actual existence of the baby. When this has not been done, mothers have regretted the ethereal nature of the loss. Some may combine a memorial service with the christening or baptism ceremony for the other twin.

10. I/we would like to notify _____ of the death by the following means _____.

    Make a list of the people whom you would like to notify immediately for support while you are in the hospital. When one twin has died, the timing of birth and death announcements may be awkward. Some couples send them out together or write a joint announcement.

11. I do not want general anesthesia in the case of a baby who dies before birth.

    Well-intentioned doctors may believe that knocking out the mother "spares" her the experience of delivery. However, the "nothingness" quality that may accompany the birth of a baby (or babies) who dies before or during labor is accentuated if anesthesia is used, making it difficult for the mother to perceive the event concretely and grieve for an actual person. Death also causes confusion in the staff, who may be overwhelmed. Stand up for your rights — the baby belongs to you, not the hospital — and you will never regret having done so.

12. I wish to cancel a tubal ligation (if one was planned).

Guidelines for Hospital Personnel in the Event of Loss

Emanuel Lewis has written extensively on the subject of infant death. He observed that death in obstetric situations tends to "de-skill" hospital staff. Personnel often are unable to overcome their own reactions to the stillbirth and suppress their feelings of failure and grief. Thus, professional staff tend to avoid discussion of the loss that would be entailed by listening and supporting the parents. (It is unfortunate that there are so few efforts to provide healing for healers, such as staff mutual support groups and private rooms for expression of feelings that mount up in a highly charged environment.) Much of the following guidelines are based on Lewis's advice.

1. Do not ask a mother/father if they want to see the baby. This unintentionally communicates the concept that they have created something that they possibly cannot bear to look at. Numerous studies have shown that mothers imagine that their baby's deformities and condition to be far worse than they actually are. Rather than regretting having seen and held their baby, parents usually deeply grieve the lost opportunity to do so.

   The dead baby should be handed to the mother and/or father, wrapped, and later dressed, appropriately. Staff can help by discussing the appearance and characteristics of the baby and referring to the baby by name, thus making the birth and death real so that parents can more easily mourn the loss they are experiencing. Substantiation of these monumental life events by others is a big help. The baby should be available to the whole family throughout the mother's hospital stay as often as they wish.

   Expect mothers and fathers to mourn the death differently and counsel them with regard to these differences. In general, mothers prefer other people to open a conversation with them about the baby who died. Depressed fathers, on the other hand, may also feel this way but worry that people do not like to discuss death. Fathers usually feel compelled to suppress their feelings in order to give the mother support. Personal sadness and individual reactions to the loss may make it difficult for spouses to be mutually helpful.

2. If the mother or father cannot hold the baby until she dies, reassure them that one of the staff will. Sometimes a baby is critically ill and not expected to live more than a few hours. Remember that handing their baby back to the nurse is the hardest thing parents may ever have to do, so receive the infant with great sensitivity.

3. Never attempt to reassure the mother that she was lucky to have one live twin, or another healthy baby, or not to have a disabled baby, or to have avoided more than she could handle, or present other rationalizations of the tragedy. Even if the dead baby had severe abnormalities, Lewis points out, "her dead baby will always be im-

portant to her, and she will never forgive you, even though she may have had similar thoughts herself." Well-meaning health professionals, like others, often underestimate the grief and loss felt by parents of multiples.

4. Do not separate the parents. This may imply that women are stronger or that a father's grieving is less significant.

5. Ask the mother her wishes with regard to a private hospital room. Sometimes it is better not to make any arrangements which may reinforce feelings of guilt or isolation or lead to feelings that others need to be protected from feeling upset over the loss. At least provide an appropriate place for private time with family members.

6. Help the parents deal with practical events. Guide bereaved parents through their haze to make whatever decisions are necessary, such as the details of burial. Help them get in touch with a grief support network. Sit down, offer parents a cup of tea or coffee, and give them your undivided attention. Avoid talking over an incubator because you may give the impression that there are more important things to do than to listen to the mother's fears and worries. It would be expedient to have a copy of Appendix 3, Part 1, "Parents' Action Plan in the Event of Loss," in all maternity units.

7. Do not direct the mother to focus on the living infant or infants. Instead help the mother integrate the duality of her birth/death experience. Recall details of the birth before they are forgotten, to acknowledge not only the existence of the dead twin but also the need to grieve. At the same time, the mother needs to bond with the living infant(s). Multiples that are separated from mothers as a result of Caesarean section run a greater risk of rejection, especially if there are problems with the baby/ies.

8. Answer questions clearly, simply, gently, and, above all, truthfully. Do not answer a question with another question. There is nothing that anyone can say or do that will take away the loss. Instead of advice, opinions, and comments, simply listen and affirm the feelings that are expressed and ask what you can do.

Glossary

amnion: The inner sac enclosing the fetus within the uterus. Also called *amniotic sac*. See also *chorion*.

anemia: A condition in which the blood contains a reduced number of red blood cells.

breech extraction: Manual assistance by the doctor when delivery is not spontaneous.

breech presentation: See *presentation*.

Braxton-Hicks contractions: Normal, irregular contractions of pregnancy.

Caesarean section: Surgical delivery of the baby through an incision in the abdominal and uterine walls.

cervical dilation: The opening of the cervix during labor (measured in centimeters; 10 centimeters is fully dilated).

cervical effacement: Thinning of the cervix before and during labor (measured in percentage).

cervical incompetence: Premature opening of the cervix, generally in the second trimester.

chorion: The outer sac enclosing the fetus within the uterus.

cord prolapse: A rare emergency that occurs when the umbilical cord drops out of the uterus into the vagina before the baby, leading to cord compression and oxygen deprivation by the after-coming head.

dichorionic: Having two chorions. See *chorion*.

dilation: See *cervical dilation*.

dizygotic: Referring to twins who result from the union of two eggs and two sperm. Also called *binovular*.

Down's syndrome: A genetic disorder (trisomy 21) that results in physical anomalies and mental retardation.

ectopic pregnancy: A pregnancy that grows outside the uterus, usually in the Fallopian tube.

epidural: A regional anesthetic administered during labor around the nerve roots outside the spinal cord. Also see *spinal anesthetic*.

episiotomy: An incision made in the vaginal opening for birth.

external version: A procedure in which the doctor turns the baby or babies in the uterus by applying manual pressure in the vagina or on the outside of the mother's abdomen.

fraternal twins: See *dizygotic*.

fundus: Body of the uterus. Fundal height (the distance from the pubic bone to the top of the uterus) is measured at prenatal visits.

hydramnios: See *polyhydramnios*.

hypertension: High blood pressure. See *pregnancy-induced hypertension*.

hypoglycemia: An abnormally low level of sugar in the blood.

identical twins: See *monozygotic*.

internal version: A procedure in which the doctor manually brings the feet of the second baby down to perform a breech extraction. See also *presentation*.

in vitro fertilization (IVF): Union of egg and sperm in a glass dish in a laboratory.

let-down reflex: Hormonal release of milk stored in the breasts.

membranes: The sacs that enclose the fetus in the uterus. See *chorion* and *amnion*.

monochorionic: Having one chorion. See *chorion*.

monozygotic: Referring to twins who result from the union of one egg and one sperm that divides in two. Also called *monovular*.

palpation: Examination by touch.

perineum: The area between the vagina and the anus.

placenta: The structure formed in the wall of the uterus composed of maternal and fetal tissue through which nutrients and waste products are transferred between the mother's and the fetus's circulations.

placental abruption: Premature detachment of the placenta from the wall of the uterus.

placenta previa: A condition in which the placenta is attached low down on the uterine wall and partially or completely blocks the cervical opening.

polyhydramnios: An excess of amniotic fluid in the uterus. Also called *hydramnios*.

pregnancy-induced hypertension: A combination of high blood pressure, protein in the urine, and fluid retention, which causes swelling throughout the body. If the brain is involved in the swelling, convulsions can result. (Previously called toxemia.)

presentation: The part of the baby's body that is against the cervix at the time of labor and delivery. Possible presentations are *vertex* (headfirst); *breech* (lower part of the body first); *transverse lie* (baby's body across the mother's pelvis).

prolapsed cord: See *cord prolapse*.

proteinuria: Protein in the urine. See *pregnancy-induced hypertension*.

spinal anesthetic: A regional anesthetic administered into the spinal fluid surrounding the nerve roots. It is given at the end of the second stage of labor to facilitate an instrumental or Caesarean delivery. See also *epidural*.

superfecundation: The phenomenon whereby two eggs are released from the ovaries and are fertilized at two separate times.

superfetation: The phenomenon whereby two eggs are fertilized in two different menstrual cycles, resulting in marked difference in the weight of the twins at birth.

supertwins: Triplets, quadruplets, and other higher-order multiples.

toxemia: See *pregnancy-induced hypertension*.

transverse lie: See *presentation*.

twin transfusion syndrome: A rare condition in which one twin develops at the expense of the other when they share a monochorionic placenta.

ultrasound: Technology that uses sound waves to view the fetuses within the uterus (diagnostic use) or to treat muscles and ligaments (therapeutic use).

vanishing twin: The phenomenon in which one twin fails to develop beyond the first trimester.

vernix: The creamy white substance (made of layers of dead skin cells) that protects the baby's skin in the fluid-filled uterus.

vertex presentation: See *presentation*.

Organizations

You can help some of these individuals and organizations by filling out questionnaires about your multiples.

Organizations in the United States

Boklage, Charles E., Ph.D., Professor and Director, Genetics Program, East Carolina University School of Medicine, Greenville, NC 27858-4354. Research into the "third type of twin," using triplets.

Center for the Study of Multiple Birth, 333 E. Superior Street, Suite 476, Chicago, IL 60611.

Greer, Jane, Ph.D., twin consultant, 42–36 235th, Douglaston, NY 11363. (718) 423-9703.

Indiana University Twin Studies, Department of Medical Genetics, Riley Research 129, 702 Barhill Drive, Indianapolis, IN 46223. (317) 274-5743.

International Society for Twin Studies (ISTS), c/o Louisville Twin Study, Health Sciences Center, School of Medicine, University of Louisville, P.O. Box 35260, Louisville, KY 40292.

International Twins Association (ITA), c/o Judy Kirk and Julie Stillwagon, 114 N. Lafayette Drive, Muncie, IN 47303.

International Twins Foundation (ITF), P.O. Box 6043, Providence, RI 02904. (401) 274-8946.

"Miss Helen" Kirk (supertwin statistician), P.O. Box 254, Galveston, TX 77553. (409) 762-4792.

Louisville Twin Study, Child Development Unit, Health Sciences Center, School of Medicine, University of Louisville, P.O. Box 35260, Louisville, KY 40232. (502) 588-5184.

Minnesota Center for Twin and Adoption Research, University of Minnesota, Department of Psychology, 75 E. River Road, Minneapolis, MN 55455. (612) 625-4067. Minnesota Study of Twins Reared Apart, Minnesota Twin Registry, Twin Loss Project, Minnesota Adoption Project, Medical and Psychological Longitudinal Follow-up of Twins Reared Apart, new studies of twins and twin relationships.

National Organization of Mothers of Twins Clubs, Inc. (NOMOTC), 12404 Princess Jeane, N.E. Albuquerque, NM 87112-4640. (505) 275-0955.

Single Triplet Moms Network, Linda Willis, 408 Holden Avenue, Lafayette, LA 70506, (318) 235-7697; Diana Vincelli, 809 Westover Hills Blvd., Richmond VA 23225, (804) 233-0099.

Triplet Connection, P.O. Box 99571, Stockton, CA 95209, (209) 474-3073/0885; Mary Kay Sainsbury, 590 Marigold Drive, Fairfield, CA 94533, (707) 427-2018. Triplet research.

Twin Services, P.O. Box 10066, Berkeley, CA 94709. (415) 524-0863. The Twinline, free counseling and referral service, Monday–Friday, 10 A.M.–4 P.M., Pacific time. (After October 7, 1991, the area code will change to 510.) Services and publications for parents of twins and triplets on pregnancy, care, development, disabilities, and loss. A network of resources and training for health and family service providers and self-help organizations.

Twins Day Committee, 10075 Ravenna Road, Twinsburg, OH 44087. (216) 425-7161.

The Twins Foundation, P.O. Box 9487, Providence, RI 02940-9487. (401) 274-8946.

Vietnam Experience Twin Study, Dr. Seth Eisen, VA Medical Center, 151 A-JB, St. Louis, MO 63125.

Organizations Abroad

ABC Club, International Society for Families with Triplets and Higher Multiples in German-language countries, c/o Helga Grützner, Strohweg 55, D-6100 Darmstadt, West Germany, 6151 59 58 57.

Association d'Entraide des Parents de Naissances Multiples (ANEPNM), 8 Place Alfred Sisley, 95430 Auvers sur Oise, France (16-1) 30-36 29 67.

Australian Multiple Birth Association, Inc. (AMBA), P.O. Box 105, Coogee, NSW 2034 Australia.

Australian National Twin Registry, 151 Barry Street, Carlton 3054, Victoria, Australia.

Combined Organization of Multiple Birth Organizations (COMBA), c/o Judi Linney, 27 Woodham Park Road, Woodham, Weybridge, Surrey, UK.

Disabled Multiples Parent Registry, Parents of Multiple Births Association (POMBA), P.O. Box 2200, Lethbridge, Alberta, Canada T1J 4K7. (403) 381-6868.

European Multiple Birth Study (EMBS), c/o R. Vlietinck, Centre of Human Genetics, Catholic University of Leuven, Heurestraat 49, B-3000 Leuven, Belgium.

Gregor Mendel Institute of Medical Genetics and Twin Studies, Piazza Galeno 5, 00161 Rome, Italy.

Japanese Association of Twins' Mothers, c/o Hukiko Amua, 5-20 Minami Aoyama, Minatoku, Tokyo, Japan.

LaTrobe Twin Study, c/o David Hay, Department of Psychology, LaTrobe University, Bundoora, Victoria 3083, Australia. The program offers a series of information leaflets. Support is provided only to families involved in LaTrobe's research because of limited staff time. Consult the Australian Multiple Birth Association (AMBA) instead. Lone Twin Register at same address.

Multiple Births Foundation, c/o Dr. Elizabeth Bryan, Queen Charlotte and Chelsea Hospital, Goldhawk Road, London W60X G. (01) 748 4666, ext. 5201. Lone Twin Register at same address.

New Zealand Multiple Birth Association, Lee Thornburn, 29 Nelson Street, Greymouth, New Zealand.

Parents of Multiple Births Association (POMBA), P.O. Box 2200, Lethbridge, Alberta, Canada T1J 4K7. (403) 381-6868.

South African Multiple Birth Association (SAMBA), P.O. Box 72260, Lynwood Ridge 0040, Republic of South Africa.

TAMBA Triplets and Higher Multiples, c/o Wendy Varley, 95 Calvert Road, Greenwich, London SE10 0DG, England.

Twins Foundation "Nakula-Sadewa," c/o Seto Mulyadi.Jl. Teuku Cik Ditiro 32, Jakarta 10310, Indonesia. (021) 769-4299, 310-6177.

Twins and Multiple Births Association (TAMBA); TAMBA groups for Supertwins, Bereavement Support and Special Needs, Adopted Twins, Single Parent Families, 41 Fortuna Way, Aylesby Park, Grimsby, South Humberside DN37 9SJ England; 1 Victoria Place, Stirling FK8 2QX, Scotland, UK.

UK National Study of Triplet and Higher Order Births, National Perinatal Epidemiology Unit, Radcliffe Infirmary, Oxford 0X2 6HE, UK.

Volunteer Twin Register, Alison McDonald, Room 147, Institute of Psychiatry, De Cresigny Paris, London SE5 8AF, England. Study of the contribution of genes and environment in mental and physical health.

General Resources

American Academy of Pediatrics, Public Education Division, Box 1034, 1801 Hinman Avenue, Evanston, IL 60204.

American Adoption Congress, Cherkoee Station, P.O. Box 20137, New York, NY 10028-0051. For open records in adoption.

American College of Nurse-Midwives, 1522 K Street, NW, Suite 1120, Washington, DC 20005.

American College of Obstetricians and Gynecologists, 409 12th Street, SW, Washington, DC 20024-2188.

American Gentle Birthing Association, Robert Doughton, M.D., 1804 SW Oak Knoll Court, Lake Oswego, OR 97034. (503) 636-7823.

Association for the Care of Children's Health (ACCH), 3615 Wisconsin Avenue, NW, Washington, DC 20016. (202) 244-8922.

AuPair in America, American Institute of Foreign Study, Dept. P-2, 102 Greenwich Avenue, Greenwich, CT 06830. (800) 727-2437. Live-in child care.

AuPair–Homestay USA: The Experiment in International Living, 114 K Street, NW, Suite 1100, Washington, DC 20005.

Cesarean Prevention Movement, P.O. Box 152, Syracuse, NY 13210. (315) 424-1942.

Cheek, David, M.D., Santa Barbara, California. (805) 569-7161. Retired obstetrician offering free telephone hypnosis to expectant mothers with preterm labor contractions, pregnancy-induced hypertension, and other prenatal complications.

Consumer Product Safety Commission, Washington, DC 20207. (800) 638-2772; (800) 628-8326 in Maryland and Alaska; (800) 492-8363 in Hawaii.

Division of the Food and Nutrition Service, USDA, 3010 Park Center Drive, Alexandria, VA 22303. (703) 756-3730. Supplemental food programs.

DPT: Dissatisfied Parents Together, Box 563, 1377 K Street, NW, Washington, DC 20005. Immunization victims.

EF AuPair, EF Foundation, One Memorial Drive, Cambridge, MA 02142. (800) 333-6506.

EurAuPair, 250 North Coast Highway, Laguna Beach, CA 92651. (800) 333-3804.

Infant Stimulation Education Association (ISEA), Susan Luddington-Hoe, Ph.D., Director, UCLA Medical Center, Factor 5-942, Los Angeles, CA 90024.

International Association of Infant Massage Instructors, P.O. Box 298, Peck Slip Station, New York, NY 10272.

International Primal Association (IPA), 2742 Fernwood Avenue, Roslyn, PA 19001. (215) 887-9168.

International Society for Prenatal and Perinatal Psychology and Medicine (ISPPM), Peter Fedor-Freybergh, M.D., Ph.D., Engelbrektsgatan 19, S-11432, Stockholm, Sweden.

Klaus, Phyllis H., Berkeley, California. (415) 528-1525. Marriage, family, and child counselor offering telephone counseling and hypnosis to expectant mothers with preterm labor contractions, pregnancy-induced hypertension, and other prenatal complications.

Maternal and Child Health Center, 2464 Massachusetts Avenue, Cambridge, MA 02140. Founded by Elizabeth Noble, specializes in educational and therapeutic programs for childbearing families.

National Maternal and Child Health Clearinghouse, 38th and R Streets, NW, Washington, DC 20057. Publishes a directory of voluntary and professional organizations in *Maternal and Child Health* (Publication #G-30) and *Starting Early: A Guide to Federal Resources in Maternal and Child Health* (Publication #H-100).

National Organization of Circumcision Information Resource Centers (No-Circ), P.O. Box 2512, San Anselmo, CA 94960.

National Passenger Safety Association, 1050 17th Street, NW, Suite 770, Washington, DC 20036. Information about infant car seats.

National Society of Genetic Counselors, 233 Canterbury Drive, Wallingford, PA 19586. (215) 872-7608.

Northrup, Christiane, M.D., Women-to-Women, 1 Pleasant Street, Yarmouth, ME 04096. (207) 846-6163. Gynecologist specializing in holistic health, with emphasis on nutrition.

Obstetrics and Gynecology Section, American Physical Therapy Association, 111 North Fairfax, Alexandria, VA 22314. Referrals to physical therapists who specialize in obstetrics and gynecology.

Parents Anonymous, 2230 Hawthorne Boulevard, Suite 208, Torrance, CA 90505. (800) 421-0353 (hot line). National agency with state and local chapters providing assistance for stressed parents to avoid abusive behavior.

Parents Without Partners, Inc. (PWP), 7910 Woodmont Avenue, Bethesda, MD 20814. (800) 638-8078. Social and educational network for single parents through divorce, death, choice.

Peterson, Gayle, Ph.D., 1749 Vine Street, Berkeley, CA 94703. (415) 527-6216. Social worker offering individual therapy and professional training in body-centered hypnosis for preterm labor and other pregnancy complications. Phone consultation available.

Pre and Perinatal Psychology Association of North America (PPPANA), 13 Summit Terrace, Dobbs Ferry, NY 10522.

Right Start Catalog, Right Start Plaza, 5334 Sterling Center Drive, Westlake Village, CA 91361. (800) LITTLE-1 (800 548-8531). Mail order catalog for innovative items including baby care acessories, childhood safety devices, and the "Tummy Rest" pregnancy pillow.

Vaginal Birth After Cesarean (VBAC), 10 Great Plain Terrace, Needham, MA 02191. For information packet, send $10 to Nancy Cohen at this address.

Zoll, Stuart, acupuncture physician and Vegatest instructor, Centre for Preventive Medicine, 7015 Bera Casa Way, Boca Raton, FL 33433.

Equipment

Baby RV, 209 S. Clark Drive, Beverly Hills, CA 90211. (213) 652-9021. Mobile "playpen" stroller.

Bulrey Lite Trailer holds two or three children when biking. Check your local bicycle store.

Bumkins, BNM, 1945 E. Watkins, Phoenix, AZ 85034. (800) 533-5302. Waterproof washable diapers.

Coop Bike Buddy Trailer, Recreational Equipment Inc., P.O. Box C-88125, Seattle, WA 98188.

Cuddle Carriers, 21 Potsdam Road, Unit 61, Downsview, Ontario M3N 1N3 Canada. (416) 663-7143.

DoubleTalk. Stocks baby carriers, strollers: McLaren Majestic, Royalty, and Brittany Double Strollers, Double Buggy, Jane Turista, and Barcelona Double Strollers. Also books; publishes a newsletter (see periodicals).

Gemini baby carrier, Tot Tenders, Inc., 30441 S. Highway 34, Suite 7A & B, Albany, OR 97321. (800) 634-6870.

The Glass Rainbow, 10022 Winzag, Cincinnati, OH 45242. Double rocker.

Home Health Products, Inc., 1160-A Millers Lane, Virginia Beach, VA 23451. (800) 284-9123. Natural health products including castor oil and wool flannel.

KidKuff, 5608 N. Roosevelt, Loveland, CO 80538. (303) 669-4568. Restraint system for two.

Kinder Carrier, Good Gear for Little People, Washington, ME 04574. Front attaching bike seat, for one on the back and one on front.

The National Baby Company, RD 1, Box 160S, Titusville, NJ 08560. Diaper covers of cotton and wool, diapers, cotton sleepwear, nursing bras.

Perego Twin and Triplet strollers available at greatly reduced cost from Janet Bleyl, 2618 Lucile Avenue, Stockton, CA 95209. (209) 474-3073.

Racing Strollers, Inc., 516 N. Bronx Avenue, Box 16, Yakima, WA 98902. (800) 548-7230. "Twinner" all-terrain stroller.

Rock-a-Crib Springs, N.K.R. Precision Manufacturing Corporation, P.O. Box 33, Harriman, NY 10926. A set of four springs to replace castors on cribs so that infants experience movement as they sleep. Parents can attach a string to the crib to rock one or more babies while taking care of another.

Runabout stroller/jogging cart with two seats, UNI-USA. (800) 832-2376.

Spurlin Distributors, Inc., 4694 Aviation Parkway, Suite L, Atlanta, GA 30349. (800) 235-0792. Manufactures a foam wedge support for the abdomen when the pregnant mother is lying on her side.

Stimobil, Pam Swing, 68 Chandler Street, Arlington, MA 02174.

Tricycle Built for Two, TwoHearts, 501 SE 2nd Street, Gainesville, FL 32601.

Twins Carriages, 5935 W. Irving Park Road, Chicago, IL 60634. (312) 794-CRIB.

Twice upon a Time, National Organization of Mothers of Twins Clubs (NOMOTC), 12404 Princess Jeane, N.E. Albuquerque, NM 87112-4640. (505) 275-0955. Magnetized wipe-off schedule board for twins.

Velcro Safety Strap by Ambassador. Three Velcro strips to keep doors closed on refrigerator, medicine cabinets, toilets.

Free Samples of Baby Products

Beechnut Food Corporation, P.O. Box 127, Fort Washington, PA 19034. (800) 523-6633. Baby foods.

Dundee Mills, Inc., Baby Products Division, 11 W. 40th Street, New York, NY 10018.

Evenflo, P.O. Box 1206, Ravenna, OH 44266. (800) 356-BABY. Nursing products.

Gerber, 445 State Street, Remont, MI 49412. (800) 4-GERBER. Baby foods.

Glenbrook Laboratories, Box 1750, Elm City, NC 17898.

Heinz. (800) USA-BABY. Baby foods.

Johnson & Johnson, 6 Commercial Street, Hicksville, NY 11801. (800) 526-3967.

Kimberly Clark, 2100 Winchester Road, Nunah, WI 54956. (800) 544-1847. Huggies disposable diapers.

Lehn and Fink Products, P.O. Box 1758, Clinton, IA 52734.

Mead and Johnson Co., 2404 Pennslanvia, Evansville, IN 47721. (812) 426-6000.

Monterey Laboratories, Inc., P.O. Box 15129, Las Vegas, NV 89114.

Playtex, 215 College, Paramus, NJ 07652. (800) 222-0453. Products for nursing mothers and babies.

Procter & Gamble, P.O. Box 599, Cincinnati, OH 452011. (800) 543-0480. Pampers, Luvs disposable diapers.

Ross Laboratories, 625 Cleveland Avenue, Columbus, OH 43216. (614) 227-3333. Formula.

Maternity Support Girdles and Hose

BabyHugger, Trennaventions, 909 4th Avenue, Suite 610, Seattle, WA 98104.

Glori-Us! Mary Jane Company, 5510 Cleon Avenue, North Hollywood, CA 91609.

Gottfried Medical, P.O. Box 8996, Toledo, OH 43623. (800) 537-1968/328-5216.

Jobst Support Hose, Box 653, Toledo, OH 43694. (800) 537-1063.

Loving Lift and Action Life, Moor Products, P.O. Box 647, Belmont, CA 94002.

Maternal Cradle, Merlin Medical Enterprise, P.O. Box 823, Corte Madera, CA 94925. Maternity support belt to reduce back pain.

Maternity Lumbo-Pelvic Support, IEM Orthopedics, P.O. Box 592, Ravenna, OH 44266.

Medi Support Hose, 76 W. Seegers Road, Arlington Heights, IL 60005. (800) 633-6334.

Warm'n Form. Jerome Medical, 102 Gaither Drive, Mt. Laurel, NJ 08054. (800) 257-8440.

Breast-Feeding Resources

Babe Too! Route 2, Box 3D, Inman, KS 67546. Clothing patterns designed for the breast-feeding mother.

International Lactation Consultants Association, P.O. Box 4031, University of Virgnia Station, Charlottesville, VA 22903. Certified consultants to help with breast-feeding.

Lactaid International, Inc., P.O. Box 1066, Athens, TN 37303. (800) 228-1933; (615) 744-9090. Nursing trainers for relactation.

La Leche League International (LLL), 9616 Minneapolis Avenue, Franklin Park, IL 60131. Breast-feeding information and support.

Medela, P.O. Box 386, Crystal Lake, IL 60014. (800) 435-8316. Breast pumps, nursing aids, video.

Motherwear, Box 114, Northampton, MA 01061. Catalog for the nursing mother.

Nursemate, Four Dee Products, Dept NN, 6014 Lattimer, Houston, TX 77035. (800) 526-2594; (713) 728-0389. Special pillow to "nurse twogether."

White River Breast Pump. (800) 824-6351. Rental pump with flexible flange.

Videos

BabyJoy. Exercises and activities for parents and infants, with Elizabeth Noble and Leo Sorger. Available from New Life Images, 448 Pleasant Lake Avenue, Harwich, MA 02645.

Channel for a New Life. Elizabeth Noble and Leo Sorger. Outdoor waterbirth of Carsten Noble Sorger. Available from New Life Images, 448 Pleasant Lake Avenue, Harwich, MA 02645.

Diary of Twin Development. National Organization of Mothers of Twins Clubs (NOMOTC), 12404 Princess Jeane, N.E. Albuquerque, NM 87112-4640. (505) 275-0955.

It's Twins! From Pregnancy to Birth. Bounty Service Videos, P.O. Box 3, Diss, Norfolk IP22 3HH, UK.

Polymorph Films, 118 South Street, Boston, MA 02111. Films about twins, premature infants, and newborn death.

The Twin Film. In progress with Greer and Associates, 905 Park, Minneapolis, MN 55404. (612) 338-6171. A documentary by identical twin producers Jill Greer and Judy Freeman that will include research on twins reared apart, Holocaust twin survivors, experience of twin loss, and the rearing of twins. Interviews with Thomas Bouchard, Ph.D., and Nancy Segal, Ph.D., of the Minnesota Center for Twin and Adoption Research.

Periodicals

Double Feature. Parents of Multiple Births Association (POMBA), P.O. Box 2200, Lethbridge, Alberta, Canada T1J 4K7. (403) 381-6868. Quarterly newsletter.

DoubleTalk. P.O. Box 412, Amelia, Ohio 45102. (513) 231-TWIN. Quarterly newsletter. Also stocks equipment (see Equipment).

MOTC Notebook. National Organization of Mothers of Twins Clubs (NOMOTC), 12404 Princess Jeane, N.E. Albuquerque, NM 87112-4640. (505) 275-0955.

Mothering magazine. P.O. Box 1690, Santa Fe, NM 87504. (800) 443-9637; (800) 354-8400 in California. Articles, poems, and resources for alternative parenting.

Twin Services Reporter. Twin Services, P.O. Box 10066, Berkeley, CA 94709. (415) 524-0863 (area code changes to 510 after October 1991). Quarterly newsletter included in membership.

Twins magazine. P.O. Box 12045, Overland Park, KS 66212. Bimonthly magazine.

Miscellaneous Resources

ABC Creations, 5101 East Keresan, Phoenix, AZ 85044. Clothing for premies, 1–6 pounds.

Birth and Life Bookstore, P.O. Box 70625, Seattle, WA 98107-0625. Mail order books and supplies.

Birth Samplers, 3937 West Good Hope Road, Milwaukee, WI 53209; 1813 E. Wood, Shorewood, WI 53211.

Mrs. R. A. Burger, 85 W. Shore Drive, Massapequa, NY 11758. Magnets.

Buttons, Carla Hall Pyeatt, 2709 Glenarbor, Santa Ana, CA 92704.

Cards by Sulti, P.O. Box 686, Slidell, LA 70459. (504) 649-4696.

Care Team Management Services, 911 Burnett, Wichita Falls, TX 76301. (817) 723-1601. Skilled nursing care at home for critically or chronically ill infants. Nanny help for mothers and newborn multiples without medical problems. Services available in Florida, Texas, New Mexico, Kansas, and North Carolina and covered by most insurance companies.

Gentle Care (Upjohn Health Care Services). (800) 345-8427; (800) 462-6603 in Michigan. Home help care for mothers and newborns with medical problems or special needs. Light household help as well as nursing care is offered, and most insurance plans provide coverage.

Greater Fort Worth Mothers of Twins Clubs, P.O. Box 331911, Fort Worth, TX 76163-1991. Poems, bumper stickers, iron-ons.

International Childbirth Education Association (ICEA), P.O. Box 20048, Minneapolis, MN 55420. (612) 854-8660. Mail order bookstore.

Kards by Kristin, P.O. Box 7146, Moreno Valley, CA 92303. Special birth announcements, NICU bonding and sympathy cards, for premies, multiples.

MJ Family Promotions, 450 Lakeville Street, Dept 301-2, Pataluma, CA 94952. (615) 744-9090. Novelties and gifts.

Multiples Choice, 11376 Route 503N, Lewisburg, OH 45338. Gifts for twins and their families.

Precious Pairs. P.O. Box 1961, Brandon, Manitoba, Canada R7A 6S8.

T-Topshop, 1808 Hoover Drive, Normal, IL 61761. T-shirts and sweatshirts for mothers of twins.

Twice as Nice, McGills's, 4965 Center, Omaha, NE 68106. Gifts and novelties.

Twozies Plus, P.O. Box 462, West Hempstead, NY 11552. (516) 486-6135. Gifts with twins insignia.

Sterling College, Sterling, KS 67579. College offering to enroll twins for price of one tuition.

Bibliography and Suggested Reading

Twins and Higher-Order Multiples

Abbe, Kathryn McLaughlin, and Frances McLaughlin Gill. *Twins on Twins.* New York: Clarkson Potter, 1980.

Ainslie, Ricardo. *The Psychology of Twinship.* Omaha: University of Nebraska Press, 1985.

Anderson, K., and J. Robinson. *Full House: The Story of the Anderson Quintuplets.* Boston: Little, Brown, 1986.

Bryan, Elizabeth. *Twins in the Family.* London: Constable, 1984.

———. *The Nature and Nurture of Twins.* London: Balliere Tindall, 1983.

Bulmer, M. G. *The Biology of Twinning in Man.* Oxford: Clarendon Press, 1970.

Burch, Sue. *Triple Trouble, Triple Treat.*

———, and Mary Fiebelkor. *Survey of 30 Mothers of Triplets.* 1983. Available from Sue Burch, 3075 Red Fox Circle, Colgate, WI 53017.

Burlingham, D. *Twins: A Study of Three Pairs of Identical Twins.* New York: International Press, 1952

Campbell, D. M., and I. MacGillivray. *Twinning and Twins.* Chichester, UK: Wiley, 1988.

Cassill, Kay. *Twins: Nature's Amazing Mystery.* New York: Atheneum, 1982.

Claridge, G., S. Canter, and W. I. Hume. *Personality Differences and Biological Variations: A Study of Twins.* Elmsford, NY: Pergamon Press, 1973.

Clegg, Avril, and Anne Woollett. *Twins from Conception to Five Years.* Century, 1988.

Collier, Herbert. *The Psychology of Twins.* 1977. 4227 North 32nd Street, Phoenix, AZ 85018.

Cunningham, Marci. *Twin Care.* Gibbon Glade, PA: Backwooods Books, 1987.

Fort Worth Mother of Twins Club. *Poems About Twins.* Available from Center for the Study of Multiple Birth, 333 E. Superior Street, Suite 476, Chicago, IL 60611.

Friedrich, Elizabeth, and Cherry Rowland. *The Parents' Guide to Raising Twins.* New York: St. Martin's Press, 1984.

Gaddis, Margaret, and V. Gaddis. *The Curious World of Twins.* New York: Warner, 1973.

Gedda, Luigi. *Twins in History and Science.* Springfield, IL: Thomas, 1961.

———, Paolo Parisi, and W. E. Nance, eds. *Twin Research 3.* Proceedings of the Third International Congress on Twin Studies, June 16–20, 1980. New York: Alan R. Liss, 1981.

Gehman, Betsy. *Twins: Twice the Trouble, Twice the Fun.* Philadelphia: Lippincott, 1965.

Gregory, Mollie. *Triplets.* New York: Watts, 1988.

Gromada, K. K. *Mothering Multiples.* Publication #52, 1981. La Leche League International, Franklin Park, IL 60131.

Hagedorn, Judy W., and J. W. Kizziar. *Gemini: The Psychology and Phenomena of Twins.* 2nd ed. Chicago: Center for Study of Multiple Birth, 1983.

Helms, D. *Twins.* Bullville, NY: Unltd, 1987.

Koch, Helen. *Twins and Twin Relations.* Chicago: University of Chicago Press, 1966.

Leigh, Gillian. *All About Twins.* London: Routledge & Kegan Paul, 1983.

Linney, J. *Multiple Births: Preparation-Birth-Management.* New York: Wiley, 1983.

Lytton, H. *Parent-Child Interaction: The Socialization Processs Observed in Twin and Singleton Families.* New York: Plenum, 1980.

McClamroch, M. *Two by Two: Twins' Stories.* Hadley, MA: Abundance Press, 1989.

McDonald, Di. *More than One.* New York: State Mutual, 1988.

MacGillivray, Ian, P. P. S. Nylander, and G. Corney. *Human Multiple Reproduction.* Philadelphia: Saunders, 1975.

Mountain Plains TMC. *Helpful Hints for New Mothers of Twins.* Box 351, Scotch Plains, NJ 07076.

Parents of Multiple Births Association, Canada. *Special Delivery: The Handbook for Parents of Triplets and Quads.* 5th ed., 1987. P.O. Box 2200, Lethbridge, Alberta, Canada T1J 4K7.

Pottker, J., and B. Speziale. *Dear Ann, Dear Abby.* New York: Paperjacks, 1988.

Nance, Walter E., ed. *Proceedings of the Second International Congress on Twin Studies.* Washington, DC, 1977. New York: Alan R. Liss, 1978.

Newman, Horatio H. *Twins: The Study of Heredity and Environment.* Chicago: University of Chicago Press, 1982.

Novotny, Pamela. *The Joy of Twins.* New York: Crown, 1988.

Osborne, R. T. *Twins: Black and White.* 1980. Foundation for Human Understanding, P.O. Box 5712, Athens, GA 30601.

Rosambeau, Mary. *How Twins Grow Up.* Bodley Head, 1987.

Rosenberg, Maxine B. *Being a Twin, Having a Twin.* New York: Lothrop, Lee, and Shepherd, 1985.

Scheinfeld, Amram. *Twins and Supertwins.* Baltimore: Penguin, 1973.

Theroux, R., and J. Tingley. *The Care of Twin Children: A Common Sense Guild for Parents.* Chicago: Center for the Study of Multiple Birth, 1984.

Vital Statistics of the United States. Natality and *Mortality.* Hyattsville, MD: U.S. Department of Health and Human Services, 1985, 1987.

Wallace, Irving, and A. Wallace. *The Two*. New York: Simon and Schuster, 1978.

Wallace, Marjorie. *The Silent Twins*. New York: Prentice-Hall, 1986.

Walters, H., and A. Hapgood. *The Twin Bond*. London: Heineman, 1983.

Watson, Peter, *An Investigation into the Strange Coincidences in the Lives of Separated Twins*. London: Hutchinson, 1981.

Wolnewr, T., and H. Stein. *Parallels: A Look at Twins*. New York: Dutton, 1978.

Zentner, Carola. *Twins: The Parents' Survival Guide*. Edinburgh: Mcdonald, 1984.

Ziner, Feeni. *A Full House*. Chicago: Center for Study of Multiple Birth, 1983.

Nutrition

Ballentine, Rudolph. *Diet and Nutrition*. 2nd ed. Honesdale, PA: Himalayan Institute, 1978.

———. *Transition to Vegetarianism*. Honesdale, PA: Himalayan Institute, 1987.

Brewer, Gail Sforza, and Tom Brewer. *What Every Pregnant Woman Should Know: The Truth About Diet and Drugs in Pregnancy*. Rev. ed. Baltimore: Penguin, 1985.

———. *The Brewer Medical Diet for Normal and High Risk Pregnancy: A Leading Obstetrician's Guide to Every Stage of Pregnancy*. New York: Fireside, 1983.

Brewer, Thomas, M.D. *Metabolic Toxemia of Late Pregnancy: A Disease of Malnutrition*. New Canaan, CT: Keats, 1982.

Brody, Jane. "Huge Study of Diet Indicts Fat and Meat." *New York Times*, 8 May 1990.

Colbin, Annemarie. *Food and Healing*. New York: Ballantine, 1986.

Diamond, Harvey, and Marilyn Diamond. *Fit for Life*. New York: Warner, 1985.

Elliott, Rose. *The Vegetarian Mother and Baby Book*. New York: Pantheon, 1987.

Erasmus, Udo. *Fats and Oils*. Burnaby, BC: Alive Books, 1986.

Food and Nutrition Board. *Recommended Dietary Allowances*. Washington, DC: National Academy of Sciences, 1989.

Goldbeck, Nikki and David. *American Wholefoods Cuisine*. New York: New American Library, 1983.

———. *The Goldbecks' Guide to Good Food*. New York: New American Library, 1987.

Kushi, Aveline, and Alex Jack. *Aveline Kushi's Complete Guide to Macrobiotic Cooking*. New York: Warner, 1985.

Kushi, Michio, and Aveline Kushi. *Macrobiotic Pregnancy and Care of the Newborn*. Tokyo: Japan Publications, 1983.

Lappe, Frances Moore. *Diet for a Small Planet*. New York: Ballantine, 1982.

McConnaughey, Evelyn. *Sea Vegetables: Harvesting Guide and Cookbook*. Happy Camp, CA: Naturegraph, 1985.

Robertson, Laurel, Carol Flinders, and Brian Ruppenthal. *The New Laurel's

Kitchen: A Handbook for Vegetarian Cooking and Nutrition. Berkeley: Ten Speed Press, 1986.

Sattilaro, A. *Recalled by Life*. Boston: Houghton Mifflin, 1982.

Shannon, Sara. *Diet for an Atomic Age*. Wayne, NJ: Avery, 1987.

U.S. Department of Agriculture, Consumer Nutrition Center. *Nutritive Value of Foods*. Home and Garden Bulletin #72. Washington, DC: Government Printing Office, 1986.

Yntema, Sharon K. *Vegetarian Baby*. Rev. ed. Ithaca, NY: McBooks, 1984.

Pregnancy and Birth

Baker, Jeannine P., Frederick Baker, and Tamara Slayton. *Conscious Conception*. Monroe, UT: Freestone Publishing, 1986.

Better Babies Series. Low-cost pamphlets on bed rest, Caesarean birth, gestational diabetes, jaundice, care of uncircumcised boys, and so on. From Birth and Life Bookstore, P.O. Box 70625, Seattle, WA 98107-0625.

Blatt, J. R. Robin. *Prenatal Tests: What They Are, Their Benefits and Risks, and How to Decide Whether to Have Them or Not*. New York: Random House, 1988.

Brewer, Gail Sforza. *The Very Important Pregnancy Program: A Personal Approach to the Art and Science of Having a Baby*. Emmaus, PA: Rodale, 1988.

Chamberlain, David. *Babies Remember Birth*. Los Angeles: Tarcher, 1989.

Gaskin, Ina May. *Spiritual Midwifery*. Summertown, TN: The Book Publishing Company, 1978.

Kelly-Buchanan, Christine. *Peace of Mind During Pregnancy: An A–Z Guide to the Substances That Could Affect Your Unborn Baby*. New York: Facts on File, 1988.

Marnie, Eve. *Love Start: Pre-Birth Bonding*. Santa Monica, CA: Hay House, 1989.

McGarey, Gladys. *Born to Live*. Phoenix, AZ: Gabariel Press, 1980.

Noble, Elizabeth. *Childbirth with Insight*. Boston: Houghton Mifflin, 1983.

———. *Essential Exercises for the Childbearing Year*. 3rd ed. Boston: Houghton Mifflin, 1988.

———. *Inside Experiences: From Conception Through Birth*. New York: Simon and Schuster, forthcoming (1991).

———. *Marie Osmond's Exercises for Mothers-to-Be* and *Marie Osmond's Exercises for Mothers and Babies*. These two titles are available only from Maternal and Child Health Center, 2464 Massachusetts Avenue, Cambridge, MA 02140, or from Elizabeth Noble, 448 Pleasant Lake Avenue, Harwich, MA 02645.

Odent, Michel. *Birth Reborn*. New York: Pantheon, 1984.

Peterson, Gayle. *Birthing Normally*. Rev. ed. Berkeley: Mindbody Press, 1984.

———, and L. Mehl. *Pregnancy as Healing*. Berkeley: Mindbody Press, 1984.

Rothman, B. K. *The Tentative Pregnancy: Prenatal Diagnosis and the Future of Motherhood*. New York: Viking, 1986.

Simkin, P., and C. Reinke. *Kaleidoscope of Childbearing.* Proceedings of the Tenth Biennial Convention of the International Childbirth Education Association, Kansas City, 1978.

Verny, T., and J. Kelly. *The Secret Life of the Unborn Child.* New York: Dell, 1981.

———, eds. *Pre- and Perinatal Psychology.* New York: Human Sciences Press, 1987.

White, G. *Emergency Childbirth.* Franklin Park, IL: Police Training Foundation, 1958.

Healing

Earnshaw, Avril. *Family Time.* 1983. A & K Enterprises, 13 Cawarrah Road, Middle Cove, Sydney, NSW 2068, Australia.

Grof, Stanislav. *Realms of the Human Unconscious.* New York: Dutton, 1976.

Hay, Louis. *Heal Your Body.* Santa Monica, CA: Hay House, 1988.

Mackarness, Richard. *Not All in the Mind.* London: Pan, 1976.

Rossi, E., & D. Cheek. *Mind-Body Therapy.* New York: Norton, 1988.

Steadman, Alice, *Who'se the Matter with Me?* Marina Del Rey, CA: De Vors, 1977.

Wambach, Helen. *Life Before Life.* New York: Bantam, 1984.

Zoll, Stuart. *The Bridge Between Acupuncture and Modern Bioenergetic Medicine.* Baden Baden, Western Germany: Kern Pharma, 1990.

Caesarean Birth

Cohen, N. W., and L. Estner. *Silent Knife: Cesarean Prevention and Vaginal Birth After Cesarean.* South Hadley, MA: Bergin and Garvey, 1983.

English, Jane. *Different Doorway: Adventures of a Cesarean Born.* Earth Heart, Box 7, Mt. Shasta, CA 96067, 1985.

Peterson, Gayle, and Lewis Mehl. *Cesarean Birth: Risk and Culture.* Berkeley: Mindbody Press, 1985.

Richards, L. *The Vaginal Birth After Cesarean Experience.* South Hadley, MA: Bergin and Garvey, 1987.

Young, D., and C. Maham. *Unnecessary Caesareans: Ways to Avoid Them.* Rev. ed. 1989. ICEA Publications, P.O. Box 20048, Minneapolis, MN 55420.

Breast-Feeding

Fleming, Nora B. "Breastfeeding Is Possible . . . Even Weeks After Delivery." *Twins,* May/June 1989.

Keith, D., S. McInnes, and L. Keith, eds. *Breastfeeding Twins, Triplets, and*

Quadruplets: 195 Practical Hints for Success. Chicago: Center for the Study of Multiple Birth, 1982.

Kitzinger, Sheila. *Breastfeeding Your Baby*. New York: Knopf, 1989.

La Leche League. *The Womanly Art of Breastfeeding*. 4th ed. 1987.

Mason, Diane, and Diane Ingersoll. *Breastfeeding and the Working Mother*. New York: St. Martin's, 1986.

Pryor, Karen. *Nursing Your Baby*. New York: Bantam, 1991.

Child Care

Baldwin, Rahima. *You Are Your Child's First Teacher*. Berkeley: Celestial Arts, 1989.

Colfax, David and Nikki. *Homeschooling for Excellence*. New York: Warner, 1988.

Colter, H. L., and P. L. Fisher. *DPT: A Shot in the Dark*. New York: Harcourt Brace Jovanovich, 1985.

Crimes of Genital Mutilation. *The Truth Seeker*. July/August 1989. P.O. Box 2832, San Diego, CA 91112-2832.

Faber, Adele, and Elaine Mazlish. *How to Talk so Kids Will Listen and Listen so Kids Will Talk*. New York: Avon, 1980.

———. *Siblings Without Rivalry*. New York: Avon, 1979.

Gaskin, Ina May. *Babies, Bonding, and Breastfeeding*. South Hadley, MA: Bergin and Garvey, 1986.

Growing Without Schooling, 2269 Massachusetts Avenue, Cambridge, MA 02140. (617) 864-3100.

James, Walen. *Immunization: The Reality Behind the Myth*. South Hadley, MA: Bergin and Garvey, 1988.

Klaus, Marshall, and John Kennell. *Parent-Infant Bonding*. St. Louis: Moseby, 1982.

La Leche League. *In Hospital: The Child and the Family*. Publication #143. La Leche League, 9616 Minneapolis Avenue, Franklin Park, IL 60131.

Liedloff, J. *The Continuum Concept*. Reading, MA: Addison-Wesley, 1986.

McMahon, Peggy. *Immunization: Mothering Special Edition*. Mothering magazine, 1987.

Mendelsohn, R. *How to Raise a Healthy Child . . . In Spite of Your Doctor*. New York: Ballantine, 1987.

Montagu, A. *Touching: The Human Significance of the Skin*. New York: Harper and Row, 1986.

Moss, Stephen. *Your Child's Teeth*. Boston: Houghton Mifflin, 1979.

Pearce, J. C. *Magical Child*. New York: Bantam, 1977.

———. *Magical Child Matures*. New York: Bantam, 1986.

Solter, Aletha J. *The Aware Baby*. Shining Star, 1984.

Schreiber, Linda, and JoAnne Stang. *Marathon Mom: The Wife and Mother Running Book*. Boston: Houghton Mifflin, 1980.

Thevenin, T. *The Family Bed*. Rev. ed. Wayne, NJ: Avery, 1987.

Wycoff, Jerry, and Barbara C. Unell. *Discipline Without Shouting or Spanking*. Deephaven, MN: Meadowbrook, 1984.

Children's Books

Abolafia, Yossi. *My Three Uncles*. New York: Greenwillow, 1984.

Albertsen, June. *Two Are Twins*. Available from DoubleTalk, P.O. Box 412, Amelia, OH 45102.

Aliki. *Jack and Jake*. Numerous other titles, published by Greenwillow Books and available from DoubleTalk, P.O. Box 412, Amelia, OH 45102.

Brennan, Jan. *Born Two-Gether*. Available from DoubleTalk, P.O. Box 412, Amelia, OH 45102.

Cleary, Beverly. *Two Dog Biscuits*. New York: Dell, 1987. Cleary is a mother of twins.

———. *The Real Hole*. New York: Dell, 1980.

———. *Mitch and Amy*. New York: Dell, 1980.

Cole, J., and Edmondson, M. *Twins: The Story of Multiple Birth*. New York: Morrow, 1972.

DeClements, Barthe, and Christophere Grimes. *Double Trouble*. New York: Penguin, 1987.

Firer, B. *Twins*. Spring Valley, NY: Feldheim, 1983.

Hagedorn, J., and J. Kizziar. *What Is a Twin?* Chicago: Center for Study of Multiple Birth, 1983.

Larson, Claudine. *Twins' Surprise and Other Stories*. New York: Carlton, 1988.

Lerner, Marguerite. *Twins: The Story of Twins*. Minneapolis: Lerner Pubs, 1961.

Ross, Pat. *M and M and the Bad News Babies*. New York: Pantheon Books, 1983.

Maidat, Rita. *Twins Visit Israel*. Brooklyn: Shulsinger, 1978.

Pascal, Francine. *Sweet Valley Twins*. Series. New York: Bantam.

Reich, Ali. *The Care Bear and the Terrible Twos*. New York: Random House, 1983.

Vogel, Ilse-Margaret. *My Twin Sister Erika*. New York: Harper and Row, 1976.

Williams, H. *Twins of Ceylon*. Chester Springs, PA: Dufour, 1965.

Articles

Acker, D. et al. "Delivery of the Second Twin." *Obstetrics and Gynecology* 59:710, 1982.

Allen, G. "Differential Method for Estimation of Type Frequencies in Triplets and Quadruplets." *American Journal of Human Genetics* 12:210–24, 1960.

Allen, M. G., et al. "Parental Perceptions of Twins." *Psychiatry* 39:65–71, February 1979.

Anand, K.J.S., et al. "Pain and Its Effects in the Human Neonate and Fetus." *New England Journal of Medicine* 317:1321, 19 November 1987.

Anderson, A., and B. Anderson. "Mothers' Beginning Relationship with Twins." *Birth* 14(2):92–94, June 1987.

Banchi, M. T. "Triplet Pregnancy with Second Trimester Abortion and Delivery of Twins at 35 Weeks' Gestation." *Obstetrics and Gynecology* 64(5):728–30, November 1984.

"Bed Rest in Obstetrics." Editorial. *Lancet* 1:1137–38, 1981.

Begley, Sharon, et al. "All About Twins." *Newsweek* 23 November 1987.

Beit-Hallahmi, B., and M. Paluszny. "Twinship in Mythology and Science: Ambivalence, Differentiation, and the Magical Bond." *Psychiatry* 18:4, July-August 1974.

Bell, D., et al. "Birth Asphyxia, Trauma, and Mortality in Twins: Has Cesarean Section Improved Outcome?" *American Journal of Obstetrics and Gynecology* 154:235–39, 1986.

Bernabei, R., and G. Levi. "Psychopathologic Problems in Twins During Childhood." *Acta Geneticae Medicae et Gemellologiae,* 1976.

Bernstein, B. A. "Siblings of Twins." *Psychoanalytic Study of the Child* 35:134–154, 1980.

Blake, D. M., and M. I. Lee. "Twin Pregnancy in Adolescents." *Obstetrics and Gynecology* 75(2):172, February 1990.

Blecker, P. G. "Counseling Families with Twins: Birth to 3 Years of Age." *Pediatrics in Review* 8:3, September 1986.

Blickstein, I., and M. Lancet. "The Growth Discordant Twin." *Obstetrical and Gynecological Survey* 43(9):509, 1988.

Blickstein, I., et al. "Growth Discordancy in Appropriate for Gestational Age Term Twins." *Obstetrical and Gynecological Survey* 72(4):582–84, October 1988.

Blickstein, I., et al. "Vaginal Delivery of the Second Twin in Breech Presentation." *Obstetrics and Gynecology* 69(5):774–76, May 1987.

Boklage, C. E. "Interactions Between Opposite Sex Dizygotic Fetuses and the Assumptions of Weinberg Difference Method Epidemiology." *American Journal of Human Genetics* 37:591–605, 1985.

Brady, K., and J. A. Read. "Vaginal Delivery of Twins After Previous Cesarean Section." Letter. *New England Journal of Medicine* 319(2):118–19, 14 July 1988.

Brennan, J. N., et al. "Fetofetal Transfusion Syndrome: Prenatal Ultrasonographic Diagnosis." *Radiology* 143:535–36, 1982.

Bryan, E. M. "The Intrauterine Hazards of Twins." *Archives of Diseases of Children* 61:1044–45, 1986.

Campbell, D. M., and I. MacGillivray. "The Importance of Plasma Volume Expansion and Nutrition in Twin Pregnancy." *Acta Geneticae Medicae et Gemellologiae* 33:19–24, 1984.

Cardwell, M. S., et al. "Triplet Pregnancy with Delivery on Three Separate Days." Part 2. *Obstetrics and Gynecology* 71(3):448–49, March 1988.

Carlson, Nancy J. "Discordant Twin Pregnancy: A Challenging Condition." *Contemporary OB/GYN* 34(2):100–16, August 1989.

Cetrulo, C. L. "The Controversy of Mode of Delivery in Twins: The Intrapartum Management of Twin Gestation." Part 1. *Seminars in Perinatology* 10:39–43, 1986.

Chervenak, F. A., et al. "Twin Gestation: Antenatal Diagnosis and Perinatal

Outcome in 385 Consecutive Pregnancies." *Journal of Reproductive Medicine* 29(10):727–30, October 1984.

———. "Intrapartum Management of Twin Gestation." *Obstetrics and Gynecology* 65(1):119–24, January 1985.

———. "Adjunctive Use of Ultrasound in the Intrapartum Management of Twin Gestation." *Female Patient* 12:52–68, November 1987.

———. "Is Routine Cesarean Section Necessary for Vertex-Breech and Vertex-Transverse Twin Gestation?" *American Journal of Obstetrics and Gynecology* 148:1, 1984.

———. "Intrapartum External Version of the Second Twin." *Obstetrics and Gynecology* 62:160, 1983.

Chescheir, N. C., and J. W. Seeds. "Polyhydramnios and Oligohydramnios in Twin Gestations." Part 1. *Obstetrics and Gynecology* 71(6):882–84, June 1988.

Collins, J. W., Jr., et al. "The Northwestern University Triplet Study," III: "Neonatal Outcome." *Acta Geneticae Medicae et Gemellologiae* 37(1):77–80, 1988.

Committee to Study the Prevention of Low Birthweight, Division of Health Promotion and Disease Prevention, Institute of Medicine. "Preventing Low Birthweight." Washington, DC: National Academic Press, 1986.

Corey, L. A., et al. "Analysis of Timing Similarities in Marital and Pregnancy History of Twins." *American Journal of Human Genetics* 425, 1980.

Creinin, M., and L. G. Keith. "The Yoruban Contribution to the Understanding of the Twinning Process." *Journal of Reproductive Medicine*, 1989.

Dallapiccola, B., et al. "Discordant Sex in One of Three Monozygotic Triplets." *Journal of Medical Genetics* 22:6–11, 1985.

D'Alton, M. E., and D. K. Dudley. "The Ultrasonographic Prediction of Chorionicity in Twin Gestation." *American Journal of Obstetrics and Gynecology* 160(3):557–61, March 1989.

Degani, S., et al. "Fetal Internal Carotid Artery Flow Velocity Time Waveforms in Twin Pregnancies." *Journal of Perinatal Medicine* 16(5–6):405–9, 1988.

Depp, R., et al. "The Northwestern University Twin Study," VII: "The Mode of Delivery in Twin Pregnancy: North American Considerations." *Acta Geneticae Medicae et Gemellologiae* 37(1):11–18, 1988.

Derom, C., et al. "Increased Monozygotic Twinning Rate After Ovulation Induction." *Lancet* 1:1236, 1987.

Devoe, L. D. "Simultaneous Antepartum Testing of Twin Fetal Heart Rates." *Southern Medical Journal* 78(4):380–83, April 1985.

Doherty, J.D.H. "Height of Women, Twinning, and Breast Cancer: Epidemiological Evaluation of a Relationship." *Acta Geneticae Medicae et Gemellologiae* 37(3–4):263–76, 1988.

Dor, J., et al. "Elective Cervical Suture of Twin Pregnancies Diagnosed Ultrasonically in the First Trimester Following Induced Ovulation." *Gynecologic and Obstetric Investigation* 13(1):55–60, 1982.

Doyle, L. W., et al. "Mode of Delivery of Preterm Twins." *Australian and New Zealand Journal of Obstetrics and Gynaecology* 28(1):25–28, February 1988.

Elstein, I. D., et al. "Cardiac Output Measurements During and After Triplet Gestation." Part 2. *Obstetrics and Gynecology* 74(3):452–53, September 1989.

Emery, A. E. H. "Identical Twinning and Oral Contraception." *Biology and Society* 3(1):23–27, 1986.

Erkkola, R. et al. "Growth Discordancy in Twin Pregnancies: A Risk Factor Not Detected by Measurement of Biparietal Diameter." *Obstetrics and Gynecology* 66(2):203–6, August 1985.

Evrard, J. R., and E. M. Gold. "Cesarean Section for Delivery of the Second Twin." *Obstetrics and Gynecology* 57(5):581–83, May 1981.

Filkins, K., et al. "Genetic Amniocentesis in Multiple Gestation." *Prenatal Diagnosis* 4:223–26, 1984.

Flamm, B. L., et al. "Vaginal Birth After Cesarean Section: Results of a Multicenter Study." *American Journal of Obstetrics and Gynecology* 158:1079–84, 1988.

Fleigner, J. R., and T. R. Eggers. "The Relationship Between Gestational Age and Birthweight in Twin Pregnancy." *Australian and New Zealand Journal of Obstetrics and Gynaecology* 24:192–97, 1984.

Gilbert, L., et al. "The Management of Multiple Pregnancy in Women with a Lower Segment Caesarean Scar." *British Journal of Obstetrics and Gynaecology* 95:1312–16, December 1988.

Giles, W. B., et al. "Umbilical Artery Flow Velocity Waveforms and Twin Pregnancy Outcome." *Obstetrics and Gynecology* 72(6):894–97, December 1988.

Gilstrap, L. C. 3rd, and C. E. Brown. "Prevention and Treatment of Preterm Labor in Twins." *Clinical Perinatology* 15(1):71–77, March 1988.

———, et al. "Twins: Prophylactic Hospitalization and Ward Rest at Early Gestational Age." *Obstetrics and Gynecology* 69:578, 1987.

Gocke, S. E. "Management of the Nonvertex Second Twin: Primary Cesarean Section, External Version, or Primary Breech Extraction." *American Journal of Obstetrics and Gynecology* 161(1):29, July 1989.

Goldberg, H. J., et al. "Timely Diagnosis by Cardiotocography of Critical Fetal Reserve due to Fetofetal Transfusion Syndrome." *Australian and New Zealand Journal of Obstetrics and Gynaecology* 26(3):182–84, August 1986.

Golding, J. "Social Class and Twinning." *Acta Geneticae Medicae et Gemellologiae*, Abstracts 35:29, 1986.

———. "Season of Conception and Risk of Twinning." *Acta Geneticae Medicae et Gemellologiae*, Abstracts 35:26, 1986.

Gonsoulin, W., et al. "Outcome of Twin-Twin Transfusion Diagnosed Before 28 Weeks of Gestation." *Obstetrics and Gynecology* 75(2):214, February 1990.

Goshen-Gottstein, E. R. "The Mothering of Twins, Triplets, and Quadruplets." *Psychiatry* 43:189–204, 1980.

Gromada, K. K. "Maternal-Infants Attachment: The First Step Toward Individualizing Twins." *American Journal of Maternal Child Nursing* 6:2, March/April 1981.

Groothuis, J. R. "Child Abuse and Twins." *Twins* 1(6):22–25, 1985.

———. "Twins and Twin Families: A Practical Guide to Outpatient Management." *Clinical Perinatology* 12:459, 1985.

———, et al. "Increased Child Abuse in Families with Twins." *Pediatrics* 70:769, 1982.

Grothe, W., and H. Rutgers. "Twin Pregnancies: An 11-Year Review." *Acta Geneticae Medicae et Gemellologiae* 34:49, 1985.

Haire, Doris. "Drugs in Labor and Birth." *Childbirth Educator*, Spring 1987, p. 26.

Halfar, M. M. "Collaborative Management of Twins: Two Case Studies." *Journal of Nurse-Midwifery* 32(3):140–48, May–June 1987.

Harlap, S., et al. "Overripe Ova and Twinning." *American Journal of Human Genetics* 37:1206–15, 1985.

Hartikainen-Sorri, A. L., et al. "Factors Related to an Improved Outcome for Twins." *Acta Obstetrica and Gynecologica Scandinavica* 62(1):23–25, 1983.

———. "Is Routine Bed Rest Needed in Antenatal Care of Twin Pregnancy?" *Journal of Perinatal Medicine* 12(1):31–34, 1984.

———. "Is Routine Hospitalization in Twin Pregnancy Necessary? A Follow-up Study." *Acta Geneticae Medicae et Gemellologiae* 34:149, 1985.

Hashimoto, B., et al. "Ultrasound Evaluation of Polyhydramnios and Twin Pregnancy." *American Journal of Obstetrics and Gynecology* 154(5):1069–72, May 1986.

Hay, D. A. "Children at Risk." *Australian Journal of Early Childhood* 11(4):6–10, 1986.

———. "The LaTrobe Twin Study: A Genetic Approach to the Structure and Development in Preschool Twins." *Child Development* 54:317–30, 1983.

———, et al. "The Older Sibling of Twins." *Australian Journal of Early Childhood* 13:25–28, 1988.

———, et al. "Speech and Language Development in Preschool Twins." *Twin Research* 36:213–23, 1987.

———, and P. J. O'Brien. "The LaTrobe Twin Study: A Genetic Approach to the Structure and Development of Cognition in Twin Children." *Child Development* 54:317–30, 1983.

Heluin, G., and E. Papiernik. "Spontaneous or Systematically Induced Labor for the Termination of Twin Pregnancies." *Acta Geneticae Medicae et Gemellologiae* 30(4):285–88, 1981.

Holczberg, G., et al. "Outcome of Pregnancy in 31 Triplet Gestations." *Obstetrics and Gynecology* 59(4):472–76, April 1982.

Hughey, M. J., and D. L. Olive. "Routine Ultrasound Scanning for the Detection and Management of Twin Pregnancies." *Journal of Reproductive Medicine* 30(5):427–30, May 1985.

Itzakowic, D. "A Survey of 59 Triplet Pregnancies." *British Journal of Obstetrics and Gynaecology* 86:23–28, 1979.

James, W. H. "Coitus-Induced Ovulation and Its Implications for Estimates of Some Reproductive Parameters." *Acta Geneticae Medicae et Gemellologiae* 33:547–55, 1984.

———. "Dizygotic Twinning, Birthweight, and Latitude." *Annals of Human Biology* 12:441–47, 1985.

———. "Hormonal Control of Sex Ratio." *Journal of Theoretical Biology* 118:427–41, 1986.

Johnson, C., M. Prior, and D. A. Hay. "Predictions of Reading Disability in Twin Boys." *Developmental Medicine and Child Neurology* 26:588–95, 1984.

Johnson, S. F., and S. G. Driscoll. "Twin Placentation and Its Complications." *Seminars in Perinatology* 10:9–13, 1986.

Katz, V. L., et al. "A Comparison of Bed Rest and Immersion for Treating the Edema of Pregnancy." *Obstetrics and Gynecology* 75(2):147–51, February 1990.

———, and A. M. Brown. "The Behavior of Twins: Effects of Birth Weight and Birth Sequence." *Child Development* 42:251–57, 1981.

Keith, L. G., et al. "The Northwestern University Triplet Study," II: "Fourteen Triplet Pregnancies Delivered Between 1981 and 1986." *Acta Geneticae Medicae et Gemellologiae* 37(1):65–75, 1988.

Khoury, M. J., et al. "Congenital Malformations and Intrauterine Growth Retardation: A Population Study. *Pediatrics* 82(1):83, July 1988.

Laros, R. K., Jr., and B. J. Dattel. "Management of Twin Pregnancy: The Vaginal Route Is Still Safe." Part 1. *American Journal of Obstetrics and Gynecology* 158:1330–38, June 1988.

Leonard, L. "Postpartum Depression in Mothers of Twins" *Maternal Child Nursing* 10:99–109, 1981.

Lodeiro, J. G., et al. "Fetal Biophysical Profile in Twin Gestations." *Obstetrics and Gynecology* 67:824, 1986.

Loucopoulos, A., et al. "Multiple Gestations: Management of Pregnancy and Delivery." *Acta Geneticae Medicae et Gemellologiae* 31(3–4):263–66, 1982.

———. "Management of Multifetal Pregnancies: Sixteen Years Experience in the Sloane Hospital for Women." *American Journal of Obstetrics and Gynecology* 143:902–5, 1982.

Macourt, D. C., et al. "Multiple Pregnancy and Fetal Abnormalities in Association with Oral Contraceptive Usage." *Australian and New Zealand Journal of Obstetrics and Gynaecology* 22:25–28, 1982.

Majsky, A., and M. Kout. "Another Case of Occurrence of Two Different Fathers of Twins by HLA Typing." *Tissue Antigens* 20:305, 1982.

Malmstrom, Patricia M., and R. Biale. "Recommendations for Policies and Psychosocial Services for Multiple Birth Families." Paper presented at the Sixth International Congress on Twin Studies, August 1989. Forthcoming in *Acta Geneticae Medicae et Gemellologiae.*

———, and M. Silva. "Twin Talk: Manifestations of Twin Status in the Speech of Toddlers." *Journal of Child Language* 13:293–304, 1986.

———, et al. Parent Education Series. Handouts covering pregnancy and twin care and development from birth through adolescence. Available from Twin Services, P.O. Box 10066, Berkeley, CA 94709.

Manning, F. A., et al. "Fetal Assessment based on Fetal Biophysical Profile Scoring: Experience in 12,260 Referred High-risk Pregnancies." *American Journal of Obstetrics and Gynecology* 151:343–50, 1985.

Martin, N. G., et al. "Gonadotrophin Levels in Mothers Who Had Two Sets of DZ Twins." *Acta Geneticae Medicae et Gemellologiae* 33:131-9, 1984.

Matheny, A. P., and C. Bruggemann. "Articulation Proficiency in Twins and Singletons from Families of Twins." *Journal of Speech and Hearing Research* 15:645–51, 1972.

——, and A. M. Brown. "The Behavior of Twins: Effects of Birth Weight and Birth Sequence." *Child Development* 42:251–57, 1981.

McCulloch, K. "Neonatal Problems in Twins." *Clinics in Perinatology* 15(1):141–58, March 1988.

Montan, S., et al. "Amniocentesis in Treatment of Acute Polyhydramnios in Twin Pregnancies." *Acta Obstetrica Gynecologica Scandinavica* 64(6):537–39, 1985.

Morales, W. J., et al., "The Use of Antenatal Vitamin K in the Prevention of Early Neonatal Intraventricular Hemorrhage." *American Journal of Obstetrics and Gynecology* 159:774–79.

"Multiple Births: An Upward Trend in the United States." *Statistical Bulletin*, January–March 1988.

Neilson, J. P., et al. "Tape Measurement of Symphysis-Fundal Height in Twin Pregnancies." *British Journal of Obstetrics and Gynaecology* 95(10):1054–599, October 1988.

——. "Cervical Assessment in the Management of Twin Pregnancy." *Acta Geneticae Medicae et Gemellologiae*, Abstracts 35:68, 1986.

Newton, E. R. "Antepartum Care in Multiple Gestation." *Seminars in Perinatology* 10(1):19–29, January 1986.

O'Brien, Diane. "The Twins Who Made Their Own Language." *Family Health/Today's Health*, September 1978.

O'Connor, M. C., et al. "The Merits of Special Antenatal Care for Twin Pregnancies." *British Journal of Obstetrics and Gynaecology* 88(3):220–30, March 1981.

O'Grady, J. P. "Clinical Management of Twins." *Contemporary OB/GYN* 29:126–42, April 1987.

O'Leary, J. A. "Prophylactic Tocolysis of Twins." *American Journal of Obstetrics and Gynecology* 154:904, 1986.

Olofsson, R., and H. J. Rydhstrom. "Twin Delivery: How Should the Second Twin Be Delivered?" *American Journal of Obstetrics and Gynecology* 153:479, 1985.

Papiernik, E. "The Social Cost of Twinning." Presented at Sixth International Congress on Twin Studies, Rome, August 1989.

Parisi, P. "Incidence of Twinning: Variability and Interpretations." *Acta Geneticae Medicae et Gemellologiae*, Abstracts 35:28, 1986.

Pedersen, I. K., et al. "Monozygotic Twins with Dissimilar Phenotypes and Chromosome Complements." *Acta Obstetrica and Gynecologica Scandinavica* 59(5):459–62, 1980.

Peterson, Gayle. "Prenatal Bonding, Prenatal Communication, and the Prevention of Prematurity." *Pre- and Peri-Natal Psychology* 2(2):87–92, Winter 1987.

Philippe, P. "The End of Reproductive Life in Mothers of Twins: Epidemiologic Analysis of a Large Data Base." *Acta Geneticae Medicae et Gemellologiae* 37(3–4):249–62, 1988.

Pijpers, L., et al. "Genetic Amniocentesis in Twin Pregnancies." *British Journal of Obstetrics and Gynaecology* 95:323–26, 1988.

Polin, J. I., and W. L. Frangipane. "Current Conceptions in Management of Obstetric Problems for Pediatricians," II: "Modern Concepts in the Management of Multiple Gestation." *Pediatric Clinics of North America* 33(3):649–61, June 1986.

Pons, J. C., et al. "Management of Triplet Pregnancy." Presented at Sixth International Congress on Twin Studies, Rome, August 1989.

———. "Quadruplet Pregnancy." Presented at Sixth International Congress on Twin Studies, Rome, August 1989.

"A Pregnant Woman's Self-Help Guide to Quit Smoking." Health Promotion Group, Inc., P.O. Box 58687, Homewood, AL 35259.

Price, J. H., and M. Marivate. "Induction of Labour in Twin Pregnancy." *South African Medical Journal* 70(3):163–65, 2 August 1986.

Pschera, H., and A. Jonasson. "Is Cesarean Section Justified for Delivery of the Second Twin?" *Acta Obstetrica and Gynecologica Scandinavica* 67(4):381–82, 1988.

Rabinovici, J., et al. "Intrapartum Management of Second Twin: Internal Podalic Version with Unruptured Membranes." Letter. *American Journal of Obstetrics and Gynecology* 155(4):914–14, October 1986.

Rattan, P. K., et al. "Cesarean Delivery of the Second Twin After Vaginal Delivery of the First Twin." *American Journal of Obstetrics and Gynecology* 154(40):936–99, April 1986.

Rayburn, W. F., et al. "Multiple Gestation: Time Interval Between Delivery of the First and Second Twins." *Obstetrics and Gynecology* 63(4):502–6, April 1984.

Rivera-Alsina, M. E., et al. "Fetal Growth Sustained by Parenteral Nutrition in Pregnancy." *Obstetrics and Gynecology* 64(1):138–41, July 1984.

Rodis, J. F., et al. "Antenatal Diagnosis and Management of Monoamniotic Twins." *American Journal of Obstetrics and Gynecology* 157(5):1255–57, November 1987.

Ron-El, R., et al. "Triplet and Quadruplet Pregnancies and Management." *Obstetrics and Gynecology* 57(4):458–63, April 1981.

Rydhstrom, H., et al. "Routine Hospital Care Does Not Improve Prognosis in Twin Gestation." *Acta Obstetrica and Gynecologica Scandinavica* 66(4):361–64, 1987.

Sakala, E. P., and B. C. Branson. "Prolonged Delivery-Abortion Interval in Twin and Triplet Pregnancies: A Report of Two Cases." *Journal of Reproductive Medicine* 32(1):79–81, January 1987.

Salat-Baroux, J., et al. "The Management of Multiple Pregnancies After Induction for Superovulation." *Human Reproduction* 3(3):339–401, April 1988.

Samueloff, A., et al. "Fetal Movements in Multiple Pregnancy." *American Journal of Obstetrics and Gynecology* 146:789–92, 1983.

Samuels, P. "Ultrasound in the Management of the Twin Gestation." *Clinical Obstetrics and Gynecology* 31(1):110–22, March 1988.

Saunders, M. C., et al. "The Effects of Hospital Admission for Bed Rest on the Duration of Twin Pregnancy: A Randomized Trial." *Lancet* 2(8459):793–95, 12 October 1985.

Schneider, K. T. M., et al. "Acute Polyhydramnios Complicating Twin Pregnancies." *Acta Geneticae Medicae et Gemellologiae* 34:179–84, 1985.

Scialli, A. R. "Intrapartum Management of Twin Gestation." Letter. *Obstetrics and Gynecology* 67(1):149–50, January 1986.

Secher, N. J. "Intrauterine Growth in Twin Pregnancies: Prediction of Fetal Growth Retardation." *Obstetrics and Gynecology* 66(1):63–68, July 1985.

Segal, Nancy. "Cooperation, Competition, and Altruism Within Twin Sets: A Reappraisal." *Ethology and Sociobiology* 5:153–77, 1984.

———. "Monozygotic and Dizygotic Twins: A Comparative Analysis of Mental Ability Profiles." *Child Development* 56:1051–58, 1985.

———. "Holocaust Twins: Their Special Bonds." *Psychology Today* 19:52–58, 1985.

———. "Origins and Implications of Handedness and Relative Birthweight for Intelligence in Monozygotic Twin Pairs." *Neuropsychologica* 27:549–61, 1989.

Showers, J., and J. T. McCleering. "Research on Twins: Implications for Parenting." *Child Care, Health, and Development* 10:391–404, 1984.

Simpson, C. W., et al. "Delayed Interval Delivery in Triplet Pregnancy: Report of a Single Case and Review of the Literature." *Obstetrics and Gynecology* 64(3 Suppl):8S–11S, September 1984.

Spellacy, W. N., et al. "A Case-Control Study of 1253 Twin Pregnancies from a 1982–87 Perinatal Data Base." *Obstetrics and Gynecology* 75(2):168, February 1990.

Strong, T. H., Jr., et al. "Vaginal Birth After Cesarean Section in the Twin Gestation." *American Journal of Obstetrics and Gynecology* 161(1):25, July 1989.

Sutter, J., et al. "Monoamniotic Twins: Antenatal Diagnosis and Management." *American Journal of Obstetrics and Gynecology* 155(4):830–36, October 1986.

Swarttjes, J. M., and H. P. van Geijan. "Maternal Perception of Fetal Movements: The Optimal Duration of a Recording Period." *European Journal of Obstetrics, Gynecology, and Reproductive Biology* 25:97–103, 1987.

Syrop, C. H., and M. W. Varner. "Triplet Gestation: Maternal and Neonatal Implications." *Acta Geneticae Medicae et Gemellologiae* 34:81–88, 1985.

Tabsh, K. "Genetic Amniocentesis in Multiple Gestation: A New Technique to Diagnose Monoamniotic Twins." *Obstetrics and Gynecology* 75(2):296, February 1990.

Terasaki, P., et al. "Twins with Two Different Fathers Identified by HLA." *New England Journal of Medicine* 299:11, 14 September 1978.

Thiery, M., G. Kermans, and R. Derom. "Triplet and Higher Order Births: What Is the Optimal Delivery Route?" *Acta Geneticae Medicae et Gemellologiae* 37:89–98, 1988.

Thompson, S. A., et al. "Outcomes of Twin Gestations at the University of Colorado Health Sciences Center, 1973–83." *Journal of Reproductive Medicine* 32(5):328–29, May 1987.

Trofatter, K. F., Jr. "Twin Pregnancy: Management of Delivery." *Clinical Perinatology* 15(1):93–105, March 1988.

Vintzileos, A. M., et al. "The Use and Misuse of the Fetal Biophysical Profile." *American Journal of Obstetrics and Gynecology* 156:527–33, 1987.

Vlietinck, R., et al. "The European Multiple Birth Study (EMBS)." *Acta Geneticae Medicae et Gemellologiae* 37(1):27–30, 1988.

Vollmar, Alice. "How the World Views Twins." *Twins,* January/February 1987.

Webster, F., and J. M. Elwood. "A Study of the Influence of Ovulation Stimulants and Oral Contraception on Twin Births in England." *Acta Geneticae Medicae et Gemellologiae* 34:105–8, 1985.

Weissman, A., et al. "Sonographic Growth Measurements in Triplet Pregnancies." Part 1. *Obstetrics and Gynecology* 75(3):324–28, March 1990.

Wernstrom, K. D., et al. "Incidence, Mortality, and Diagnosis of Twin Gestations." *Clinical Perinatology* 15(1):141–58, March 1988.

Wilson, R. S. "Growth Standards for Twins from Birth to Four Years." *Annals of Human Biology* 21(2):175–88, 1974.

Wittman, B. K., et al. "Antenatal Diagnosis of Twin Transfusion Syndrome by Ultrasound." *Obstetrics and Gynecology* 58:123–27, 1981.

Woolfson, J., et al. "Twins with 54 Days Between Deliveries: Case Report." *British Journal of Obstetrics and Gynaecology* 90(7):685–6, July 1983.

Wu, I. H., et al. "Successful Management of a Quadruplet Pregnancy: A Case Report." *Journal of Reproductive Medicine* 28(2):163–66, February 1983.

Wyshak, G. "Menopause in Mothers of Multiple Births and Mothers of Singletons Only." *Social Biology* 25:52–61, 1978.

———, and C. White. " A Genealogical Study of Human Twinning." *American Journal of Public Health* 55:586–93, 1965.

Yarkoni, S., et al. "Estimated Fetal Weight in the Evaluation of Growth in Twin Gestations: A Prospective Longitudinal Study." *Obstetrics and Gynecology* 69(4):636–39, April 1987.

Zazzo, R. "The Twin Condition and the Couple Effect on Personality Development." *Acta Geneticae Medicae et Gemellologiae* 25:343–52, 1979.

Special Resources

Prematurity

Organizations and Equipment

William Carter Co., Needham Heights, MA 02194. Clothing for premature babies.

Children in Hospitals (CIH), 31 Wilshire Park, Needham, MA 02192. (617) 482-2915.

GentleCare. (800) 462-6603 in Michigan; (800) 462-6603 elsewhere.

Health Dyne Perinatal Services. (800) 548-3591. Home monitors.

Parent Care, University of Utah Health Sciences Center, Room 2A210, 50 North Medical Drive, Salt Lake City, UT 84132. (801) 581-5323.

Parent Care, Inc., 101 1/2 S. Union Street, Alexandria, VA 22314. Parent support groups in neonatal intensive care.

Parenting Premies, P.O. Box 530, Stevens Point, WI 54481.

Parents of Premature and High Risk Infants International, Inc., Sherri Nance, M.O.M., 22940 W. Frisca Drive, Valencia, CA 91355. (805) 254-2426.

Premature and High Risk Infant Association, P.O. Box 37114, Peoria, IL 61614.

Premature Inc., Suite 100, 10200 Old Katy Road, Houston, TX 77043.

Termguard home monitors, Tokos Medical Corporation, 821 E. Dyer Road, Santa Ana, CA 92705. (800) 258-6567 in California; (800) 248-6567 elsewhere.

Books

Erling, Susan. *Newborn Intensive Share: Poems for the NICU.* Centering Corporation, Box 3367, Omaha, NE.

Gunther, Kristine. *The Babies: Portraits of Fragile Lives.* Shorewood, WI: Main Street, 1986.

Gustaitis, Rosa, and Ernie Young. *A Time to Be Born, A Time to Die: Conflicts and Ethics in an Intensive Care Nursery.* Reading, MA: Addison-Wesley, 1986.

Harrison, Helen. *The Premature Baby Book: A Parents' Guide to Coping and Caring in the First Years.* New York: St. Martin's Press, 1983. Periodically updated. A new edition is in progress.

Hynan, Michael R., and Lauren Leslie-Hynan. *The Pain of Premature Parents: A Psychological Guide for Coping.* Lanham, MD: University Press of America, 1987.

Katz, Michael, et al., eds. *Preventing Preterm Birth: A Parent's Guide.* Health Publishing Company, 3700 California Street, San Francisco, CA 94118, 1988.

Nance, Sherri. *Premature Birth: A Handbook for Parents.* New York: Berkeley, 1984.

Pankow, Valerie. *No Bigger than My Teddy Bear.* Nashville, TN: Abingdon, 1987.

Robertson, Patricia, M.D., and Peggy Berlin, Ph.D. *The Premature Labor Handbook.* Garden City, NY: Doubleday, 1986.

Articles

Bronsteen, R., et al. "Classification of Twins and Neonatal Morbidity." *Obstetrics and Gynecology* 74(1):98, July 1989.

Crowther, G. A. "Preterm Labour in Twin Pregnancies: Can It Be Prevented by Hospital Admission?" *British Journal of Obstetrics and Gynaecology* 96(7):850, July 1989.

Freeman, Roger K. "Symposium: Home Monitoring of Uterine Contractions." *Contemporary OB/GYN* 32(5):173, November 1988.

Gilstrap, L. C. III, and C. E. Brown. "Prevention and Treatment of Preterm Labor in Twins." *Clinical Perinatology* 15(1):71–77, March 1988.

Harrison, Helen. "How to Treat Respiratory Distress Syndrome." *Twins,* January/February 1987.

———. "Neonatal Intensive Care: Parents' Role in Ethical Decision-Making." *Birth* 13(3):165–75, September 1986.

Houlton, M. C., et al. "Factors Associated with Pre-term Labour and Changes in the Cervix Before Labour in Twin Pregnancy." *British Journal of Obstetrics and Gynaecology* 89(3):190–94, 1982.

Kosasa, T. S., et al. "Ritodrine and Terbutaline Compared for the Treatment of Preterm Labor." *Acta Obstetrica Gynecologica Scandinavica* 64(5):421–26, 1985.

Leveno, K. J., and F. G. Cunningham. "Dilemmas in the Management of Preterm Birth," Part 2: "Interventions." *Williams Obstetrics.* Supplement #15. 17th ed. Ed. Pritchard, McDonald, Gant. New York: Appleton and Lange, 1987.

Londner, Ronnie. "A Tour of the NICU." *Twins,* July/August 1988.

———. "Siblings' Special Adjustments." *Twins,* May/June 1989.

Mazor, M., et al. "Delivery of Premature Twins." Letter. *American Journal of Obstetrics and Gynecology* 155(4):915, October 1986.

McCoy, Rebecca, et al. "Nursing Management of Breastfeeding for Preterm Infants." *Journal of Perinatal and Neonatal Nursing* 2(1):47, July 1988.

McCulloch, Kristine. "Neonatal Problems in Twins." *Clinical Perinatology* 15(1), March 1988.

Meier, P. "Responses of Small Pre-term Infants to Bottle and Breastfeeding." *American Journal of Maternal Child Nursing* 12:97–105, March/April 1987.

———. "Bottle and Breastfeeding: Effects on Transcutaneous Oxygen Pressure and Temperature in Preterm Infants." *Nursing Research* 37(1):36, January–February 1988.

Morales, W., et al. "The Effect of Mode of Delivery on the Risk of Intraventricular Hemorrhage in Nondiscordant Twin Gestations Under 1500 g." *Obstetrics and Gynecology*, January 1989.

Neilson, J. P., et al. "Preterm Labor in Twin Pregnancies: Prediction by Cervical Assessment." *Obstetrics and Gynecology* 72(5):719–23, November 1988.

Neukrug, Linda. "Mother Kept Us in Our Own Shoebox." *Twins,* January/February 1987.

O'Connor, M. C., et al. "Double Blind Trial of Ritodrine and Placebo in Twin Pregnancy." *British Journal of Obstetrics and Gynaecology* 86:706, 1979.

O'Shea, R. T. "Twin Pregnancy: Prematurity and Perinatal Mortality." *Australian and New Zealand Journal of Obstetrics and Gynaecology* 26(3):156–57, August 1986.

Polin, J. I., and W. L. Frangipane. "Modern Concepts in the Management of Multiple Gestation." *Pediatric Clinics of North America* 33(3), June 1986.

"Preterm Labor." ACOG Technical Bulletin #133, October 1989. American College of Obstetricians and Gynecologists, 409 12th Street, SW, Washington, DC 20024-2188.

Puissant, F., and F. Leroy. "A Reappraisal of Perinatal Mortality Factors in Twins." *Acta Geneticae Medicae et Gemellologiae* 31(3–4):213–19, 1982.

Thiele, Janice K., et al. "Inside a Neonatal Intensive Care Unit." *International Journal of Childbirth Education* 3(3):12, August 1988.

Valentine, P. H., et al. "Increased Survival of Low Birth-Weight Infants: Impact on Incidence of Retinopathy of Prematurity." *Pediatrics* 84:442, 1989.

Watson, P., and D. M. Campbell. "Preterm Deliveries in Twin Pregnancies in Oxford." *Acta Geneticae Medicae et Gemellologiae* 35(3–4):193–99, 1986.

Whitelaw, A., and K. Sheath. "The Myth of the Marsupial Mother: Home Care of Very Low Birth-Weight Babies in Bogotá, Colombia." *Lancet* 1:1206–9, 1985.

Special Needs

Organizations

American Guild for Infant Survival, Inc., 1565 Laskin Road, Virginia Beach, VA 23451. (804) 463-3845. Prescreening test for infants at high risk for SIDS and other disorders.

American Speech-Language-Hearing Association (ASHA), 10801 Rockville Pike, Rockville, MD 20852. (800) 638-6868. Publishes a booklet, *Partners in Language: A Guide for Parents.*

Association for Children with Down Syndrome, 2616 Martin Avenue, Bellmore, NY 11710. (516) 221-4700.

Association for the Help of Retarded Children, Dr. Edmund Haddad, Sibling

Network Coordination, 200 Park Avenue South, New York, NY 10003. (212) 254-8203.

Association for Parents of Children with Learning Disabilities, 1456 Library Road, Pittsburgh, PA 15236.

Association for Retarded Children of the U.S. (ARC), 2501 Avenue J, Arlington, TX 76011. (800) 433-5255.

Bittersweet Beginnings, c/o Terri Koelling, 5700 E. Greenwood Place, Denver, CO 80222. (303) 759-3979. A support network for parents experiencing loss of a multiple.

Canadian Association for the Mentally Retarded, 8605 Rue Berri, Bureau 300, Montreal, Quebec H2P 2G5 Canada. (514) 281-2307.

Cleft Parent Guild, c/o Crippled Children's Society, 7120 Franklin Avenue, Los Angeles, CA 90046.

Closer Look, P.O. Box 1492, Washington, DC 20013. Parents of disabled children.

Exceptional Parent magazine, 605 Commonwealth Avenue, Boston, MA 02215.

Mothers United for Moral Support (MUMS), c/o Julie Gordon, 150 Custer Court, Green Bay, WI 54301.

National Center for Clinical Infant Programs, 733 15th Street, NW, Suite 912, Washington, DC 20005.

National Down Syndrome Congress, 1800 Dempster Street, Park Ridge, IL 60608-1146. (800) 232-6372.

National Down Syndrome Society, 141 Fifth Avenue, New York, NY 10010. (800) 221-4602.

National Foundation of March of Dimes, P.O. Box 2000, White Plains, NY 10602. Birth defects.

National Genetics Foundation, Inc., 9 W. 57th Street, New York, NY 10019. Genetic counseling and referrals.

National Information System. (800) 922-9234. A computerized database of information on specialized services for developmentally disabled and chronically ill children.

Parents of Twins with Disabilities, 2129 Clinton Avenue East, Alameda, CA 94501.

Video

The Birth of a Sick or Handicapped Baby: Impact on the Family. Infant-Parent Institute, Inc., 328 N. Neil Street, Champaign, IL 61820. 57 min.

Books

Buscaglia, Leo. *The Disabled and Their Parents.* Rev. ed. New York: Holt, 1983.
Equals in This Partnership: Parents of Disabled and At-risk Infants and Toddlers Speak to Professionals. National Center for Clinical Infant Programs, 733 15th Street, NW, Suite 912, Washington, DC 20005.

Meyer, Donald, et al. *Living with a Brother or Sister with Special Needs: A Book for Sibs.* Seattle: University of Washington Press, 1986.

Simons, Robin. *After the Tears: Parents Talk About Raising a Child with a Disability.* New York: Harcourt Brace Jovanovich, 1987.

Thompson, Charlotte E. *Raising a Handicapped Child: A Helpful Guide for Parents of the Physically Disabled.* New York: Ballantine, 1987.

Articles

Biale, Rachel. "Counseling Families of Disabled Twins." *Social Work* 34(6):531–35, November 1989.

———. "Twins Have Unique Developmental Aspects." *Brown University Child Behavior and Development Letter* 5(6), June 1989.

Boklage, C. E. "Twinning, Nonrighthandedness, Fusion Malformations: Evidence for Heritable Causal Elements Held in Common." *American Journal of Medical Genetics* 28(1):67–84, September 1987.

Bryan, E., et al. "Congenital Anomalies in Twins." *Clinical Obstetrics and Gynecology* 1(3):697–721, September 1987.

"Congenital Anomalies and Birth Injuries Among Live Births: United States, 1973–74." Hyattsville, MD: National Center for Health Statistics.

David, T. J. "Vascular Basis for Malformations in a Twin." *Archives of Diseases of Children* 60:166–67, 1985.

Gericke, G. S. "Genetic and Teratological Considerations in the Analysis of Concordant and Discordant Abnormalities in Twins." *South African Medical Journal* 69(2):111–14, January 1986.

Schinzel, et al. "Monozygotic Twinning and Structural Defects." *Journal of Pediatrics* 95(6):921–30, December 1979.

Windham, G. C. "Neural Tube Defects Among Twin Births." *American Journal of Human Genetics* 34:988–98, 1982.

Loss

Organizations

American Sudden Infant Death Syndrome Institute, 1220 SW Morrison, Suite 625, Portland, OR 97205. (503) 228-9121.

Bereavement Support Services, Cope/Outreach Department, National Organization of Mothers of Twins Clubs (NOMOTC), 12404 Princess Jeane, N.E. Albuquerque, NM 87112-4640. (505) 275-0955.

Bittersweet Beginnings, c/o Terri Koelling, 5700 E. Greenwood Place, Denver, CO 80222. (303) 759-3979. A support network for parents experiencing loss of a multiple.

Compassionate Friends, Inc., P.O. Box 1347, Oak Brook, IL 60521. (708) 990-0010. Support for bereaved parents.

Life, Death, and Transition Workshop, Elisabeth Kübler-Ross Center, South Route 616, Head Waters, VA 24442. (702) 396-3441.

Miscarriage, Infant Death, and Stillbirth, Inc. (MIDS), 16 Crescent Drive, Parsippany, NJ 07054.

National Center for the Prevention of Sudden Infant Death Syndrome, 330 N. Charles Street, Baltimore, MD, 21201. (301) 547-0300; (800) 638-SIDS. Free booklet.

National Sudden Infant Death Syndrome Foundation, 2 Metro Plaza, Suite 205, 8240 Professional Place, Landover, MD 20785. (301) 459-3388.

Our Newsletter, Jean Kollantai, P.O. Box 1064, Palmer, AK 99645, (907) 745-2706; Patti Dubler, (907) 344-0925; Lisa Fleischer, (907) 333-2935. A network by and for parents who have experienced the death of a baby during a multiple pregnancy, birth, or infancy.

Pregnancy and Infant Loss Center, 1421 E. Wayzata Boulevard, #40, Wayzata, MN 55391. (612) 473-9372.

Sharing Our Caring, P.O. Box 400, Milton, WA 98354.

Shattered Dreams, 21 Potsdam Road, Unit 61, Downsview, Ontario M3N 1N3 Canada. (416) 663-7143. Miscarriage.

Spiritual Emergence Network (SEN), 2250 Oak Grove Avenue, Menlo Park, CA 04025. (415) 327-2776.

Films/Videos

Empty Arms: Coping After Miscarriage, Stillbirth, and Infant Death. Pregnancy and Infant Loss Center, 1415 E. Wayzeta Blvd., Suite 122, Wayseta, MN 55391. (512) 472-9372. Video for bereaved parents, especially while in the hospital.

Some Babies Die. University of California Extension Media Center, 2176 Shattuck Avenue, Berkeley, CA 04704. An Australian documentary featuring pediatrician Peter Barr and a family with unrestricted opportunities to say good-bye to their dead baby.

Books

Barr, Peter, and D. de Wilde. *Stillbirth and Newborn Death.* Royal Alexandra Hospital for Children, Camperdown, NSW 2050, Australia, 1987.

DeFrain, John D. *Coping with Sudden Infant Death.* South Hadley, MA: Bergin and Garvey, 1982.

———. *Stillborn: The Invisible Death.* New York: Lexington, 1986.

Fritsch, J., and S. Ilse. *The Anguish of Loss.* Long Lake, MN: Wintergreen Press, 1988.

Ilse, Sherokee, and Linda Burns. *Miscarriage: A Shattered Dream.* Long Lake, MN: Wintergreen Press, 1985.

———. *Empty Arms: Coping After Miscarriage, Stillbirth, and Infant Death.* 2nd ed. Long Lake, MN: Wintergreen Press, 1990.

Johnson, J. and M. *Death of an Infant Twin.* Centering Corp., Box 3367, Omaha, NE 68103-0367.

Johnson, Marvin and Joy. Centering Series. Booklets such as "Katie's Premature Brother," "Miscarriage," "She Was Born, She Dies," "Where's Jess?," "Why Mine?," "Difficult Decisions." Birth and Life Bookstore, P.O. Box 70625, Seattle, WA 98107-0625.

Kübler-Ross, Elisabeth. *On Children and Death.* New York: Macmillan, 1983.

Levine, Stephen. *Who Dies?* New York: Doubleday, 1982.

Millar, Christopher. *The Second Self: Consequences of the Intra-uterine Death of One of Twins.* Holistikon Publishing, P.O. Box 74, Creswick, VIC 3363, Australia.

Peppers, L. G., and R. J. Knapp. *How to Go on Living After the Death of a Baby.* Atlanta: Peachtree Publications. 1985.

Schaefer, D., and C. Lyons. *How Do We Tell the Children?* Newmarket, 1988.

Schiff, Harriet. *The Bereaved Parent.* Baltimore: Penguin, 1978.

———. *Living Through Mourning.* Baltimore: Penguin, 1987.

Articles

Baskett, T. A., et al. "Fetal Biophysical Profile and Perinatal Death." *Obstetrics and Gynecology* 70:357–60, 1987.

Berman, S. M. "Assessing Sex Differences in Neonatal Survival: A Study of Discordant Twins." *International Journal of Epidemiology* 16(3):436–40, September 1987.

Botting, B. J., et al. "Recent Trends in the Incidence of Multiple Births and Associated Mortality." *Archives of Diseases of Children* 62(9):941–50, September 1987.

Bourne, S., and E. Lewis. "Pregnancy After Stillbirth or Neonatal Death: Psychological Risks and Management." *Lancet* ii:31–33, 1984.

Boyle, G. and G. "A Special Relationship." *Twins,* March/April 1985.

Bryan, E. "No Longer a Twin." *British Journal of Obstetrics and Gynaecology,* 1987.

———. "The Death of a Newborn Twin: How Can Support for Parents Be Improved?" *Acta Geneticae Medicae et Gemellologiae* 5:115–15, 1986.

Carlson, N., and C. V. Towers. "Multiple Gestation Complicated by the Death of One Fetus." Part 1. *Obstetrics and Gynecology* 73(5):685–89, May 1989.

Casey, J. L., and K. F. Rogers. "When Sudden Infant Death Syndrome Strikes a Twin: Coping with the Tragedy and Mystery of SIDS." *Twins,* July/August 1986.

Cherouny, P. H., et al. "Multiple Pregnancy with Late Death of One Fetus." Part 1. *Obstetrics and Gynecology* 74(3):318–20, September 1989.

Crowther, C. A. "Perinatal Mortality in Twin Pregnancy: A Review of 799 Twin Pregnancies." *South African Medical Journal,* 1987.

Doherty, J. "Perinatal Mortality in Twins, Australia, 1973–1980," I and II: "Maternal Age, Lethal Congenital Malformations, and Sex." *Acta Geneticae Medicae et Gemellologiae,* 1988.

Dudley, D. K., and M. E. D'Alton. "Single Fetal Death in Twin Gestation." *Seminars in Perinatology* 10(1):65–72, January 1986.

Engel, G. L. K. "The Death of a Twin: Mourning and Anniversary Reactions. Fragments of a 10-Year Self-Analysis." *International Journal of Psycho-Analysis* 56:24–42, 1975.

Evans, M. I., et al. "Selective First-Trimester Termination in Octuplet and Quadruplet Pregnancies: Clinical and Ethical Issues." Part 1. *Obstetrics and Gynecology* 71(3):289–96, March 1988.

Fabia, J., and M. Drolette. "Twin Pairs, Smoking in Pregnancy, and Perinatal Mortality." *American Journal of Epidemiology*, 1980.

"Facing Up to a Twin's Death Is a 10-year Trial." *People*, 30 May 1983.

Ghai, Vetch. "Morbidity and Mortality Factors in Twins: An Epidemiological Approach." *Clinical Perinatology* 15(1):123–40, March 1988.

Golbus, M. S., et al. "Selective Termination of Multiple Gestations." *American Journal of Medical Genetics* 31(2):339–48, October 1988.

Gonen, R., et al. "The Outcome of Triplet Gestations Complicated by Fetal Death." *Obstetrics and Gynecology* 75(2), February 1990.

Grether, J., et al. "Sudden Infant Death Syndrome Among Asians in California." *Pediatrics* 116(4):525, April 1990.

Guneroth, W., et al. "Risk of Sudden Infant Death Syndrome in Subsequent Siblings." *Pediatrics* 116(4):520, April 1990.

Hagay, Z. J., et al. "Multiple Pregnancy Complicated by a Single Intrauterine Fetal Death." (Letter.) *Obstetrics and Gynecology* 66(6):837–38, December 1985.

Hanna, J. H., and J. M. Hill. "Single Intrauterine Fetal Demise in Multiple Gestation." *Obstetrics and Gynecology* 63(1):126–30, January 1984.

Hendel, J. "The Death of a Twin." *Bereavement*, July/August 1989.

Jeanty, P., et al. "The Vanishing Twin." *Ultrasonics* 2:25–31, 1981.

Johannsen, L. "As Birth and Death Coincide." *American Journal of Maternal-Child Nursing*, March/April 1989.

Kahn, A., et al. "Sudden Infant Death Syndrome in a Twin." *Pediatrics* 78(1):146–50, July 1986.

Keith, L. G., et al. "The Northwestern University Multi-Hospital Twin Study," 1: "A Description of 588 Twin Pregnancies and Associated Pregnancy Loss, 1971–1975." *American Journal of Obstetrics and Gynecology* 138:781–89, 1 December 1980.

Kerenyi, T. D., and U. Chitkara. "Selective Birth in Twin Pregnancy with Discordancy for Down Syndrome." *New England Journal of Medicine* 304:1525–27, 1981.

Kiley, K. C. "Umbilical Cord Stricture Associated with Intrauterine Fetal Demise." *Journal of Reproductive Medicine* 65(2):172–75, February 1986.

Knuppel, R. A., et al. "Intrauterine Fetal Death in Twins After 31 Weeks of Gestation." *Obstetrics and Gynecology* 65(2):172–75, February 1985.

Landy, H. J. "Management of a Multiple Gestation Complicated by an Antepartum Fetal Demise." *Obstetrical and Gynecological Survey*, 1989.

———, et al. "The Vanishing Twin." *Acta Geneticae Medicae et Gemellologiae* 31(3–4):179–94, 1982.

———, et al. "The Vanishing Twin: Ultrasonographic Assessment of Fetal Disappearance in the First Trimester." *American Journal of Obstetrics and Gynecology* 155:14, 1986.

Landy, H., and A. Weingold. "Management of a Multiple Gestation Complicated by an Antepartum Fetal Demise." *Obstetrical and Gynecological Survey* 44(3):171–76, March 1989.

Lewis, E. "Inhibition of Mourning by Pregnancy: Psychopathology and Management." *British Medical Journal* 2:27–28, 1979.

———. "Management of Stillbirth: Coping with an Unreality." *Lancet* ii:619–20, 1976.

———. "Mourning by the Family After a Stillbirth or Neonatal Death." *Archives of Diseases of Children* 54:303, 1979.

———. "Stillbirth: Psychological Consequences and Strategies of Management." In *Advances in Perinatal Medicine*, ed. A. Milunsky, E. A. Friedman, and L. Gluck. New York: Plenum, 1983.

———, and D. Bryan. "Management of Perinatal Loss of a Twin." *British Medical Journal* 297:1321–23, 19 November 1988.

Lewis, E., and A. Page. "Failure to Mourn a Stillborn: An Overlooked Catastrophe." *British Journal of Medicine and Psychology* 51:247–51, 1978.

Lumme, R., and S. Saarikoski. "Antepartal Fetal Death of One Twin." *International Journal of Gynaecology and Obstetrics* 25(4):331–36, August 1987.

McInnes, S. "Death of a Twin." *Twins* 47:31–33, March–April 1985.

McKenna, James J. "An Anthropological Perspective on the Sudden Infant Death Syndrome: A Testable Hypothesis on the Possible Role of Parental Breathing Cues in Promoting Infant Breathing Stability." Part 1. *Pre- and Peri-Natal Psychology* 2(2):93–135, Winter 1987.

Meehan, F. P. "Perinatal Mortality in Multiple Pregnancy Patients." *Acta Geneticae Medicae et Gemellologiae* 37:331, 1988.

Mulcahy, M. T., et al. "Chorion Biopsy, Cytogenetic Diagnosis, and Selective Termination in a Twin Pregnancy at Risk of Hemophilia." *Lancet* ii:866–67, 1984.

Noble, Elizabeth. "Resolution of Habitual Abortion in the Survivor of a 'Vanishing Twin' Pregnancy." *International Journal of Prenatal and Perinatal Studies* 1(1):117–120, 1989.

Prager K., et al. "Smoking and Drinking Behavior Before and During Pregnancy of Married Mothers of Live Born Infants and Stillborn Infants." *Public Health Report* 99:117, 1984.

Puckett, J. D. "Fetal Death of Second Twin in Second Trimester." *Obstetrics and Gynecology*, September 1988.

Redwine, F. O., and P. M. Hays. "Selective Birth." *Seminars in Perinatology* 10:73–81, January 1986.

Reveley, A. M., et al. "Mortality and Psychosis in Twins." In W. Nance et al., eds., *Twin Research 3: Epidemiological and Clinical Studies*. New York: Alan R. Liss, 1981.

Rogers, J. G., et al. "Monozygotic Twins Discordant for Trisomy 21." *American Journal of Medical Genetics* 11:143–46, 1982.

Segal, N. L. "Research on Twin Loss." *Twins*, March/April 1985.

———. "Twins of the Holocaust." *Twins*, 2(3):28–31, 1985.

———. "Who Is a Twin?" *Twins*, July/August 1989.

Sehgal, N. "Perinatal Death in Twins." *Postgraduate Medicine* 68(5), November 1980.

Smialek, J. E. "Simultaneous Sudden Infant Death Syndrome in Twins." *Pediatrics*, June 1986.

Swanson-Kauffman, K. "There Should Have Been Two: Nursing Care of Parents Experiencing the Perinatal Death of a Twin." *Journal of Perinatal and Neonatal Nursing* 2(2):78–86, 1988.

Syzmonowicz, W., et al. "The Surviving Monozygotic Twin." *Archives of Diseases of Children* 61:454–58, 1986.

Uchida, I. A., et al. "Twinning Rate in Spontaneous Abortions." *American Journal of Human Genetics* 35:787–93, 1983.

Walker, E. M., and N. B. Patel. "Maternal Serum Alphafetoprotein, Birthweight, and Perinatal Death in Twin Pregnancy." *British Journal of Obstetrics and Gynaecology* 93(11):1191–93, November 1986.

Warrier, U., et al. "Pregnancy Outcome at 24–31 Weeks' Gestation: Mortality." *Archives of Diseases of Children* 64(5):670–67, May 1989.

Wessel, J., and K. Schmidt-Gollwitzer. "Intrauterine Death of a Single Fetus in Twin Pregnancies." *Journal of Perinatal Medicine* 16(5–6):467–76, 1988.

Wilson, A. L. "Death of a Newborn Twin: An Analysis of Parental Bereavement." *Pediatrics* 70(4):587–91, October 1982.

Woodward, J. "The Bereaved Twin." *Acta Geneticae Medicae et Gemellologiae* 37:173–80, 1988.

Wyshak, G. "Pregnancy Loss in Mothers of Multiple Births and in Mothers of Singletons Only." *Annals of Human Biology* 12:85–89, 1985.

Zahalkova, M., and Z. Zudova. "Spontaneous Abortions and Twinning." *Acta Geneticae Medicae et Gemellologiae* 33:25–26, 1984.

Index